Methods in Medical Ethics

SECOND EDITION

Jeremy Sugarman
and Daniel P. Sulmasy
Editors

Georgetown University Press/Washington, D.C.

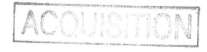
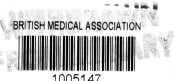

Library of Congress Cataloging-in-Publication Data
Methods in medical ethics / Jeremy Sugarman and Daniel P. Sulmasy, editors. — 2nd ed.
    p. ; cm.
  Includes bibliographical references and index.
  ISBN 978-1-58901-701-6 (pbk. : alk. paper)
1. Medical ethics. 2. Medical ethics—Research—Methodology. I. Sugarman, Jeremy. II. Sulmasy, Daniel P., 1956–
  [DNLM: 1. Ethics, Medical. 2. Research—methods. W 50 M592 2010]
  R724.M43 2010
  174'.2—dc22
     2010003709

15 14 13 12 11 10   9 8 7 6 5 4 3 2
First printing

Printed in the United States of America

The following chapters are not subject to U.S. copyright:

Chapter 12, "Qualitative Methods," by Holly A. Taylor, Sara Chandros Hull, and Nancy E. Kass
Chapter 14, "Quantitative Surveys" by Robert A. Pearlman and Helene E. Starks
Chapter 15, "Experimental Methods" by Marion Danis, Laura Hanson, and Joanne M. Garrett
Chapter 16, "Economics and Decision Science" by David A. Asch, excluding the following material for which the publisher attained permission to reprint:
    Asch, D. A., J. C. Hershey, M. L. DeKay, M. V. Pauly, J. P. Patton, M. K. Jedrziewski, F. X. Frei, R. Giardine, J. A. Kant, and M. T. Mennuti. 1998. Carrier screening for cystic fibrosis: Costs and clinical outcomes. *Medical Decision Making* 18:202–12.
    Asch, D. A., J. C. Hershey, M. V. Pauly, J. P. Patton, M. K. Jedrziewski, and M. T. Mennuti. 1996. Genetic screening for reproductive planning: Methodologic and conceptual issues in policy analysis. *American Journal of Public Health* 86:684–90. © 1996 by the American Public Health Association.

For David M. Levine, MD, MPH, ScD, our fellowship director, who was a generous mentor. His commitment to our careers made work on this book possible.

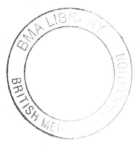

Contents

Contents

Contents

∾ Part III: Applications

Illustrations

∾ Tables

℘ Figures

Preface

Medical ethics is a field of scholarly inquiry that uses a wide variety of methods. These methods derive from the humanities and the social sciences, including anthropology, economics, epidemiology, health services research, history, law, literature, medicine, nursing, philosophy, psychology, sociology, and theology. Although specific problems in medical ethics continue to be addressed in the literatures of all of these disciplines, the first edition of *Methods in Medical Ethics* took up the challenge of systematically examining many of these disciplines and their multiple methods of inquiry across the broad field of medical ethics (Sugarman and Sulmasy 2001).

Both of us, the editors, are physicians trained in empirical research methods as well as in philosophy. We live in a multidisciplinary academic world yet continue to believe that excellent scholarship in medical ethics requires immersion in one or more of the disciplines that contribute to the field. Moreover, sound training in different disciplines helps to make interdisciplinary work more productive, relevant, and exciting.

It has been nine years since the first edition of *Methods in Medical Ethics* was published. In that time, educational programs in medical ethics have proliferated. New on-campus and online master's degree programs have sprung up at a number of universities. Doctoral degrees and postgraduate professional programs are offering specializations in medical ethics. We are grateful that many of these programs make use of our book and have found it to be a helpful pedagogical tool. A book on methodology can only remain useful to educators, however, if it is revised periodically in order to take stock of the evolution of the field of inquiry. Since this book is also a resource tool for those contemplating further training in one or more of the disciplines that contribute to medical ethics, updating changes in those educational resources and opportunities is also important.

Moreover, the volume of literature in medical ethics has grown enormously in all of the relevant disciplines since the first edition of *Methods in Medical Ethics*. The methods employed by scholars in all of the disciplines working in medical ethics have continued to grow and evolve, and it is therefore important for a book on multiple methodologies to be revised in order to stay current with the state of scholarship in all of the various disciplines. The scholars who have contributed chapters to this book are well-equipped to survey their own disciplines and provide such updates.

In organizing the first edition we struggled with the question of which methods to include. In the end we settled on approaches that we believed played the most significant role in shaping the contemporary field of medical ethics. These were philosophy, religion and theology, professional codes, law, casuistry, history, qualitative research, ethnography, quantitative surveys, experimental methods, and economics and decision science. While we tried to be comprehensive, setting the boundaries the way we did was not perfectly satisfactory. Given the way the field has evolved, we have rethought some of these boundary decisions in bringing forth a second edition.

First, we have expanded our coverage of the range of philosophical methods. While method is itself one of the contested questions in philosophy, and a book such as this one cannot possibly cover every unique philosophical perspective, we have included in the second edition a chapter that challenges the dominant philosophical views that have comprised work in medical ethics in the United States. We have also expanded the scope of the chapter on codes to include its relationship to virtue theory.

Second, while we do not believe that all medical humanities are subsumed under the umbrella of medical ethics, the discipline of literary studies is becoming even more important as a tool for teaching and exploring questions in medical ethics. For example, the U.S. President's Council on Bioethics has produced an extensive compendium of Western literary sources regarding medical ethics titled *Becoming Human* (President's Council 2003). We therefore thought it important to include a new chapter on literature and medical ethics in the second edition.

Third, we have added one new empirical chapter, covering the discipline of sociology.

Fourth, some chapters in the first edition were more abstract than others, describing the scholarly methods of their respective disciplines in a manner too detached from its application to medical ethics to be useful to some readers. We have worked with the authors in the second edition to help make sure that the connections between each methodology and the field of medical ethics are clear.

The second edition of *Methods in Medical Ethics* begins, once again, with two introductory chapters. In chapter 1, we examine the many methods of scholarship in medical ethics as well as their relationship to one another. We go on to a more robust discussion than in the first edition of some of the norms governing the relationship between descriptive and normative ethics. Chapter 2 is an update on the empirical research literature in medical ethics. The particular methods of medical ethics outlined above are addressed in chapters 3 through 16. To provide sufficient expertise in each of these methods, we once again assembled a team of authors based upon their scholarly training and work in medical ethics. Some authors have changed for some topics, but most are written by returning authors who have generously agreed to contribute revised chapters. While this provides a strong continuity between the editions, we have asked all of the returning authors to update the methodological considerations in their fields and we have asked the new authors to dramatically rethink their topics. We feel quite fortunate to have so many talented scholars working with us. As in the first edition, in each chapter dealing with a particular method, the author(s) generally provide a description of the method, a critique of the method, and then notes on resources and training in the method.

The concluding chapters are designed to illustrate how these methods can relate to one another and how to assess the quality of scholarship in medical ethics.

Specifically, chapter 17 uses the topic of decision making by surrogates on behalf of patients at the end of life as an example of the richness of multidisciplinary work in medical ethics regarding a single issue. This replaces the chapter on physician-assisted suicide in the first edition. Finally, as in the first edition, the last chapter uses the information gleaned from the preceding chapters to offer a proposed approach to being a critical reader of scholarship in medical ethics.

We continue to define our field of inquiry as "medical ethics" and not "bioethics." We do this because we take bioethics to be an extremely broad field, encompassing such topics as environmental ethics, animal rights, and pure biological research. The focus of this book is more narrowly centered on the methods used to study the ethical issues surrounding the provision of health care to human beings. While this certainly includes the ethics of being a physician, we do not take the phrase medical ethics to exclude, in any way, the ethics of being a patient, a nurse, a psychologist, or a member of any of the other health professions allied with medicine.

We are grateful to the authors of the contributed chapters for their considerable efforts and to Margie Cummins for her help in preparing the manuscript for publication.

Our hopes for the second edition of *Methods in Medical Ethics* are to continue to introduce students to the many methods of medical ethics, to renew our call for scholars to strive for the standards of methodological excellence described in the book, and to provide readers of the medical ethics literature with a better appreciation of the methods employed by disciplines other than their own. Medical ethics is a multi-disciplinary field that we hope will become ever more interdisciplinary. To the extent that this book helps any of this to happen it is worth having expended the effort to produce it.

✎ References

President's Council on Bioethics. 2003. *Being human: Readings from the President's Council on Bioethics.* Washington, DC: U.S. Government Printing Office.

Sugarman, J., and D. P. Sulmasy, eds. 2001. *Methods in medical ethics.* Washington, DC: Georgetown University Press.

PART I

Overview

CHAPTER I

The Many Methods of Medical Ethics

(Or, Thirteen Ways of Looking at a Blackbird)

DANIEL P. SULMASY AND

JEREMY SUGARMAN

The range of scholarship falling under the umbrella of medical ethics is astounding. For instance, the disciplines of anthropology, economics, epidemiology, health services research, history, law, literature, medicine, nursing, philosophy, social psychology, sociology, and theology all have scholars working in the field of medical ethics. Some employ unique methods. Others use similar methods but have different theoretical orientations. However, it is not always clear whether, or how appropriately, work done in many of these disciplines is considered scholarship in medical ethics. Neither is it always clear how these methods and disciplines relate to each other. In this chapter we provide a general orientation to the scope of these many methods and offer what we take to be proper interdisciplinary relationships in medical ethics.

Types of Ethical Inquiry

Philosophers hold that there are three basic types of ethical inquiry: normative ethics, metaethics, and descriptive ethics (Frankena 1973). Normative ethics is the branch of philosophical or theological inquiry that sets out to give answers to the following questions: What ought to be done? What ought not to be done? What kinds of persons ought we strive to become? Normative ethics sets out to answer these questions in a systematic, critical fashion, and to justify the answers that are offered. In medical ethics normative ethics is concerned with arguments about such topics as the morality of physician-assisted suicide or whether it is morally proper to clone human beings.

Metaethics is the branch of philosophy that investigates the meaning of moral terms, the logic and linguistics of moral reasoning, and the fundamental questions of moral ontology, epistemology, and justification. It is the most abstract type of ethical inquiry but one vital to normative investigations. Whether or not it is explicitly acknowledged, all normative inquiry rests upon a fundamental stance regarding metaethical questions. Metaethics asks, What does "right" mean? What does "ought" mean? What is implied by saying "I ought to do X?" Is morality objective or subjective? Are there any moral truths that transcend particular cultures? If so, how does one know what these truths are? Positions regarding all of these questions lurk below the surface of most normative ethical discussions, whether in general normative ethics or in medical ethics. Sometimes it is only possible to understand the grounds upon which people disagree by investigating questions at this level of abstraction. In many cases, however, there is enough general agreement that normative inquiry can proceed without explicitly engaging metaethical questions.

Descriptive ethics does not directly engage questions of what one ought to do or the proper use of ethical terms. Descriptive ethics asks empirical questions such as, How do people think they ought to act in this particular situation of normative concern? What facts are relevant to this normative ethical inquiry? How do people actually behave in this particular circumstance of ethical concern? In medical ethics the literature is replete with descriptive ethics studies, such as surveys concerning what patients and doctors think about the morality of late-term abortions, about attitudes toward completing advance directives, or about perceptions concerning the risk of being tested for BRCA1/2 (breast and ovarian cancer susceptibility genes).

While all these types of ethical inquiry are important, normative ethics seems to be at the core of ethical inquiry. This is not to suggest that normative ethics is more intellectual or more worthwhile than other disciplines. Rather, we suggest that while the other types of ethical inquiry are inherently interesting, they are most important, meaningful, and useful because of the normative questions that are at stake. One asks, "What does the word 'ought' mean?" because it is very interesting and important to know what one ought to do. In general one is fundamentally interested in knowing what percentage of the population thinks something ought to be done in particular circumstances or how people actually behave in such circumstances, if it is interesting and important to know how one ought to behave in such circumstances. It is relatively uninteresting to ask, "How often should men shine their shoes?" It is much more interesting to know how a physician ought to respond when a patient asks, "Doctor, will you help me die?"

Yet, even if normative ethics is at the core of scholarship in ethics, all these types of research are interesting and important. The methods employed to answer the three types of questions necessarily differ, but each contributes something. They all help to fill in the outlines of ethical inquiry. This can be metaphorically illustrated by the Wallace Stevens poem "Thirteen Ways of Looking at a Blackbird" (1951). Stevens's poem masterfully captures both the complexity and the advantages of looking at anything from a multiplicity of perspectives. Medical ethics is like this poem. Each of the thirteen stanzas of the poem illustrates a view of the blackbird. Each view tells us something about the viewer as well as something about the blackbird. No single view tells us what a blackbird is. But in sum, at the end of the poem, the reader has a better sense of the blackbird. That sense is ineluctably incomplete. But it is ever richer and fuller after thirteen views. As Stevens writes:

The blackbird whirled in the autumn winds.
It was a small part of the pantomime.

So it is, we suggest, with medical ethics. Neither the methods employed by philosophy nor theology nor anthropology nor history nor law nor any other methods that contribute to scholarship in medical ethics describe the blackbird called medical ethics in its entirety. But by examining a moral question from the vantage point of several different methods, one gains a richer understanding of that moral question and a better grasp of an answer. Under ideal circumstances, each method of medical ethics contributes something that is of importance for scholars who employ other methods to investigate the same questions. Each method looks at the blackbird from a different perspective. And ultimately, in health care, such research is vital not only to scholars, but above all to those practicing the healing professions. After all, medical ethics is, in large part, about what these people ought to do. And what these people do obviously has profound implications for individuals when they are sick.

❧ One Field, Many Disciplines, Many Methods

Is medical ethics a discipline in its own right? Jonsen (1998) has suggested that in a simple sense it is, but in the strictest sense it is not. Some might suggest that medical ethics is now really a single, unified discipline in which any scholar can employ any of the methods described in this book to address the question at hand, jettisoning the disciplinary boundaries and theoretical assumptions that otherwise keep these disciplines from communicating with each other. Witness, for example, the growth of graduate programs that offer degrees in "bioethics." Others might suggest that the scholarly product would be better if each discipline were to use the methods proper to that discipline to practice medical ethics without ever bothering to examine how other disciplines examine questions in medical ethics, even if these other disciplines employ the same methods. The result is confusion over what medical ethics scholarship really is, or ought to be.

We would like to bring further conceptual clarity to this discussion by carefully distinguishing between field, discipline, and method. Borrowing from the *Oxford English Dictionary*, we define a field of inquiry as a subject matter or set of phenomena or questions addressed by a scholar or scholars. By contrast we define a discipline as a department of learning or knowledge, a community of scholars who share common assumptions about training, modes of inquiry, the kind of knowledge that is sought, and the boundaries of the subject matter proper to the discipline. Finally, we define a method as a systematic procedure, technique, or mode of inquiry that is employed in examining research questions.

We take the view that medical ethics is a single field of inquiry of great interest to many disciplines rather than a discipline in its own right. What medical ethicists share is a common subject matter, not a common disciplinary mode of investigating that subject. Their common subject matter is the normative aspect of health care. This is the medical ethicists' blackbird. It is their field. However, they view it through the eyes of a wide variety of disciplines. These disciplines employ a wide variety of methods, some shared by several disciplines and some unique to a particular discipline. Medical ethics is one field that embraces a variety of disciplines and methods. Thus, one conducts research in medical ethics as a philosopher or as a health services researcher or as a historian. One can certainly be cross-trained in more than one of these disciplines. But the quality of scholarship, in our view, will generally be best when investigators have a disciplinary home base. This will ensure a firm understanding of the assumptions and the limitations of the methods proper to these disciplines, as well as ensuring rigor and appropriate peer review of the research.

Childress (2007) has criticized our argument that all the various types of scholarship in this field can properly be called medical ethics. Childress would limit the use of the term to describing normative work, and the methods of medical ethics to the philosophical and theological methods described in chapters 3 through 7 in this book. In a certain sense the use of a term such as "medical ethics" is stipulative, and one can stipulate that it cover whatever set of studies one wishes. Narrowing the use of the term "medical ethics" to normative work alone, however, seems to deny the reality of the rich, complex, and multidisciplinary field that medical ethics has become. Many of the scholars whose work is described in this book, while using the techniques of nonnormative disciplines, describe themselves as medical ethicists. Many have worked as part of multidisciplinary teams, informing theory with data and orienting descriptive studies to help find solutions to knotty normative questions. What else should all this research be called? "Sociological studies contributing in a descriptive and cooperative way to the normative work of real medical ethics"? It seems simpler and truer to reality to call it all medical ethics. Further, a narrow approach, such as the one proposed by Childress, flies in the face of the standard division we have outlined between metaethics, normative ethics, and descriptive ethics, a description of the types of ethical inquiry that Childress has espoused in every edition of the famous textbook that he coauthored with Beauchamp (Beauchamp and Childress 2009, 2).

We agree with Childress that the normative questions are central, but if it is standard usage to call all this work forms of ethical investigation, and those who use these various methods are in serious dialogue with one another, sometimes even collaborating as part of the same multidisciplinary team, then it is unclear what is gained by restricting the use of the term to normative methods. While not denying the primacy of the normative, medical ethics has become an extraordinarily multidisciplinary field.

❧ Medical Ethics as an Interdisciplinary Field

Multidisciplinarity, however, is not interdisciplinarity. Although there is constant chatter about interdisciplinary research on university campuses, medical ethics is a field of inquiry with enormous potential to make that chatter real. Normative questions, as stated above, are inherently interesting. These questions are of interest to scholars in many disciplines. Sadly, however, what often seems to be missing is genuine interchange between these scholars. For example, the eyes of a lawyer or philosopher often glaze over when someone describes the statistical methods used in a research project about informed consent. Or a health services researcher can be overheard muttering something about "fluff" when a theologian begins to expatiate about the relationship between the concepts of dignity and justice in health care. In this book we hope to move beyond these stereotypes. We realize that we cannot make a casuist into a decision-scientist in a few pages. However, part of what we hope to make possible for medical ethicists is enough of a rudimentary understanding of the other disciplines in the field to help facilitate a richer, genuinely interdisciplinary conversation in medical ethics.

If we are correct in our contention that medical ethics is an interdisciplinary field, then it is incumbent upon us to suggest how these various disciplines and methods should relate to one another. The focus of this discussion will be on the relationship between normative and descriptive methods. Although metaethical questions are important in medical ethics and often lie just beneath the surface of important normative arguments, metaethics is more part of ethics in general than part of the field of medical ethics. We therefore do not discuss metaethics further. We instead describe the proper role and the limitations of some of the methods commonly employed in normative and descriptive ethics, a topic that has received scant attention in the literature.

We begin by discussing the fact/value distinction. We believe it is critical to understand this distinction if one is to understand the role and limits of various kinds of medical ethics scholarship. We then propose a series of guidelines for the proper conduct of genuinely interdisciplinary scholarshp among the various empirical and normative disciplines that contribute to medical ethics. In so doing we hope to spark further conversation, collaboration, and investigation.

❧ The Fact/Value Distinction

There is probably no single principle in ethics that is more important to discuss with respect to the relationship between descriptive and normative studies in medical ethics than the so-called fact/value distinction (Beauchamp 1982). Most (but not all) ethicists subscribe to this distinction, which is also called "the naturalistic fallacy" and the "is/ought distinction." It was originally proposed by David Hume in *Treatise of Human Nature*, in which he noted that many ethical arguments, particularly in scholastic philosophy, consisted of a series of factual statements using the verb "is," leading to a conclusion using the verb "ought" (Hume 1978). This struck Hume as peculiar. He wondered whether any set of facts ever added up, by itself, entailing any normative conclusion.

Over the ensuing centuries there have been many discussions of this principle. Some who have attacked the fact/value distinction have noted that certain social facts do appear to entail normative conclusions. For example, Searle (1969) points out that the fact that one has made a promise to do something does seem to imply a normative conclusion, namely, that one ought to do it. Others have argued that certain facts about the role and purpose of something or someone also seem to entail normative conclusions. MacIntyre (1984), for example, points out that the fact that something is a knife does entitle one to draw certain conclusions about what an object said to be a knife ought to be like. What makes a knife good has to do with such characteristics as sharpness and sturdiness. Likewise, he argues, the fact that someone occupies a role as the practitioner of a certain human practice does entitle one to draw conclusions about what makes that individual a good practitioner (e.g., the fact that someone is a soldier implies that if he or she is a good soldier, one can expect courage, loyalty, dependability, and so forth). Similarly, one might say that the fact that someone is a physician entitles one to draw certain conclusions about what makes that person a good physician (e.g., competence, compassion, respectfulness, and so on).

One counterargument to both Searle and MacIntyre might be that these human purposes and social facts are already implicitly moral. These sorts of facts are different from brute facts about the world that seem to entail no normative conclusions. On this view social facts and human purposes would not truly violate the fact/value distinction because these sorts of facts already contain implicit moral premises. In reply it could be argued that there really is a purpose to being a physician. If one could better understand what it means to be an excellent physician, one would be well on one's way to having a system of medical ethics (see, for example, Pellegrino and Thomasma 1981). Although this discussion cannot be concluded here, it is important to note that questions of fact and value enfold discussions about the relationship between normative and descriptive work in medical ethics (Pellegrino 1995).

∾ Illicit Inference in Medical Ethics Research

Putting these arguments aside, even defenders of the possibility of drawing normative conclusions from certain special facts would tend to agree that the fact/value distinction holds over a variety of important sets of facts. This allows one to conclude that there are some kinds of inferences in medical ethics research that are illicit and can be avoided.

HISTORICAL FACTS DO NOT ENTAIL NORMATIVE CONCLUSIONS

One might call this the historicist version of the naturalistic fallacy. The historicist fallacy in moral argument differs from the mistakes of anachronism and essentialism in historical research (Baker and McCullough 2009). Anachronism means interpreting past events as if they had occurred in the present context. Essentialism means treating certain ideas as if they were timeless and ahistorical. The historicist fallacy, by contrast, means concluding that the moral judgments of the historical past are true merely because they are old. For example, the mere fact that infanticide was practiced in the early Mediterranean world does not entitle one to conclude that all societies should be free to decide for themselves whether to permit this practice. Likewise, the mere fact that payment for health care has never before been organized with financial incentives for physicians to provide fewer services does not entitle one to conclude that such payment structures are immoral. Whether something has or has not been done in the past does not mean that it is moral or immoral.

MAJORITY OPINIONS AND BEHAVIORS DO NOT ENTAIL NORMATIVE CONCLUSIONS

The opinion survey, which is a commonly used empirical technique in medical ethics, should never be construed to give "the answer." For example, 75 percent of young physicians in a poll might approve of sexual relationships occurring between physicians and patients provided the physician–patient relationship, as such, is ter-minated once it turns sexual. However, this would not imply that the practice ought to be considered morally permissible. Likewise the fact that many physicians are willing to endorse or justify the falsification of medical insurance claims to obtain medically indicated treatments for patients does not imply that such practices are morally appropriate (Freeman et al. 1999; Wynia et al. 2000). The mere fact that almost everyone says that something is proper, or that almost everyone acts in a cer-tain way, does not make it proper to act that way. The appeal to popular opinion can sometimes amount to an example of the informal logical fallacy of the *argumentum ad populum* (see also chapter 6).

As described in chapter 14, quantitative surveys are best viewed as tools to exam-ine what clinical or social factors might be associated with particular opinions about moral issues, pointing out, for example, significant cultural divides. For instance, African Americans are less likely to want to forgo life-sustaining treatment than are Caucasian Americans (Barnato et al. 2009; Blackhall et al. 1999). But it is critical to understand the limitations of such survey research in ethics. Individuals may not share group beliefs, and whole cultures can be mistaken in their moral beliefs.

THE MERE FACT THAT SOMETHING IS LEGAL OR ILLEGAL DOES NOT MAKE IT MORAL OR IMMORAL

In general the moral goodness of a just society will be reflected in its laws. Even Thomas Aquinas, however, thought it unwise for a government to pass laws regarding all aspects of the moral life (*Summa Theologia* I-II, q.94, a.4, c). Such an effort would probably be impossible. And so, questions about the proper relationship between law and morality will be operative even in morally homogeneous societies.

In an increasingly multicultural democratic republic like the United States, how-ever, in which the rule of law is predicated upon majority rule, it sometimes can be forgotten that laws do not give normative answers. Democratic procedures such as referenda, majority votes of elected representatives, or judicial decisions might settle the legal aspects of certain moral questions, but not everything that is legal is moral, and not everything that is moral is legal. Laws can be immoral. Segregation in the United States was once legal, but this does not mean that the practice was moral once and then became immoral after the law changed. Majority rule, even by free election, can commit moral error. Adolf Hitler, for example, was made chancellor of Germany by the vote of elected representatives in a democratic republic. Ethics judges the law; the law does not judge ethics.

Neither does the fact that one might be sued constitute a moral argument. The threat of a lawsuit does not render a proposed course of action moral or immoral. Legal consequences should be given the same moral weight that one generally gives to other types of consequences in making moral decisions. For instance, if one is a strict deontologist, which is basing decisions solely upon doing one's duty, legal con-sequences will have no bearing on the decision whatsoever. For others, the threshold might vary for taking a moral stand depending upon practical concerns. For example, under threat of lawsuit, one might not want to make a moral issue out of a patient's refusal to be weighed daily, even though one might beneficently think that from a moral point of view, daily weighings are in the patient's best interest. On the other hand, fidelity to patients and professional integrity do sometimes demand doing what one thinks morally correct even under threat of lawsuit. Legal liability concerns are not a reliable guide to morally correct action.

To illustrate this, there are cases in which one can be sued no matter which course one pursues. For example, if a patient clearly expresses her wishes not to be placed on a ventilator and then goes into a coma, and her husband the lawyer then demands that she be intubated when she develops respiratory distress, one could be sued no matter what course one were to pursue. Successfully resuscitating the patient could invite legal action for battery. Failure to attempt resuscitation could invite legal action for negligence. The law does not settle the moral matter. One must rely on moral analysis and do what one determines to be morally right.

THE OPINIONS OF EXPERTS DO NOT NECESSARILY ENTAIL MORAL CONCLUSIONS

As Edmund Pellegrino argues in chapter 6, under certain specified conditions, tradition and opinion can form important parts of sound moral arguments. There is practical value to reliance upon expertise and tradition. But it is sometimes appropriate to be certain that reliance upon this authority is justified. For example, the mere fact that a clinical ethics consultant has recommended a course of action does not mean that this is the morally correct course of action. Expert advice can and should be obtained in morally troubling cases. The opinions of experts should be taken quite seriously. But experts often disagree, and experts can be wrong. So-called expertise among ethicists, for example, is limited by their training, knowledge, practical wisdom, and potential biases. Appeal to expert opinion represents the informal logical fallacy of the *argumentum ad verecundiam*. At times it is appropriate to challenge expertise.

THE MERE FACT THAT SOMETHING IS BIOLOGICALLY TRUE DOES NOT ENTAIL AUTOMATIC MORAL CONCLUSIONS

The mere fact that human beings do not have wings does not imply that it is immoral for human beings to fly. Likewise, the mere fact that brain wave activity begins at a certain stage of fetal development does not, in itself, imply anything about the morality of abortion at one stage of development or another.

An often-misunderstood moral theory relevant to this issue is known as natural law. It is a misconstrual of natural law theory to think that it states that morality is to be read off human biology as if one were reading a script. Properly understood, natural law ethics has more to do with a broad understanding about what it means to be a good human being and what constitutes human flourishing (Finnis 1980). Brute biological facts do not imply immediately clear moral truths.

❧ Empirical Studies and Normative Ethics

Carefully conducted empirical studies can help elucidate facts. But as discussed in detail above, the fact/value distinction precludes moral inference from brute facts. This might appear to make empirical studies irrelevant. However, such a conclusion would be premature. There are at least eight ways in which empirical studies can be important in medical ethics.

PURELY DESCRIPTIVE STUDIES

Purely descriptive studies of what human beings believe about morality, how their beliefs change with time, and how they behave in situations of moral concern can be of enormous intellectual interest in and of themselves. Anthropological studies of how human societies differ with respect to the treatment of elderly people, for instance, can be fascinating. Differences in sexual morality can be interesting. Differences in the ways in which cultures pay for medical care, whether by government insurance, private for-profit managed care organizations, or the payment of chickens to the local shaman, can be very stimulating to learn about. Such studies need have no normative purpose.

Yet descriptive ethics studies are interesting precisely because they illuminate human responses to normative questions. To study how different cultures grow rice would be of interest to an anthropologist but not necessarily to an ethicist. When anthropologists or other social scientists apply their techniques to the study of normatively interesting questions, they are doing descriptive ethics. In many cases the relationship between normative ethics and descriptive ethics is only that normative ethics has raised the questions of interest for empirical study.

It is of interest to know, for example, why certain persons have the opinions they do about certain disputed normative questions even if the answers one gathers through survey research are acknowledged to have no normative implications. If Southerners, for example, were to be less concerned than Northerners about the ethics of vaccinating military recruits with an experimental vaccine without their consent, and this were to be found independent of race and religion, this would be an interesting empirical fact. It might lead one to ask further empirical questions or further normative questions. It deals with an interesting normative issue about research ethics but has no normative implications in itself.

An important new area of investigation in descriptive ethics is neuroethics (Illes 2005). Neuroethicists are examining the psychology, neurology, and genetics of moral decision making, especially by making use of new brain-imaging techniques. Whether these studies will have an ultimate impact on normative ethics, especially with respect to issues such as mind/brain reductionism, or freedom and determinism, is a matter of intense debate (Glannon 2009; Reichlin 2007).

A good deal of empirical research in ethics is of this nature, carefully describing anthropological, sociological, psychological, neurological, and epidemiological facts that are of interest. They are of interest because the subject is normative. But the techniques are descriptive, and the conclusions have no immediate normative implications. Nevertheless, empirical findings may introduce facts not already being considered in reaching normative conclusions, thereby better informing this work.

TESTING ESTABLISHED OR NEW NORMS

Another way in which descriptive studies can be related to normative ethics is through studies that describe compliance with existing moral norms. Again, such studies do not answer the normative question. But provided there is widespread acceptance of a moral norm, it is of interest to study actual behavioral adherence to this norm. In studies of this type, there is no question about the norm itself. What is of interest is the extent to which human beings live up to it or the extent to which it is legally or socially enforced. For example, in the United States today, almost everyone thinks that if patients do not wish to be connected to a ventilator, they should not receive ventilator therapy. Yet, a multicenter study of critically ill patients has shown that patients' preferences are often overlooked and they frequently receive therapy they do not want (SUPPORT 1995).

In other cases new policies or procedures designed to operationalize certain moral norms are introduced into clinical settings. Descriptive studies can help to decide whether or not the plan for operationalizing the norm has been successful. For example, studies have shown that between 11 percent and 29 percent of scientific authors and presenters at conferences fail to disclose publicly discoverable financial conflicts of interest (Mayer 2006; Okike et al. 2009). This does not imply that conflicts of interest are either morally trivial or a profound moral evil. It does suggest that if one considers them morally wrong and wishes to reduce them, voluntary disclosure may be an ineffective means of doing so.

DESCRIPTIONS OF FACTS RELEVANT TO NORMATIVE ARGUMENTS

Good ethics depends upon good facts. Failure to understand thoroughly the facts of a situation will clearly lead to perils in moral decision making. Further, many normative arguments depend upon factual information, even though these facts themselves do not confer normative status upon the arguments. For example, one might argue that liver transplantation should be withheld from alcoholics because the chances of relapse of alcoholism are so high that the prognosis will be poor. In fact, it turns out that the survival of alcoholic patients who have been sober for six months and undergo liver transplantation is equivalent to that of patients transplanted for other conditions (Berlakovich et al. 1994; Björnsson et al. 2005; Hwang et al. 2006). The moral argument against transplants for alcoholics, based on a presumption of poor prognosis, is thus falsified by the facts disclosed in a descriptive study.

Reliance upon the facts in these sorts of arguments does not violate the fact/value distinction. The premises in these arguments are moral and factual, not simply factual. Such arguments are not only permissible but essential to moral reasoning.

Ethics is concerned with what to do (Aristotle *Nichomachean Ethics* 1 103b.28–31). Ethics is, in this sense, the most practical of all branches of philosophy. Moral premises relate facts to duties and virtues. Moral arguments often take forms such as the following:

1. Whenever situation X occurs, it is permissible to do Y.
2. If Z is true, then I am in situation X.
3. Therefore, if Z is true, it is permissible to do Y.

Proposition 1 is a moral premise. Proposition 2 is empirical. Empirical studies can make important contributions to ethics if they can show whether a proposition in the form of proposition 2 is always true, or under what conditions Z obtains. Knowing this empirical information is critical to determining whether one is bound by the obligation in proposition 3.

For example, proposition 1 might be the moral rule known in medical ethics as therapeutic privilege (Beauchamp and Childress 2009, 124). This states that it is morally permissible to withhold information from patients (Y) if disclosing that information would cause the patient very grave harm (X). The key to applying this moral rule will be to determine under what conditions situation X is true. Someone might argue (as generations of physicians in the United States did up until the 1970s), that whenever patients have cancer, informing them would cause the patients great harm (Oken 1961). Physicians were constructing a moral argument based upon a proposition of the form of proposition 2: If the patient has cancer (Z), this is a situation in which disclosing the facts will cause the patient great harm (X).

This is precisely the sort of situation in which descriptive ethics can play an enormously important role in medical ethics. In the 1970s empirical studies were undertaken to show that patients with cancer overwhelmingly wanted to be told of their diagnosis and felt that they had the coping skills to handle it (Alfidi 1971). Further studies were then performed to demonstrate that patients, by and large, felt much better when they were informed of their diagnoses and perhaps even evidenced better cooperation with treatment and better outcomes. Descriptive ethics studies showed that proposition 2 was false when Z was cancer. Therefore, the moral conclusion, proposition 3, could not be inferred. Physicians' practices changed. By the late 1970s, 90 percent of American physicians reported that they routinely informed their patients with cancer of their diagnoses (Novack et al. 1979).

SLIPPERY SLOPE ARGUMENTS

Another way in which empirical studies can uncover facts that are relevant to normative arguments is when so-called slippery slope arguments are invoked in moral debates. Slippery slope arguments are those that suggest that if a certain moral rule is changed, other, untoward moral consequences will follow.

These sorts of moral arguments have an empirical form. The facts to which they refer, however, are facts about a possible future that has not yet been realized. Therefore, empirical studies cannot answer the question of whether or not a slippery slope *will* occur, but they can contribute to an understanding of the *likelihood* that the slippery slope will occur. Descriptive studies that can contribute to an understanding of the likelihood of slippery slopes include historical studies of similar situations, studies of other settings in which the change in moral norms has already taken place, psychological studies of those likely to be affected by the slippery slope concerns, and legal studies of statutes and case law precedents that might be relevant.

For example, important studies have been conducted about the psychology of the slippery slope. A famous example is the experiment by Milgram (1963) in which students, responding to an authority figure, were willing, gradually, to increase the voltage of what was unbeknownst to them a feigned electrical shock they delivered to a subject who responded with cries of simulated pain. This experimental evidence of a psychological slippery slope has recently been invoked to help explain how it is that psychologists or other health professionals could become involved in torture (Olson, Soldz, and Davis 2008). And while some have demurred at pursuing so-called harm-reduction strategies with respect to drug use, arguing that such strategies will lead to increased abuse, few empirical studies have been conducted regarding the effect of such programs on the attitudes of the intended audience, giving some indication of the likelihood that such a slippery slope might come to pass (Whittingham et al. 2009).

Empirical studies thus can contribute indirectly to slippery slope arguments. Slippery slope arguments often envisage a likely future so fraught with moral danger that one ought not to engage in the social experiment of finding out whether the predicted slippery slope will come to pass, so that even pilot trials might be precluded. Slippery slope arguments can be bolstered or attacked, however, by indirect examinations of related facts that help to clarify how realistic such fears might be. Descriptive studies in ethics can thus play a key role in assessing the plausibility of slippery slope arguments.

ASSESSING LIKELY CONSEQUENCES

Empirical studies can also suggest the consequences of certain courses of action in a manner that helps moral decision makers. One need not be a utilitarian to pay attention to consequences in making moral decisions. For example, if the chances of a patient surviving an operation are only one in five thousand, the argument that it would be unjust to withhold the treatment seems much less persuasive than if the chances were one in five. Similarly, data showing that cardiopulmonary resuscitation is unlikely to be effective in patients with widespread metastatic cancer may help those who must make decisions about whether it would be appropriate to use this procedure.

THE EMPIRICAL TESTING OF NORMATIVE CLAIMS

Sometimes the relationship between normative and descriptive ethics can be very tight and very direct. This is particularly the case when normative theory prescribes practices whose components can be empirically tested. One important technique for performing such tests is based upon the moral principle, attributed to Kant, that "ought implies can" (Rescher 1987). This means that a normative argument that someone "ought" to do something necessarily entails that it is possible for the person to do it. Thus, if one can demonstrate empirically that what has been proposed as normatively required is actually impossible, one can invalidate the normative claim. Say, for example, someone has argued that all premature infants must be resuscitated, regardless of how small or premature they may be. Such a norm is invalidated by the empirical findings that for infants less than twenty-two weeks' gestational age (Lorenz 2000) or less than 500 grams' birth weight (Kaiser et al. 2004), survival after attempted resuscitation is virtually impossible.

Hypothetically, an interesting empirical study might be to test whether the norm of aiming for consensus truly is, as some have argued, the best decision-making strategy to use in performing ethics consults (Dubler and Liebman 2004; Moreno 1995).

A mathematical argument can be made that this will often lead to incorrect answers (Jansen 2009). If a "gold standard" correct answer could be established, ethics consults could then be modeled under two different approaches to see which gives the gold standard answer more often.

CASE REPORTS

As in other aspects of medical practice, case reports play a role in medical ethics. Careful descriptions of unusual situations can serve as a springboard for substantial normative discussion. Others who encounter similar situations in the future can benefit from having read and considered the ethical issues in a case encountered by a colleague at another institution. Those who subscribe to the theory of casuistry (moral reasoning by analogies between cases) as their sole method of approaching cases in medical ethics depend heavily upon good case descriptions (Jonsen and Toulmin 1988). Those who appeal to narrative and care-based theories of ethics depend upon "thick" descriptions of the case, including details about interpersonal dynamics and emotions that are often excluded from more traditional case discussions. Since case reports are now generally frowned upon as anecdotal and unscientific in the standard medical literature, in some ways, the case report has experienced something of a revival with the advent of medical ethics. As Jonsen points out eloquently in chapter 7, in ethics there is no escaping the case.

DEMONSTRATION PROJECTS

Descriptive ethics studies can be conducted to demonstrate the implementation of a normative idea or standard. The empirical project thus can function as a vehicle for the promulgation of a normative idea. This happens frequently in medical ethics. It is particularly common in ethics education. Few people will argue against teaching ethics to medical students or nurses, for example. But it is sometimes important simply to demonstrate that such programs can be successfully implemented (Sulmasy et al. 1994). The content of the program might be shared so that others can benefit by comparing that content with their own program's content or that others might be inspired to start a program of their own. Pitfalls in the implementation of the program can be discussed for the benefit of others. Such empirical descriptions might also include simple survey data about the acceptability of the course and its perceived value and importance.

Similar descriptive reports can be generated regarding other programs, such as ethics consult services, ombudsperson programs for medical students experiencing ethical conflicts in relation to faculty or residents, or programs on research integrity. All of these can contribute substantially to advancing the field of medical ethics.

Finally, as described by Danis and colleagues in chapter 15, it is possible to conduct controlled trials of new policies or programs. For example, one might test the effectiveness of a new policy regarding orders not to resuscitate patients (e.g., Sulmasy et al. 2006). Causal inferences about the effectiveness of such programs are most securely made in randomized controlled trials. Even having a concurrent nonrandomized control group is much better than having no control group. Such studies represent an important contribution of empirical research to medical ethics. They provide the best way to assess the impact (including the unintended ill effects) of new programs.

∽ Normative and Descriptive Ethics: Two-way Feedback

Based on the discussion above, it should be clear that the relationship between normative and descriptive research in medical ethics is one of two-way feedback (Pearlman, Miles, and Arnold 1993). Such work is not easy. It is important for scholars from different disciplines, when engaged in interdisciplinary work of any sort, to strive to understand each other's techniques and assumptions, and to work in an integrated way, striving to avoid the pitfall of merely working in parallel while talking past each other (Leget, Borry, and De Vries 2009). It is also true that all ethical decision making is empirical in the sense that it requires attention to empirical data about the real world (Musschenga 2005). Yet the autonomy of research disciplines must always be respected and understood in authentically interdisciplinary research. Some have called for a blurring of the autonomy of the various disciplines in favor of an integrated empirical ethics (Molewijk et al. 2004). The authors, however, appear to be conflating the necessary integration of the empirical into the making of concrete ethical decisions with the proper cooperation and mutual understanding tempered by respect for boundaries that ought to guide interdisciplinary research in ethics.

Normative and descriptive scholars can work with each other in a variety of ways. Normative ethics can generate claims that are associated with empirically testable hypotheses or set normative standards that must be operationalized and can be studied in educational or practice settings. The empirical lessons gained from such studies can, in turn, feed back upon and influence normative theory. Normative arguments may also depend upon facts that can be garnered from empirical inquiry, thus sustaining or refuting the empirical basis for the normative arguments. Descriptive ethics studies can also generate new material for normative study. Anthropological and sociological studies can raise questions about the universalizability of normative claims. Surveys can identify areas of disagreement that are ripe for ethical inquiry. Case studies can give rise to new questions that have never been addressed in normative inquiry, or can supply the entire basis for casuistic, narrative, and care-based work.

The two types of ethical inquiry are thus mutually supportive. Good studies in normative ethics will be grounded in good empirical data. Good descriptive studies will be shaped by ethical theory, providing a framework in which the data will be interpreted. Ethical reflection is enhanced when these two types of investigation are undertaken in an interdisciplinary and cooperative fashion.

∽ Conclusion

In this chapter we have tried to present a broad overview of a rather extensive field of inquiry—medical ethics. We have distinguished studies in descriptive ethics from studies in normative ethics and metaethics. We have described medical ethics as a single field of inquiry that involves multiple disciplines and multiple methods. We have discussed the importance of the fact/value distinction and delineated how this distinction helps us to understand some illicit inferences in medical ethics research. We have suggested some norms governing the proper relationship between normative ethics and descriptive ethics and how empirical studies can properly contribute to medical ethics.

Scholarship in medical ethics is exciting, dynamic, and growing. If normative and descriptive work in medical ethics can be pursued in a truly synergistic fashion, we believe there will be extraordinary research opportunities that neither approach could fulfill alone (Singer, Siegler, and Pellegrino 1990). Medical ethics is among the few academic fields in which truly interdisciplinary study is flourishing. It would be wonderful if the flavor of this interdisciplinary field were enriched further.

References

Alfidi, R. J. 1971. Informed consent: A study of patient reaction. *Journal of the American Medical Association* 216:1325–39.

Aquinas, T. 1972. *Summa Theologiae*. I–II, q. 94, a.4, c. Blackfriars Edition. New York: McGraw-Hill.

Aristotle. 1985. *Nichomachean Ethics*. 1 103b.28–3 1. Trans. Terence Irwin. Indianapolis: Hackett.

Baker, R. B., and L. B. McCullough. 2009. What is the history of medical ethics? In *The Cambridge world history of medical ethics*, ed. R. B. Baker and L. B. McCullough, 1–15. Cambridge: Cambridge University Press.

Barnato, A. E., D. L. Anthony, J. Skinner, P. M. Gallagher, and E. S. Fisher. 2009. Racial and ethnic differences in preferences for end-of-life treatment. *Journal of General Internal Medicine* 24:695–701.

Beauchamp, T. L. 1982. *Philosophical ethics: An introduction to moral philosophy*. New York: McGraw-Hill, 336–79.

Beauchamp, T. L., and J. F. Childress. 2009. *Principles of biomedical ethics*. 6th ed. New York: Oxford University Press.

Berlakovich, G. A., R. Steininger, F. Herbst, M. Barlan, M. Mittlbock, and F. Muhlbacher. 1994. Efficacy of liver transplantation for alcoholic cirrhosis with respect to recidivism and compliance. *Transplantation* 58:560–65.

Björnsson, E., J. Olsson, A. Rydell, K. Fredriksson, C. Eriksson, C. Sjöberg, M. Olausson, L. Bäckman, M. Castedal, and S. Friman. 2005. Long-term follow-up of patients with alcoholic liver disease after liver transplantation in Sweden: Impact of structured management on recidivism. *Scandinavian Journal of Gastroenterology* 40:206–16.

Blackhall, L. J., G. Frank, S. T. Murphy, V. Michel, J. M. Palmer, and S. P. Azen. 1999. Ethnicity and attitudes towards life sustaining technology. *Social Science and Medicine* 48:1779–89.

Childress, J. F. 2007. Methods in bioethics. In *Oxford handbook of bioethics*, ed. B. Steinbock, 15–45. New York: Oxford University Press.

Dubler N. N., and C. B. Liebman. 2004. *Bioethics mediation: A guide to shaping shared solutions*. New York: The United Hospital Fund.

Finnis, J. 1980. *Natural law, natural rights*. Oxford: Clarendon Press.

Frankena, W. 1973. *Ethics*. 2nd ed. Englewood Cliffs, NJ: Prentice Hall, 4–5.

Freeman, V. G., S. S. Rathore, K. P. Weinfurt, K. A. Schulman, and D. P. Sulmasy. 1999. Lying for patients: Physician deception of third party payers. *Archives of Internal Medicine* 159:2263–70.

Glannon W. 2009. Our brains are not us. *Bioethics* 23:321–29.

Hume, D. 1978. *A treatise of human nature*. 3rd ed. Edited by L. A. Selby-Bigge. Oxford: Oxford University Press, 468–70.

Hwang S., S. G. Lee, K. K. Kim, K. H. Kim, C. S. Ahn, D. B. Moon, T. Y. Ha, and G. W. Song. 2006. Efficacy of 6-month pretransplant abstinence for patients with alcoholic liver disease undergoing living donor liver transplantation. *Transplant Proceedings* 38:2937–40.

Illes, J., ed. 2005. *Neuroethics: Defining the issues in theory, practice and policy*. Oxford: Oxford University Press.

Jansen, L. A. 2009. Consensus and independent judgment in clinical ethics: Or what can an eighteenth-century French mathematician teach us about ethics consultation? *Journal of Clinical Ethics* 20 (1): 56–63.

Jonsen, A. R. 1998. Bioethics as a discipline. In *The birth of bioethics*, 325–51. Oxford: Oxford University Press.

Jonsen, A. R., and S. Toulmin. 1988. *The abuse of casuistry*. Berkeley: University of California Press.

Kaiser, J. R., J. M. Tilford, P. M. Simpson, W. A. Salhab, and C. R. Rosenfeld. 2004. Hospital survival of very-low-birth-weight neonates from 1977 to 2000. *Journal of Perinatology* 24:343–50.

Lorenz, J. M. 2000. Survival of the extremely preterm infant in North America in the 1990s. *Clinics in Perinatology* 27 (2): 255–62.

Leget C., P. Borry, and R. De Vries. 2009. "Nobody tosses a dwarf!" The relation between the empirical and the normative reexamined. *Bioethics* 23:226–35.

MacIntyre, A. 1984. *After virtue*. 2nd ed. Notre Dame, IN: University of Notre Dame Press.

Mayer, S. 2006. Declaration of patent applications as financial interests: A survey of practice among authors of papers on molecular biology in nature. *Journal of Medical Ethics* 32:658–61.

Milgram, Stanley. 1963. Behavioral study of obedience. *Journal of Abnormal and Social Psychology* 67:371–78.

Molewijk, B., A. M. Stiggelbout, W. Otten, H. M. Dupuis, and J. Kievit. 2004. Empirical data and moral theory. A plea for integrated empirical ethics. *Medicine, Health Care, and Philosophy* 7:55–69.

Moreno, J. D. 1995. *Deciding together: Bioethics and moral consensus*. New York: Oxford University Press.

Musschenga, A. W. 2005. Empirical ethics, context-sensitivity, and contextualism. *Journal of Medicine and Philosophy* 30:467–90.

Novack, D. H., R. Plumer, R. L. Smith, H. Ochitil, F. R. Morow, and J. M. Bennett. 1979. Changes in physicians' attitudes toward telling the cancer patient. *Journal of the American Medical Association* 241:897–900.

Oken, D. 1961. What to tell cancer patients. *Journal of the American Medical Association* 175:1120–28.

Okike, K., M. S. Kocher, E. X. Wei, C. T. Mehlman, and M. Bhandari. 2009. Accuracy of conflict-of-interest disclosures reported by physicians. *New England Journal of Medicine* 361:1466–74.

Olson, B., S. Soldz, and M. Davis. 2008. The ethics of interrogation and the American Psychological Association: A critique of policy and process. *Philosophy Ethics and Humanities in Medicine* 3 (January 29): 3.

Pearlman, R. A., S. H. Miles, and R. M. Arnold. 1993. Contributions of empirical research to medical ethics. *Theoretical Medicine* 14:197–210.

Pellegrino, E. D. 1995. The limitations of empirical research in ethics. *Journal of Clinical Ethics* 6:161–62.

Pellegrino, E. D., and D. C. Thomasma. 1981. *A philosophical basis of medical practice: Toward a philosophy and ethic of the healing professions*. New York: Oxford University Press.

Reichlin, M. 2007. The challenges of neuroethics. *Functional Neurology* 22:235–42.

Rescher, N. 1987. *Ethical idealism*. Berkeley: University of California Press, 26–54.

Searle, J. 1969. Deriving "ought" from "is." In *Speech acts*, 175–98. Cambridge: Cambridge University Press.

Singer, P. A., M. Siegler, and E. D. Pellegrino. 1990. Research in clinical ethics. *Journal of Clinical Ethics* 1:95–99.

Stevens, W. 1951. Thirteen ways of looking at a blackbird. In *Collected Poems of Wallace Stevens*. New York: Knopf.

Sulmasy, D. P., J. R. Sood, K. Texeira, R. McAuley, J. McGugins, and W. A. Ury. 2006. Prospective trial of a new policy eliminating signed consent for do not resuscitate orders. *Journal of General Internal Medicine* 21:1261–68.

Sulmasy, D. P., P. B. Terry, R. R. Faden, and D. M. Levine. 1994. Long-term effects of ethics education on the care of patients with do not resuscitate orders. *Journal of General Internal Medicine* 9:622–26.

SUPPORT Investigators. 1995. A controlled trial to improve care for seriously ill hospitalized patients: The study to understand prognoses and preferences for outcomes and risks of treatment (SUPPORT). *Journal of the American Medical Association* 274:1591–98.

Whittingham, J. R., R. A. Ruiter, L. Bolier, L. Lemmers, N. Van Hasselt, and G. Kok. 2009. Avoiding counterproductive results: An experimental pretest of a harm reduction intervention on attitude toward party drugs among users and nonusers. *Substance Use and Misuse* 44:532–47.

Wynia, M. K., D. S. Cummins, J. B. VanGeest, and I. B. Wilson. 2000. Physician manipulation of reimbursement rules for patients: Between a rock and a hard place. *Journal of the American Medical Association* 283:1858–65.

CHAPTER 2

A Quarter Century of Empirical Research in Biomedical Ethics

JEREMY SUGARMAN,
RUTH FADEN, AND ALISON BOYCE

While philosophical, legal, and theological scholarship traditionally dominated the field of biomedical ethics, empirical, data-based research with methodological roots in the social sciences has assumed an important role in the field. In this chapter we set out to describe the empirical literature in the field of biomedical ethics beginning in the 1980s, which are the first years in which data on this question are readily available. We define empirical research in biomedical ethics as the application of research methods in the social sciences to the direct examination of issues in biomedical ethics (Sugarman, Faden, and Weinstein 2001). We provide empirical answers to the following specific empirical questions: What topics in biomedical ethics were empirically studied? How did empirical research in biomedical ethics change?

❧ Methods

After considering alternative strategies, we elected to conduct a search in Medline using the online resource PubMed. Due to resource constraints, we did not review each citation individually to ensure the accuracy of the postings. Instead, we relied upon the keywords assigned by the online index. Nevertheless, we took steps in constructing the search and analyzing the data to help ensure accuracy. As suggested by Strech and colleagues (2008), the search strategy was designed to be consistent with the underlying structure of the database. For instance, we used Medical Subject Heading (MeSH) terminology, which is the controlled vocabulary that is used by the National Library of Medicine to index citations in the Medline database.[1] Each article in Medline is reviewed by a specialist and assigned the applicable MeSH terms (Coletti and Bleich 2001).

There were three steps to the initial search. First, we determined the total number of postings in the entire database in each five-year interval from 1980 to 2005. Next, we identified all biomedical ethics publications for each time period, searching for "ethics" as a MeSH term. Note that "ethics" is used as a proxy for biomedical ethics, given the structure of the MeSH taxonomy.[2] Finally, we combined "ethics" with a search strategy designed to retrieve empirical postings.[3]

To examine additional characteristics of the empirical biomedical ethics postings we identified, we imported the entire data set into EndNote (Version XI, Thomson Reuters, New York, NY). The MeSH terms that are tagged to articles are imported into EndNote in the "keyword" field, permitting quantification of the times a particular keyword is used for all of the references in a database. We were thus able to inductively identify the frequency with which MeSH terms were assigned for topics, subjects, and methods. Given the overwhelming amount of data, we generated a list of keywords that were assigned to at least one hundred publications. We then removed keywords that were assigned to methods (e.g., questionnaires, focus groups) and subjects (e.g., patients, nurses). Since multiple keywords are typically assigned to each posting, and we wanted to get a picture of the most frequently studied topics, we then conducted a new search in PubMed for articles whose major topics included one of these frequently identified keywords and the empirical ethics search strategy described above. To analyze the data further, we then condensed this list of topics by combining terms that denote similar topics following the MeSH "tree" hierarchy where feasible (e.g., combining "professional misconduct" with "scientific misconduct," which is a subclass of professional misconduct in the MeSH taxonomy).

❧ Results

As of December 2008 there were 89,095 total ethics postings in PubMed for the period from 1980 through 2005, which represents less than 1 percent of all PubMed postings for this period. Of the total ethics postings, 11,776 (13 percent) represented empirical research (see table 2.1 and figure 2.1).

Within the total body of empirical biomedical ethics postings (n=11,776), there were 326 MeSH terms that were applied to at least one hundred publications. After removing MeSH terms that applied to methods (n=16) and subjects (n=15), the

TABLE 2.1 Ethics Postings

Time Period	Total	All Ethics	Empirical Biomedical Ethics	Empirical Biomedical Ethics/Ethics postings (%)
1980–84	1,460,276	7,667	577	8
1985–89	1,809,682	11,166	910	8
1990–94	2,059,890	18,315	2,220	12
1995–99	2,281,690	21,751	3,247	15
2000–2005	3,488,522	30,196	4,822	16
1980–2005	**11,100,060**	**89,095**	**11,776**	**13**

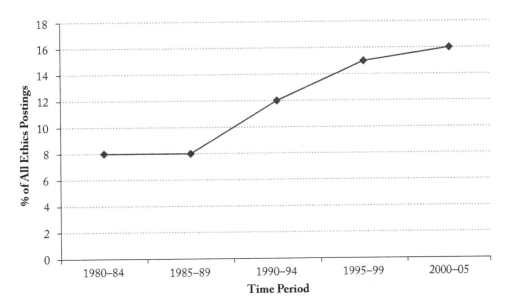

FIGURE 2.1   Proportion of Empirical Biomedical Ethics Postings over Time

Note: Percentage equals the number of empirical postings divided by the total number of ethics postings times 100.

initial topic list comprised 295 MeSH terms. The condensed list of the most frequently studied topics according to MeSH terminology as described above consisted of 92 topic terms (table 2.2).

Overall, the topics that received the most attention were quality of health care, health services, public health, professional ethics, the delivery of health care, and ethical theory. Note that most of these categories, with the exception of public health, consisted of several combined terms.[4] Quality of health care encompassed the terms "quality of health care"; "quality assessment (health care)"; "treatment outcome"; "guidelines as topic"; "patient satisfaction"; and "health care reform." Health services included the terms "health services"; "health services accessibility"; "health services needs and demands"; "nursing homes"; "rehabilitation"; "counseling"; and "hospitals." Professional ethics included "ethics, professional"; "ethics, clinical"; "ethics, dental"; "ethics, institutional"; "ethics, nursing." Ethical theory was comprised of "ethical theory"; "humanism"; "feminism"; "philosophy"; "morals"; "moral development"; "moral obligation"; and "ethical analysis."

The frequency of topics that received empirical attention has changed over time. Some topic areas that are high in absolute numbers in the overall time period, such as professional ethics, are trending downward in relative frequency over time. Similarly, informed consent is high in overall postings but more recently accounts for a smaller proportion for postings. Other topic areas, such as nursing, are increasing in proportion to other topics. Figure 2.2 shows the changing proportions over time for the most prevalent topics in each five-year interval.[5]

TABLE 2.2 Frequent Major Topics of Empirical Biomedical Ethics Postings, 1980–2005

MeSH Term		MeSH Term	
Quality of Health Care[a]	4,122	Family	369
Health Services[a]	3,956	Tissue and Organ Procurement[a]	283
Public Health	3,518	Physician–Patient Relations[a]	281
Ethics, Professional[a]	3,144	Epidemiology[a]	279
Delivery of Health Care[a]	2,827	Personal Autonomy	274
Ethical Theory[a]	2,754	Patient Advocacy	263
Bioethics[a]	2,743	AIDS[a]	244
Patient Care[a]	2,730	Social Values	243
Organization and Administration[a]	2,564	Privacy	237
Human Rights[a]	2,199	Drug Therapy[a]	222
Communication[a]	2,183	Physician's Role[a]	204
Education[a]	2,153	Social Support[a]	204
Mass Screening[a]	1,976	Industry	194
Research[a]	1,921	Value of Life[a]	191
Legislation and Jurisprudence[a]	1,833	Information Services	184
Economics[a]	1,776	Abortion[a]	181
Nursing[a]	1,486	Religion	176
Genetics[a]	1,408	Reproductive Techniques, Assisted[a]	155
Records as Topic[a]	1,257	Prejudice[a]	133
Health Knowledge, Attitudes, Practice[a]	1,200	Policymaking	128
Terminal Care[a]	1,071	Sexual Behavior	124
Psychology[a]	1,029	Advance Directive	120
Decision-Making[a]	884	Conflict of Interest	115
Attitude of Health Personnel	881	Third-Party Consent[a]	112
Health[a]	847	Liability, Legal[a]	108
Socioeconomic Factors[a]	781	Pregnancy	98
Mental Disorders[a]	767	Publishing	95
Informed Consent[a]	744	Drug Industry	93
Ethics, Research[a]	733	Public Opinion	93
Euthanasia[a]	710	Politics	92
Health Policy[a]	688	Societies	86
Psychiatry	685	Codes of Ethics	80
Confidentiality	658	Social Change	71
Government[a]	648	Mental Competency[a]	66
Prenatal Diagnosis[a]	645	Attitude to Death	63
Ethics Committees[a]	601	Leadership	51
Disclosure[a]	596	Treatment Refusal	47
Internationality[a]	528	Mandatory Programs	45
Public Policy	524	Eugenics	42
Risk[a]	511	Vulnerable Populations	40
Professional Misconduct[a]	481	Animals	37
Ethics Committees, Research[a]	437	Deception	37
Social Justice	435	Paternalism	35
Social Responsibility	434	Beneficence	22
Cultural Diversity[a]	391	Trust	22
Statistics as Topic	379	Altruism	13

[a]Term is a composite of one or more keywords; see note 4.

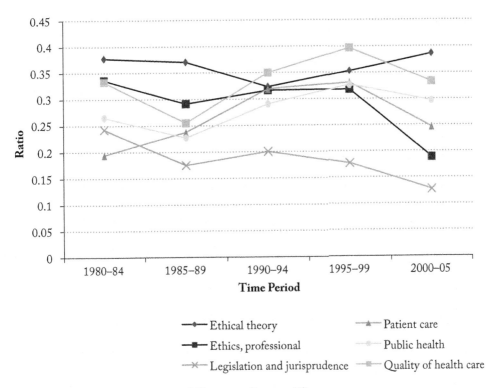

FIGURE 2.2   Topics Examined Empirically over Time

METHODS

There were 8,414 postings associated with MeSH terms that indicated the research methods employed, which accounted for 71 percent of our database (table 2.3). Within this set, the most commonly used methodology was questionnaires (n=2,037).

Figure 2.3 displays the ratio of publications tagged with particular methodological terms to the total empirical biomedical ethics publications over time. Comparative studies and questionnaires had the greatest absolute numbers in all time periods, with focus groups, ethnology, and qualitative research having none or very few postings in the first fifteen years of the twenty-five-year time period, but are more recently used in a greater proportion of postings.

SUBJECTS

There were also 6,012 postings associated with MeSH terms that indicated the subjects of empirical study, which accounted for 51 percent of our database (table 2.4). The most common research subjects identified in our search were the aged, followed by adults, physicians, newborns, and adolescents. Over time, physicians were studied to a lesser extent. In contrast, studies with adults and the aged represent a growing proportion of subjects overall. Most recently, a greater proportion of empirical attention is being focused on adolescents (figure 2.4).

TABLE 2.3 Methods[6]

Method	N	%
Questionnaires	2,037	24.2
Comparative Studies	1,752	20.8
Evaluation Studies	1,585	18.8
Trends	603	7.2
Empirical Research	372	4.4
Qualitative Research	313	3.7
Health Services Research	285	3.4
Ethnology	232	2.8
Registries	209	2.5
Behavioral Research	207	2.5
Focus Groups	201	2.4
Cross-cultural Comparison	147	1.7
Pilot Projects	139	1.7
Databases	118	1.4
Random Allocation	114	1.4
Needs Assessment	100	1.2

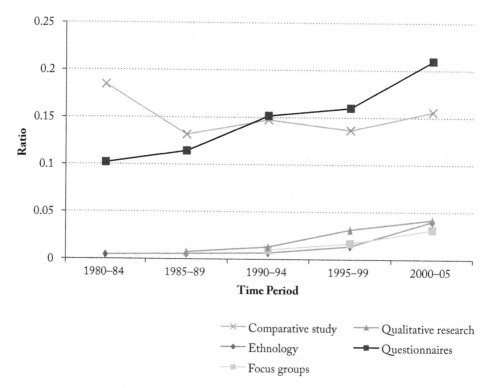

FIGURE 2.3 Empirical Methods Used over Time

TABLE 2.4   Research Subjects

Subject	N	%
Aged	1,172	19.5
Adults	1,126	18.7
Physicians	679	11.3
Infant, Newborn	610	10.1
Adolescents	456	7.6
Research Personnel	322	5.4
Patients	235	3.9
Pregnant Women	227	3.8
Parents	221	3.7
Health Personnel	208	3.5
Nurses	199	3.3
Ethicists	171	2.8
Students, Medical	155	2.6
Nursing Staff	119	2.0
Students, Nursing	112	1.9

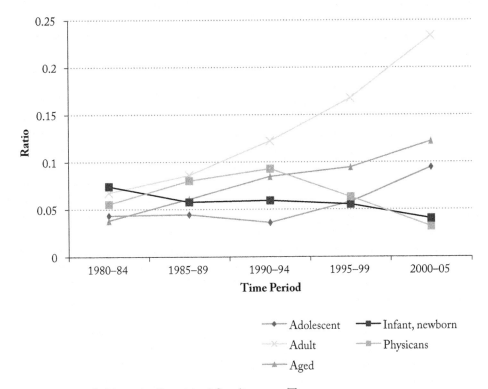

FIGURE 2.4   Subjects in Empirical Studies over Time

∾ Limitations

The main limitations of this study regard the specificity and sensitivity of the method. As a practical matter the large number of retrieved postings prohibits the examination of each individual article to ensure the accuracy of its assigned keywords, as was done in the description of the first decade of bioethics included in the first edition of *Methods in Medical Ethics* (Sugarman, Faden and Weinstein, 2001). The method we used relies considerably upon the judgment of PubMed indexers who assign keywords to publications. Previous reviews have established that interpreting data using such search methods must be done with caution, given that the actual topic of a particular study may be substantially different than suggested by keywords alone (Sugarman, McCrory, and Hubel 1998; Sugarman et al. 1999). Further, what is encompassed by a particular MeSH term can be difficult to discern in some cases. It is unclear how these indexing concerns would affect our findings. For example, some studies that would have been considered ethics studies by the authors might have been indexed as studies of decision making or quality of care but not ethics. Finally, our list of MeSH terms was not sufficiently comprehensive to capture all the empirical methods used in biomedical ethics research. This renders our method less accurate with respect to the proportion of biomedical ethics studies that employed particular empirical methods. Nonetheless, the data we present can still provide useful information about general trends and relative proportions regarding empirical work in the field of biomedical ethics over time.

∾ Discussion

The primary value of this analysis is to identify the major trends in empirical bioethics research. Our data, which span a quarter of a century, suggest that empirical research in biomedical ethics represents 13 percent of the total postings in bioethics. The proportion of biomedical ethics literature that uses empirical research methods appears to be increasing steadily, although the rate of increase appears to have slowed in recent years compared with the late 1980s to 1990s. Specifically, we found that empirical research represented 8 percent of the biomedical ethics literature in the 1980–1984 period, increasing to 16 percent in the 2000–2005 period. In terms of topics, quality of health care, health services, and public health have received substantial empirical attention. The data also suggest that there has been a proliferation of the number of topic areas examined empirically, particularly over the past decade. These findings are consistent with previous reviews of the empirical bioethics literature (Sugarman, Faden, and Weinstein 2001; Sugarman 2004), as well as reviews that used different methods (e.g., Borry, Schotsmans, and Dierickx 2006; Cohen et al. 2008).

Borry, Schotsmans, and Dierickx (2006) performed a review of all publications from 1990 to 2003 in nine selected bioethics journals. They reviewed and coded each individual article and found that overall 10 percent of studies used an empirical design, increasing from 5 percent in 1990 to 15 percent in 2003. Although the final percentage of empirical publications is similar to our findings, their strategy is incapable of capturing many empirical studies of bioethical issues (for instance, those published in medical journals). In addition, Borry et al. identified end-of-life issues as the most frequent topic of empirical study, which diverges from our results. This may be due to their use of a strategy that was limited to bioethics journals, reflecting the topics that would be of interest to bioethics journal editors or scholars electing to publish their work in these specialty journals. As in our analysis, Borry et al. found a substantial increase in nursing-related studies in recent years.

Cohen et al. (2008) examined how the topics of publications in bioethics varied from 1970 through 2004. They used the terms "ethics OR bioethics" in all fields, in the period from 1970 through 2004, when performing a search in Medline and assessed the ratio of publications about particular topics to the total bioethics postings in five-year intervals. Their search strategy did not distinguish between empirical and nonempirical postings, nor did they attempt to validate the indexing of terms on Medline. Nonetheless, they also found that the percentage of total bioethics postings in Medline was increasing over time, to about 1 percent. In addition, they too found that the relative prevalence of many topics has varied considerably over time, reflecting the changes in relative attention given to certain topics in the field of bioethics, which is consistent with our findings. Looking at particular topics, Cohen et al. reported specific data for just four topics (induced abortion, conflict of interest, AIDS, and medical education). Their findings corroborate ours, showing the same trends with respect to these four topics (i.e., decreasing, increasing, decreasing after a precipitous peak, and steady over time, respectively).

Later chapters in this book discuss the issue of whether the empirical research methods used in a study are appropriate for the questions being asked. Valid empirical studies must employ the proper method according to a carefully refined research question (Guyatt, Sackett, and Cook 1993; Levine et al. 1994). Consider the following simple hypothetical example:

Researchers are interested in determining which of two methods of obtaining informed consent is better, a video presentation about a proposed intervention or a conversation with a nurse. The optimal method to answer this research question likely would be a randomized trial comparing the two methods. Patients in each arm of the trial could be asked about their knowledge and beliefs about the proposed intervention as well as their satisfaction and attitudes toward the informed consent process and their perceptions about the voluntariness of their decisions. These data might then facilitate determining which method was better. In contrast, a simple cross-sectional survey of patients or nurses who had participated in different procedures for soliciting consent might lead to erroneous conclusions because methodological biases inherent in such a cross sectional design would likely permit factors other than the method by which consent was obtained to mask or enhance differences.

It is relevant to note that almost a quarter of all the empirical studies for which we had information on the methods employed used questionnaires. In addition, most methods were descriptive. However, other powerful research methods, such as randomized trials, were seldom used. It may be that empirical researchers coming from a variety of home disciplines were largely unfamiliar with these methods. Furthermore, as discussed in subsequent chapters in this book, these methods can demand substantial expertise and resources that may not be available to those conducting empirical research in medical ethics.

Empirical research today is an accepted and growing component of the literature in medical ethics. This work should be expected to continue to change over time, reflecting different topics and perhaps using different methods.

ꙮ Notes

1. See www.nlm.nih.gov/pubs/factsheets/pubmed.html for general characteristics of PubMed and Medline.
2. A search of "ethics" as a MeSH term gives the same results as "ethics" OR "bioethics" in PubMed, so we simply used the term "ethics." We used the term "ethics" searched as an exploded MeSH (medical subject heading) term in order to perform this study. As noted by Cohen et al. (2008, 82) this strategy includes many subject terms automatically and can therefore be considered reasonably comprehensive. The exploded term includes the following: Bioethical Issues; Bioethics; Ethics, Clinical; Complicity; Conflict of Interest; Ethical Analysis; Casuistry; Retrospective Moral Judgment; Wedge Argument; Ethical Relativism; Ethical Review; Ethics Consultation; Ethical Theory; Ethicists; Ethics, Business; Ethics Committees; Ethics Committees, Clinical; Ethics Committees, Research; Ethics, Institutional; Ethics, Professional; Codes of Ethics; Ethics, Clinical; Ethics, Dental; Ethics, Medical; Ethics, Nursing; Ethics, Pharmacy; Ethics, Research; Helsinki Declaration; Humanism; Feminism; Morals; Conscience; Moral Development; Social Responsibility; Virtues; Personhood; Principle-Based Ethics; Beneficence; Personal Autonomy; Social Justice; Professional Misconduct; Scientific Misconduct; Complicity; Double Effect; Humanism; Feminism; Morals; Conscience; Social Responsibility; Virtues; Personhood; Principle-Based Ethics; Bioethics; Physician Self-Referral.
3. The search strategy was: "ethics"[MeSH] AND ("Empirical Research"[MeSH] OR "data collection"[MeSH] OR Clinical Trial[ptyp] OR Meta-Analysis[ptyp] OR Randomized Controlled Trial[ptyp] OR Comparative Study[ptyp] OR Controlled Clinical Trial[ptyp] OR Evaluation Studies[ptyp] OR Interview[ptyp] OR Multicenter Study[ptyp] OR Validation Studies[ptyp]) AND ("1980"[PDAT] : "2005"[PDAT]).
4. Terms included in the condensed list of topics.

Topic	Terms Included
Abortion	Abortion, Induced; Abortion, Eugenic
AIDS	AIDS; HIV Seropositivity; HIV Infection
Bioethics	Bioethics, Bioethical Issues, Ethics, Medical
Communication	Communication; Interpersonal Relations; Professional Patient Relations; Information Dissemination; Interprofessional Relations; Interdisciplinary Communication; Dissent and Disputes
Cultural Diversity	Cultural Diversity; Culture; Cross-cultural Comparisons
Decision Making	Decision Making; Patient Participation; Consumer Participation; Uncertainty
Delivery of Health Care	Delivery of Health Care; Utilization; Supply and Distribution; Primary Health Care; Family Practice
Disclosure	Disclosure; Truth Disclosure
Drug Therapy	Drug Therapy; Adverse Effects; Administration and Dosage; Pharmaceutical Preparations
Economics	Economics; Health Care Rationing; Cost-Benefit Analysis; Resource Allocation

Topic	Terms Included
Education	Education; Medical Education; Patient Education; Teaching; Curriculum; Professional Competence; Clinical Competence; Internship and Residency
Epidemiology	Epidemiology; Prevalence; Severity of Illness Index; Fatal Outcome; Geriatric Assessment; Life Expectancy; Etiology; Incidence; Morbidity; Cause of Death; Infant Mortality; Survival Rate
Ethical Theory	Ethical Theory; Humanism; Feminism; Moral Development; Moral Obligations; Philosophy; Morals; Ethical Analysis
Ethics Committees	Ethics Committees; Ethics Committees, Clinical
Ethics Committees, Research	Ethics Committees, Research; Ethical Review
Ethics, Professional	Ethics, Professional; Ethics, Nursing; Ethics, Clinical; Ethics, Dental; Ethics, Institutional
Ethics, Research	Ethics, Research; Therapeutic Human Experimentation; Nontherapeutic Human Experimentation; Researcher-Subject Relations
Euthanasia	Euthanasia; Euthanasia, Passive, Euthanasia, Active, Voluntary; Euthanasia, Active; Suicide, Assisted; Right to Die
Genetics	Genetics; Genetics, Medical; Gene Therapy; Genetic Privacy; Genetic Research; Human Genome Project; Genetic Engineering
Government	Government; Government Regulation; National Institutes of Health; Federal Government; State Government; State Medicine; National Health Programs
Health	Health; Women's Health; Health Education; Health Priorities; Health Status; Health Care Surveys; Health Status Indicators
Health Knowledge, Attitudes, Practice	Health Knowledge, Attitudes, Practice; Attitude to Health
Health Policy	Health Policy; Insurance, Health; Managed Care Programs
Health Services	Health Services Accessibility; Nursing Homes; Hospitals; Counseling; Rehabilitation; Health Services Needs and Demand
Human Rights	Human Rights; Women's Rights; Civil Rights; Patients' Rights; Freedom
Informed Consent	Informed Consent; Consent Forms; Comprehension
Internationality	Internationality; International Cooperation; Developing Countries
Legislation and Jurisprudence	Legislation and Jurisprudence; Jurisprudence; Legislation as Topic; Legislation, Medical
Liability, Legal	Liability, Legal; Malpractice
Mass Screening	Mass Screening; Genetic Screening
Mental Disorders	Mental Disorders; Substance-Related Disorders; Mentally Ill Persons; Commitment of Mentally Ill
Nursing	Nursing; Nursing-Patient Relations; Nursing Methodology Research; Nurse's Role; Nursing Research; Philosophy, Nursing
Organization and Administration	Organization and Administration; Organizational Policy; Decision Making, Organizational; Computer Security; Organizational Culture
Patient Care	Patient Care; Diagnosis; Prognosis; Physician's Practice Concerns; Patient Selection; Patient Care Team; Referral and Consultation
Physician's Role	Physician's Role; Duty to Warn; Forecasting; Practice Guidelines as Topic

Topic	Terms Included
Policymaking	Policymaking; Advisory Committees
Prejudice	Prejudice; Stereotyping
Prenatal Diagnosis	Prenatal Diagnosis; Genetic Diseases, Inborn; Prenatal Counseling
Professional Misconduct	Professional Misconduct; Scientific Misconduct
Psychology	Psychology; Stress, Psychological; Adaptation, Psychological; Self-Concept; Models, Psychological; Power (Psychology); Conflict (Psychology); Motivation; Group Processes
Quality of Health Care	Quality of Health Care; Outcome Assessment (Health Care); Health Care Reform; Treatment Outcome; Patient Satisfaction; Guidelines as Topic
Records	Records as Topic; Medical Records; Medical Records System, Computerized
Reproductive Techniques, Assisted	Reproductive Techniques, Assisted; Fertilization in Vitro
Research	Research; Biomedical Research; Research Design; Research Subjects
Risk	Risk; Risk Assessment; Risk Factors
Social Support	Social Support; Social Welfare
Socioeconomic Factors	Socioeconomic Factors; Income; Social Class; Employment; Poverty
Terminal Care	Terminal Care; Palliative Care; Terminally Ill; Resuscitation Orders; Life Support Care; Withholding Treatment
Third-Party Consent	Third-Party Consent; Parental Consent
Tissue and Organ Procurement	Tissue and Organ Procurement; Tissue Donors
Value of Life	Value of Life; Quality of Life; Quality-Adjusted Life Years

5. The two tables below show the five most common topics in each interval. The results differ according to whether the term is a major topic, as assigned in PubMed, or is just a MeSH term.

Major topic only.

	1980–84	1985–89	1990–94	1995–99	2000–05
1st most common	Ethical Theory	Ethical Theory	Quality of Health Care	Quality of Health Care	Ethical Theory
2nd	Ethics, Professional	Ethics, Professional	Ethical Theory	Ethical Theory	Quality of Health Care
3rd	Quality of Health Care	Quality of Health Care	Patient Care	Patient Care	Public Health
4th	Public Health	Patient Care	Ethics, Professional	Public Health	Patient Care
5th	Legislation and Jurisprudence	Public Health	Public Health	Ethics, Professional	Ethics, Professional

MeSH term (any)

	1980–84	1985–89	1990–94	1995–99	2000–05
1st most common	Informed Consent	Ethics, Professional	Ethics, Professional	Ethics, Professional	Psychology
2nd	Research	Patient Care	Patient Care	Psychology	Ethics, Professional
3rd	Ethical Theory	Research	Psychology	Patient Care	Epidemiology
4th	Government	Ethical Theory	Economics	Economics	Patient Care
5th	Legislation and Jurisprudence	Informed Consent	Ethical Theory	Research	Nursing

6. PubMed Definition of Terms.

Term	Definition
Questionnaires	Predetermined sets of questions used to collect data—clinical data, social status, occupational group, and so on. The term is often applied to a self-completed survey instrument.
Comparative Study (publication type)	Comparison of outcomes, results, responses, and so on, for different techniques, therapeutic approaches, or other inputs.
Evaluation Studies	Works consisting of studies determining the effectiveness or utility of processes, personnel, and equipment.
Trends (subheading)	Used for the manner in which a subject changes, qualitatively or quantitatively, with time, whether past, present, or future. It excludes discussions of the course of disease in particular patients.
Empirical Research	The study, based on direct observation, use of statistical records, interviews, or experimental methods, of actual practices or the actual impact of practices or policies.
Qualitative Research	Research that derives data from observation, interviews, or verbal interactions and focuses on the meanings and interpretations of the participants (from Holloway and Wheeler, "Ethical Issues in Qualitative Nursing Research," *Nursing Ethics* 2, no. 3 [September 1995]: 223–32).
Health Services Research	The integration of epidemiologic, sociological, economic, and other analytic sciences in the study of health services. Health services research is usually concerned with relationships between need, demand, supply, use, and outcome of health services. The aim of the research is evaluation, particularly in terms of structure, process, output, and outcome (from Last, *Dictionary of Epidemiology*, 2nd ed.).
Ethnology	The comparative and theoretical study of culture, often synonymous with cultural anthropology.
Registries	The systems and processes involved in the establishment, support, management, and operation of registers, for example, disease registers.
Behavioral Research	Research that involves the application of the behavioral and social sciences to the study of the actions or reactions of persons or animals in response to external or internal stimuli (from *American Heritage Dictionary*, 4th ed.).

Term	Definition
Focus Groups	A method of data collection and a qualitative research tool in which a small group of individuals are brought together and allowed to interact in a discussion of their opinions about topics, issues, or questions.
Pilot Projects	Small-scale tests of methods and procedures to be used on a larger scale if the pilot study demonstrates that these methods and procedures can work.
Databases	Organized collections of computer records, standardized in format and content, that are stored in any of a variety of computer-readable modes. They are the basic sets of data from which computer-readable files are created (from ALA *Glossary of Library and Information Science*, 1983).
Random Allocation	A process involving chance used in therapeutic trials or other research endeavor for allocating experimental subjects, human or animal, between treatment and control groups, or among treatment groups. It may also apply to experiments on inanimate objects.
Needs Assessment	Systematic identification of a population's needs or the assessment of individuals to determine the proper level of services needed.

❧ References

Borry, P., P. Schotsmans, and K. Dierickx. 2006. Empirical research in bioethical journals. A quantitative analysis. *Journal of Medical Ethics* 32:240–45.

Cohen, C., J. A. R. Vianna, L. R. Battistella, and E. Massad. 2008. Time variation of some selected topics in bioethical publications. *Journal of Medical Ethics* 34:81–84.

Coletti, M. H., and H. L. Bleich. 2001. Medical subject headings used to search the biomedical literature. *Journal of the American Medical Informatics Association* 8:317–23.

Guyett, G. H., D. L. Sackett, and D. J. Cook. 1993. Users' guides to the medical literature. *Journal of the American Medical Association* 270:2598–2601.

Levine, M., S. Walker, H. Lee, T. Haines, A Holbrook, and V. Moyer, for the Evidence-Based Medicine Working Group. 1994. Users' guides to the medical literature. *Journal of the American Medical Association* 271:1615–19.

Strech, D., M. Synofzik, and G. Marckmann. 2008. Systematic reviews of empirical bioethics. *Journal of Medical Ethics* 34:472–77.

Sugarman, J. 2004. The future of empirical research in bioethics. *Journal of Law, Medicine, and Ethics* 32:226–31.

Sugarman, J., R. Faden, and J. Weinstein. 2001. A decade of empirical research in medical ethics. In *Methods in medical ethics*, eds. J. Sugarman and D. Sulmasy. Washington, DC: Georgetown University Press.

Sugarman, J., D. C. McCrory, and R. C. Hubal. 1998. Getting meaningful informed consent from older persons: A structured literature review of empirical research. *Journal of the American Geriatrics Society* 46:517–24.

Sugarman, J., D. C. McCrory, D. Powell, A. Krasny, B. Adams, E. Ball, and C. Cassell. 1999. Empirical research on informed consent. *Hastings Center Report* 29:S1–S42.

PART II

Methods

CHAPTER 3

Philosophy: Ethical Principles and Common Morality

DAVID DEGRAZIA AND TOM L. BEAUCHAMP

What distinctive contributions does philosophy provide to medical ethics? Philosophy's most prominent contribution, on which this chapter focuses, is to provide the critical resources of ethical theory and methodology in ethics.[1] The ambition of ethical theory is to provide an adequate normative framework for addressing the problems of moral life. Usually such a framework takes the form of a theory of right action, but it may take the form of a theory of good character. The ambition of methodology in ethics is to provide a procedure or method for producing such a normative framework, using such a framework once it has been identified, or navigating the complexities of moral life in the absence of such a framework.

This chapter examines a range of philosophical methods in medical ethics. We explore five leading methods, or models, of moral reasoning, with special attention given to the problems of medical ethics. In contrast to other approaches presented in this book, the methods discussed here place a strong emphasis on ethical principles, common morality, and ethical theory. Our discussion of particular ethical theories is relatively compressed because the application of established ethical theories represents only one of the five methods we explore.

The chapter begins with a section titled "Description of Methods of Philosophical Medical Ethics," in which each method or model is described in a subsection and then subjected to one or more important criticisms in a separate subsection. The next section provides a critique of philosophical methods in medical ethics in general. The chapter ends with a section on philosophical training in medical ethics and on leading scholarly resources in the field.

Description of Methods of Philosophical Medical Ethics

Moral philosophers have traditionally aspired to normative theories of what is right or wrong that are set out in the most general terms. But it is increasingly questioned whether such general theories can be fruitfully applied in specific cases and contexts.

It is also controversial which philosophical methods best achieve the objectives of "applied ethics" or "practical ethics"—terms that came into vogue as philosophical ethics increasingly addressed such practical issues as abortion, physician-hastened death, human research, access to health care, and genetic engineering.

Several methods have been prominent in philosophical medical ethics. Among those influential methods, we will focus on these five: medical tradition and practice standards; principles, common morality, and specification; ethical theory as the basis of applied ethics; casuistry (case-based reasoning); and reflective equilibrium (a form of coherence theory). The terrain of philosophical methods in ethics is broader than the large area that we will sketch here. We will omit, for example, feminist ethics, virtue ethics, narrative ethics, and pragmatist approaches to medical ethics. Several of these approaches are discussed elsewhere in this book. Some philosophers might regard one or more of the methods just mentioned as ethical theories that could serve as the backbone of "applied ethics," but these approaches are also widely regarded as alternatives to the "applied ethics" model.

APPEALS TO MEDICAL TRADITION AND PRACTICE STANDARDS

Among the most influential sources of medical and nursing ethics are traditions: the concepts, practices, and norms that have long guided conduct in these fields. Some scholars of medical ethics find them to be a logical starting point in reflecting on professional ethics. Great traditions such as Hippocratic ethics clearly deserve respect, but they also often fail to provide a comprehensive, unbiased, and adequately justified ethics. Philosophers ought to take this history seriously while raising questions about the moral authority of oaths, prayers, codes, published lectures, and general pamphlets and treatises on medical conduct. One approach is to reconstruct traditional norms in a more perspicuous and defensible manner while remaining largely faithful to those norms (see, e.g., Pellegrino 1985; Arras 1988). Sometimes, however, it is preferable to propose new norms.

It is sometimes unclear whether statements made in documents of great historical influence were primarily descriptive, exhortatory, or self-protective. Some writings describe, for educational purposes, conduct that conformed to prevailing professional standards. Other documents aim at reforming professional conduct by prescribing what should be established practice. Still others seem constructed to protect the physician from suspicions of misconduct or from legal liability. Accordingly, to view prescriptions in codes and similar material at face value as if they capture proper professional norms may cause moral confusion or distortion. Moreover, philosophers want to do more than understand the concepts, practices, and norms found in medical traditions. Although historical understanding is a worthy goal, it is no substitute for careful moral analysis. The ultimate philosophical goal is to defend or criticize the concepts, practices, and norms under investigation—an exercise in normative ethics.

A traditionalist might argue that appreciating the history of medicine is a crucial part of normative ethics, by enabling one to grasp the essential nature (or essence) of medicine and of the physician–patient relationship. From this perspective, one can extract an understanding of the ethics of medicine. Edmund Pellegrino, for example, has argued that the nature of illness, the historically validated fact that medical knowledge is not individually owned, and the physician's public act of taking the Hippocratic Oath together entail that physicians have an obligation to serve patients even when doing so requires effacement of self-interest (Pellegrino 1987).

PROBLEMS WITH APPEALS TO MEDICAL TRADITION AND PRACTICE STANDARDS

The essential problem with attempts to base applied ethics in practice standards and traditional oaths and guidelines is that such resources are not self-justifying. Whether a particular practice standard or oath is justified must be determined by careful ethical reflection, which may conclude that the prevailing norm is morally inadequate. Even ethicists and physicians working largely within a traditional framework accept the need for some degree of independent ethical reflection.

One variant of the traditional approach might seem less susceptible to this line of criticism. Suppose that the history of medical practice reveals the essential nature of medicine, the understanding of which allows us to extract a viable medical ethics. Pellegrino, for example, maintains that medicine must be understood entirely in terms of the end of medicine, which is healing. Accordingly, the category of medical benefits cannot include items such as fertility controls (unless for the prevention and maintenance of health and bodily integrity), purely cosmetic surgery, or active euthanasia (Pellegrino 1999, 2001).

The claim that medicine has some single, essential nature is debatable. Arguably, medicine is an evolving set of practices with no intrinsic limits to the possibility for change. Moreover, even if medicine has a fixed essence or purpose, it is doubtful that ethical norms other than highly abstract statements of general purpose can be derived from facts about this essence. It has become more apparent during the last forty years that traditional codes and practices of medical and nursing ethics are inadequate to address problems arising from modern scientific research, clinical practice, biomedical technology, health policy, and related social developments. The history of medical ethics emanating from the practices of two thousand years ago is disappointing from the perspective of today's concerns in medical ethics about the rights of patients and subjects and the ways in which society should promote the health of its members. Most topics in medical ethics that are of major concern today have been ignored or given but passing notice until the second half of the twentieth century. In conclusion, although there is no reason for philosophers to discount appeals to tradition, it is very doubtful that today's medical ethics can be reconstructed from this source alone.

PRINCIPLES, COMMON MORALITY, AND SPECIFICATION

Once many observers came to regard medical traditions of ethics as outmoded by modern developments in medicine, representatives of various disciplines sought to identify basic ethical principles that could help determine which clinical practices and human experiments are morally questionable or in need of reform. Because basic moral principles are of great interest to moral philosophers, there was a turn to philosophy to identify and analyze the principles that could serve as a moral framework for medical ethics. But on what are these principles to be based?

One possibility is that just as tradition can be a resource, so can common morality—the morality shared by morally committed persons. Common morality, so understood, is not merely *a* morality in contrast to *other* moralities; it is normative for everyone, and all persons are rightly judged by its standards. The content of common morality may be understood in various ways (which need not be mutually exclusive). It may be understood in terms of the broad ethical principles to which, as just noted, philosophers turned their attention in their dissatisfaction with medical tradition. Such principles include respect for autonomy (one ought to respect the decision-making capacities of autonomous persons) and nonmaleficence (one ought to avoid causing harm to others). Alternatively, common morality may be understood as comprising basic rules of obligation such as "do not kill," "do not cause pain or suffering," and "keep your promises" (Beauchamp and Childress 2009). In recent years the favored category to express the norms of common morality has perhaps been human rights (see, for example, Dworkin 1977, Thomson 1990, Macklin 1992).[2]

Many people, including many philosophers, are skeptical about the idea of a common morality. They think that virtually nothing is shared across cultures and different moral traditions. However, the notion of the common morality is simply intended to capture the moral norms that we all accept. Some critics also object that general principles, rules, and rights are sometimes validly overridden by other norms with which they conflict. But this well-known feature of morality does not constitute an objection to common morality theories. We should expect that general norms will be validly overridden in circumstances in which there is conflict with other moral claims. For example, one might not tell the truth in order to prevent someone from killing another person; and protecting the liberty or rights of one person may require interfering with another's autonomous choice. When a conflict of two or more principles or rules occurs, the conflict must be addressed to extract the proper content from each. Alternatively, as the context requires, one precept may be found to override the other.[3]

How, then, does one fill the gap between abstract principles and concrete judgments to guide moral decision making? The answer is that principles must be specified to suit the needs of particular contexts. Specification is the progressive filling in of the abstract content of principles, shedding their indeterminateness and thereby providing action-guiding content (Richardson 1990, 2005).[4] In managing complex cases involving conflicts, we should begin with the effort to specify norms and eradicate conflicts between them. Many already-specified norms will need further specification to handle new circumstances of indeterminateness or conflict. Incremental specification will continue to refine one's commitments, gradually reducing the circumstances of conflict to more manageable dimensions. Increase of substance (normative content) through specification is essential for decision making in clinical and research ethics, as well as for the development of institutional rules and public policy.

The famous case *Tarasoff v. Regents of University of California* (1976) illustrates specification (as well as the related concept of balancing). Psychotherapeutic practice has long honored the principle—or rule—of confidentiality, which states that the information divulged in psychotherapy by a patient to the therapist may not be shared with other individuals without the patient's prior consent. This rule is grounded in the need for the patient to trust the therapist as a condition for fully open discussion of the patient's personal difficulties and in respect for the patient's autonomy. But what if a patient divulges the intention to kill an identified third party? Another commonly accepted rule, even if less often explicitly stated, is that one should take reasonable steps to prevent or warn of major harm to another individual if one is uniquely situated to do so and can do so relatively easily. The strength of this obligation may increase if one occupies a professional role such as that of psychiatrist, psychologist, or social worker. Clearly we have a conflict, because maintaining confidentiality is inconsistent with the second rule; taking steps to warn the prospective victim would violate the rule of confidentiality.

How should one manage this conflict? Consistent with the legal judgment rendered in the case, many therapists and ethicists hold that a serious threat of consequential bodily injury to an identified third party warrants an exception to the rule of confidentiality. Efforts to balance the relevant considerations suggest that the importance of helping the endangered person is weightier than that of confidentiality. So long as balancing is understood as involving a judgment adequately supported by justifying reasons—and not as a purely intuitive act—the metaphor of balancing fits well with the idea of specification. The reason justifying the resolution can, in effect, be incorporated into a specification of one of the principles or already specified rules (assuming they are regarded as nonabsolute).

The original rule is thus modified by this process and can then be specified as follows: The information divulged in psychotherapy by a patient to the therapist may not be shared with other individuals without the patient's prior consent, unless the patient expresses an intention to cause severe harm to an identified third party. This specification eliminates the dilemma that originally existed because of a contingent conflict between two rules.

But how are particular specifications to be justified since more than one specification is always possible? In the case just described, an alternative way to remove conflict would be to preserve confidentiality as an absolute rule and revise the other norm as follows: "One should take reasonable steps to prevent major harm to another individual ... unless one's professional duties prohibit the only available means for doing so." Given that such competing specifications will often arise in practical contexts, can the resolution in terms of making a disclosure to a third party be shown to be more defensible than this competing specification? Is there always only one best specification?

A particular specification, or any revision in moral belief, can reasonably be said to be justified if it maximizes the coherence of the overall set of beliefs that are accepted upon reflection.[5] This is, admittedly, a very abstract thesis, and employment of the criteria that together constitute "coherence" in the relevant (rather broad) sense is a subtle and unresolved affair (Arras 2007). Although we believe at least some of these criteria of coherence—such as logical consistency, argumentative support, and intuitive plausibility—are implicitly accepted by nearly anyone who engages in serious moral reflection and discourse, we cannot further explore the criteria of coherence here. We note, however, that the present approach often employs the technique of "reflective equilibrium," as described below.

PROBLEMS WITH PRINCIPLES AND THE COMMON MORALITY

Several concerns about principles drawn from the common morality have been raised by contemporary writers in medical ethics. Clouser and Gert (1990), for example, maintain that general "principles" function more as book chapter headings than as directive rules or normative theories (see also Herissone-Kelly 2003).[6] Principles, they argue, highlight important moral themes by providing general labels for them but do not furnish a method for medical ethics. Receiving no clear guidance from the principle, a moral agent confronting a problem may give the principle whatever weight he or she wishes when it conflicts with another principle.

These writers allege that these deficiencies are especially pronounced in the area of justice. We know that justice is important and concerns distribution, but invoking "justice" amounts to little more than a checklist of moral concerns. Lacking any definite normative content with which to guide actions or establish policies where we have concerns about justice, the agent is free to decide what is just and unjust, without constraints. Other moral considerations besides the principle(s) of justice, such as intuitions and theories about the equality of persons, must be called upon for real normative guidance. Clouser and Gert think the same problem afflicts all general principles, which alert us to issues but, lacking an adequate unifying theory, offer no real guidance on their own (Gert 2005, 2007; Gert, Culver, and Clouser 2006).

Do principles lack specific, directive substance? The charge is most plausible in the case of unspecified principles. Any principle—and any rule, for that matter—will have this problem if the norm is underspecified for the task at hand. A basic principle is necessarily general, covering a broad range of circumstances; in this regard, principles contrast with specific norms. As the territory governed by any norm (principle, rule, paradigm case judgment, and so on) is narrowed, the conditions become more specific—for example, shifting gradually from "all persons" to "all competent patients"—such that it becomes less likely that the norm can even qualify as a principle. For example, although the principle of respect for autonomy applies to autonomous actions generally, the narrower norm of respecting informed refusals by competent patients is more likely to be considered a rule than a principle.

If general principles can be specified and rendered more useful for particular contexts, why continue to think in terms of general principles at all? One practical reason is that principles must be learned by everyone—not just philosophers, but health professionals, ethics committee members, and laypeople. If individuals thought only in terms of specified principles, the latter's specificity and proliferation would make them very difficult to remember, master, and internalize for practical use.

ETHICAL THEORY AS THE BASIS OF APPLIED ETHICS

Once the notion of "applied ethics" gained a foothold in philosophy, it was commonly understood as requiring that general moral principles or ethical theories should be applied to particular moral problems or cases. This vision suggests that ethical theory develops general principles, rules, and the like, whereas applied ethics treats particular contexts by applying these general norms—either directly to particular cases or through the intermediary of more specific norms.[7] In this account applied work does not generate novel ethical content. Applied ethics requires only a detailed knowledge of the areas to which the ethical theory is being applied (e.g., medicine, nursing, public health) and perhaps some skill in drawing out a theory's implications.

Sometimes called "deductivism" or "top-down application" of general norms, this model is inspired by justification in disciplines such as mathematics, in which claims can often be shown to follow logically (deductively) from credible premises. In ethics the parallel idea is that general principles or rules, together with the relevant facts of a situation (in the fields to which the theory is being applied), support an inference to justified moral judgments. In short, the method of reasoning involves the application of a norm to a clear case falling under the norm. One version of this approach would feature two or more basic moral principles arranged in a strict hierarchical ordering, so that conflicts between principles are always resolved in the same way. However, there is no significant example of an ethical theory that has been successfully constructed along these lines.[8]

A more prominent version of this approach features a single overarching or supreme principle that is presented as foundational for morality. The most widely discussed theory of this kind is utilitarianism, which defends the "principle of utility" as the supreme principle of ethics. According to this principle, the right action or policy is that which maximizes the balance of good (beneficial) consequences over bad (harmful) consequences. By contrast, deontological theories assert (in different ways, depending on the particular theory) that the right action or policy is to be identified by reference to one or more principles that cannot be equated with, or fully derived from, the principle of utility.[9] During the 1970s and 1980s, utilitarian and deontological approaches exerted enormous influence on the literature and discourse of medical ethics, and their characteristic patterns of reasoning are still common today. Accordingly, a closer look at these theories is warranted.

Utilitarian theories

The principle of utility demands production of the maximal balance of good consequences over bad consequences.[10] But what characteristics determine the value of particular consequences? The answer offered by a particular version of utilitarianism represents that version's value theory. These value theories (or theories of the good) point to happiness, the satisfaction of desires or preferences, and the attainment of such conditions or states of affairs as autonomy, understanding, various kinds of functioning, achievement, and deep personal relationships. Whatever its value theory, any utilitarian theory decides which actions are right entirely by reference to the consequences of the actions, rather than by reference to any intrinsic moral features the actions may have, such as truthfulness or fidelity. Finally, in the utilitarian approach all parties affected by an action must receive impartial consideration.

There has long been a dispute among utilitarians regarding how to apply the principle of utility. Act utilitarianism and rule utilitarianism are distinguished by their different attitudes towards rules of common morality such as "do not cheat" and "if someone is drowning in the vicinity, try to save him or her." Education in and compliance with such rules usually promote utility. Automatic compliance further promotes utility by obviating complex utility calculations, enabling efficient and reliable decision making. Although *act utilitarians* often follow such rules (without deliberating about utility), they also frequently apply the principle of utility directly to actions. When direct application of this principle entails breaking a moral rule, act utilitarians treat the latter as a dispensable "rule of thumb." *Rule utilitarians*, by contrast, place greater stock in these utility-promoting rules and only rarely would regard violating such a rule as worthy of consideration.[11]

Kantian theories

Deontological theories are increasingly called Kantian because of their origins in the theory of Immanuel Kant.[12] In this theory, morality provides a rational framework comprising a universal principle and derivative rules. Kant's supreme principle, called "the categorical imperative," is expressed in several ways in his writings. His first formulation may be roughly paraphrased in this way: "Always act such that you can will that everyone act in the same manner in relevantly similar situations" (Kant, 1785, sect. 421). Kant maintained that wrongful practices, such as lying, theft, cheating, and failure to help someone in distress when you can easily do so, involve a kind of contradiction. Consider cheating on exams. If everyone behaved as the cheater did, exams would not serve their essential function of testing mastery of relevant material, in which case there would effectively be no such thing as an exam: Faculty would not bother giving exams. But cheating on exams presupposes the background institution of taking exams, so the cheater cannot consistently will that everyone act as she does.

Kant also offered another formulation of his categorical imperative that is today frequently invoked in medical ethics. It may be paraphrased in this way: "Treat every person as an end and never solely as a means" (Kant, 1785, sect. 429). This principle requires us to treat persons as having their own autonomously established goals; persons may not be used as mere tools for promoting other people's or society's goals. Thus, for example, deceiving prospective subjects to obtain their consent to participate in nontherapeutic research violates this principle.

PROBLEMS WITH ETHICAL THEORY AS THE BASIS FOR APPLIED ETHICS

Ethical theories such as utilitarianism and Kantianism today hold a diminished stature in medical ethics, compared with their influence in the 1970s and 1980s. The reasons for the demotion of utilitarian and single-principle deontological theories concern the disadvantages of any approach that attempts to provide a foundation for the entire domain of morality with one supreme principle or general viewpoint. Three disadvantages are noteworthy.

First, there is a problem of authority. Despite myriad attempts by philosophers in recent centuries to justify the claim that some principle is morally authoritative—that is, correctly regarded as the supreme moral principle—no such effort at justification has persuaded a majority of philosophers or other thoughtful people. Thus, to attempt to illuminate problems in medical ethics with a single-principle theory has struck many as misguided as well as presumptuous or dogmatic.

Second, even if an individual working in this field is convinced that some such theory is correct (authoritative), he or she must deal responsibly with the fact that many other morally committed individuals do not embrace this theory. Thus, problems of how to communicate and negotiate in the midst of disagreement do not favor appeals to rigid theories or inflexible principles, which can generate a gridlock of conflicting principled positions, rendering moral discussion hostile and alienating. In our experience—and we believe generally in the experience of teachers of medical ethics—even if people disagree at the level of basic theory, they commonly agree at the level of the principles of medical ethics. These principles, then, may be a more fruitful starting point for discussion than ethical theories.

Third, there is the problem that a highly general principle functioning as the centerpiece of an entire theory is indeterminate in many contexts in which one might try to use it. The content of the principle itself will usually not identify a unique course of action as right. Single-principle theories frequently seem to depend on independent moral considerations in order to serve as effective guides to action.

CASUISTRY (CASE-BASED REASONING)

In contemporary medical ethics, clinicians and ethicists often focus not on principles or theories as the basis of their moral reasoning, but instead on practical decision making in particular cases and on the implications of those cases for other cases (Jonsen 1995, 2000).[13] We can make reliable moral judgments, some philosophers say, only when we have an intimate understanding of particular situations and an appreciation of the record of relevantly similar situations.

This approach, casuistry, proceeds by identifying the particular features of and problems present in the case. The authority operative in case law furnishes a helpful analogy. When the decision of a majority of judges becomes authoritative in a case, the decision is positioned to become authoritative for other courts hearing cases with similar facts. This is the doctrine of precedent. Defenders of casuistry see moral authority similarly: Social ethics develops from a social consensus formed around cases, which can then be extended to new cases without loss of the accumulated moral wisdom. As a history of similar cases and similar judgments grows, a society becomes more confident in its moral judgments, and the stable elements crystallize in the form of tentative generalizations about how to handle similar cases. For example, if the case at hand involves a problem of medical confidentiality, analogous cases are considered in which breaches of confidentiality were deemed justified or unjustified in order to see whether such a breach is justified in the present case. So understood, casuistry overlaps with the method of appeals to tradition: certain cases serve as the focal points of an evolving tradition of ethical reflection and practice.

The leading cases, often called "paradigm cases," become enduring, authoritative sources for reflection and decision making. Cases such as the Tuskegee syphilis study—in which a group of African American men were intentionally not treated for syphilis in order to follow the course of the disease—are invoked to illustrate unjustified biomedical experimentation. Moral judgments regarding this case provide authority for decisions in new cases. Such cases influence our standards of fairness, negligence, unjustified paternalism, and the like. Just as case law (the set of legal rules) develops incrementally from legal decisions in cases, so the moral law (the set of moral rules) develops incrementally. From this perspective, principles are less important for moral reasoning than cases. Indeed, principles may be expendable because moral authority rests in the paradigm cases and the traditions of their interpretation and extension to new cases.

Casuists sometimes write as if cases lead to moral paradigms, analogies, or judgments entirely by their facts alone, but this picture is inaccurate. No matter how many salient facts are assembled, some value premises will be needed to reach a moral conclusion. The properties that we observe to be of moral importance in cases are picked out by the values that we have already accepted as morally important. In short, the paradigm cases are value-laden.

The best way to understand paradigm cases is as a combination of facts that can be generalized to other cases—for example, "The patient refused the recommended treatment"—and settled values—for example, "Competent patients have a right to refuse treatment." For a casuist to reason morally, one or more settled values must connect the cases. Hence the necessity of what casuists sometimes call "maxims," which are moral generalizations derived from a string of relevantly similar cases.

PROBLEMS WITH CASUISTRY

Several challenges confront casuistry. First, it is less independent of principle-based reasoning than its proponents suggest. Casuists claim that moral certainty is to be found in particular cases. But grasping the ethical significance of a case may not be distinguishable from grasping a moral generalization (principle or rule) under which the case falls. When we perceive that a man's harsh slap of a child without cause is wrong, we also perceive the wrongness of some kind of action, such as harming the innocent or hurting children; after all, something about the action makes it wrong. Thus, there is no basis for claiming that judgments about particular cases are more certain than judgments about more general norms governing the cases; indeed, it is doubtful that the two kinds of judgment can be entirely separated.

Casuistry sometimes faces difficulties in justifying judgments in particular cases. For example, it is now widely accepted that a competent patient may refuse medical treatment, and courts and commentators have largely agreed that competent patients may also refuse food (nutrition) and water (hydration)—presumably because the latter refusal is relevantly similar to refusals of medical treatment. But what supports the claim of relevant similarity here? The casuist is likely to vest authority in community judgment or consensus within the evolving practices and traditions of American and other traditions of medicine. But it is not self-evident that one should accept the ethical judgments woven into these practices and traditions.

Finally, by focusing so heavily on cases, casuistry risks being both unable to make progress on controversial issues, since consensus on particular cases is elusive, and overlooking very general and fundamental issues, the resolution of which may be relevant to specific cases. As an example of the first problem, casuistry offers little help in illuminating fundamental questions regarding the moral status of animals. Since consensus about the moral status of animals is lacking, any case involving animals to which a casuist might appeal will either elicit incompatible moral judgments from those who consider the case, or elicit agreement to vague or relatively trivial judgments (for example, "It is wrong to cause animals to suffer unnecessarily"). For an example of the second problem related to focusing on cases, consider a casuist who attempts to determine, by examining relevant government funding decisions, whether some new medical treatment should be publicly funded. This approach may miss broader questions of social justice and access to health care, the resolution of which might vindicate major reform of our health care system, implying different answers to specific funding questions than the answers at which the casuist would arrive.

REFLECTIVE EQUILIBRIUM (A FORM OF COHERENCE THEORY)

Many philosophers now defend the view that the relationship between general moral norms and particular moral judgments is bilateral (neither a unilateral "application" of general norms nor a unilateral abstraction from particular case judgments). John Rawls's (1971, as revised 1999) celebrated account of "reflective equilibrium" has been the most influential model.

In developing and refining a system of ethics, he argues, we should start with the broadest possible set of considered judgments (see below) about a subject and erect a provisional set of principles that reflects them. Reflective equilibrium views investigation in ethics (and theory construction generally) as a reflective testing of moral principles, theoretical postulates, and other moral beliefs to render them as coherent as possible. Starting with paradigms of what is morally right or wrong, one searches for principles that are consistent with these paradigms and one another. Such principles and considered judgments are taken, as Rawls puts it, "provisionally as fixed points," but also as "liable to revision."

Considered judgments are judgments in which our moral capacities are most likely to be presented without a distorting bias. Examples are judgments about the wrongness of racial discrimination, religious intolerance, and sexual oppression. By contrast, judgments in which one's confidence level is low and judgments that may reflect self-interest or other forms of bias do not qualify as considered judgments. The goal is to match, prune, and adjust considered judgments and principles so that they form a coherent moral outlook.

This model seeks the best approximation to full coherence—while recognizing the possibility of unanticipated situations that force reconsideration of earlier-accepted judgments. From this perspective, just as hypotheses in science are tested, modified, or rejected through experience and experimental thinking, principles and other moral norms are tested, revised (sometimes by specification), or rejected. This outlook differs greatly from deductivism, because the method of reflective equilibrium regards ethical theories as never complete, always standing to be informed by practical contexts, and susceptible to testing by the theories' practical implications.

PROBLEMS WITH REFLECTIVE EQUILIBRIUM

The central problem with the reflective-equilibrium model is that the flexibility associated with its bilateral approach is a double-edged sword: While avoiding some difficulties associated with (top-down) application of ethical theories and with the case-focused method of casuistry, reflective equilibrium also gives relatively little specific guidance about how to engage in moral reasoning. Several philosophers have endeavored to characterize reasoning within this model in a nontrivial manner (see, for example, Rawls 1971; Daniels 1979, 1996, 2003; Holmgren 1989; Nielsen 1991, chs. 9–11; DeGrazia 1996, ch. 2; and Arras, 2007). But, theoretically, the model needs further development, and, practically, it remains uncertain how helpful this model will be to nonphilosophers seeking moral guidance.

❧ Critique

This chapter has presented an overview of several prominent philosophical methods in medical ethics. It began with a characterization of five major methods, or models, for conducting the work of moral reasoning, with special emphasis on the problems that arise in medical ethics. It is one thing to know what a method is, another to judge its adequacy. Therefore, each subsection describing a method was followed by a subsection identifying one or more leading criticisms of that method.

We now conclude the body of this chapter with a few remarks about the limits of philosophy in medical ethics and some comments indicating common ground amid the diversity of philosophical contributions to medical ethics. One limit to what philosophy can accomplish in medical ethics is implicit throughout the above discussions of methods and the criticisms they face. Despite the merit of much work in ethical theory and methodology in ethics, no approach has proved so convincing and resilient in responding to criticisms as to convince all philosophers and ethicists—or even a majority of them—to adopt it as the preferred method. This means that everyone interested in methodological issues of medical ethics must think critically about the strengths and weaknesses of leading approaches.

A second limit of philosophy derives from its nonempirical nature. Philosophy involves a critical perspective from which to evaluate theses, arguments, and viewpoints as well as (in ethics) actions, motives, practices, and institutions. Philosophy must depend on empirical disciplines in a joint effort of critically evaluating any specific domain of human knowledge and practice, whether it be medicine, law, international relations, or another. Philosophy can contribute to medical ethics through ethical theory and, more broadly, methodology in ethics (and can make other contributions [see note 1]), but philosophy can provide reliable moral guidance only to the extent that its empirical assumptions are accurate.

If, for example, one argues that physician-assisted suicide is justified—based on the conviction that currently legal means of pain control and the alleviation of suffering are ineffective for many patients—one's argument depends on clinical data that are relevant to assessing the adequacy of legal methods of pain control and alleviation of suffering. Philosophy itself cannot address the factual issues without relying on other fields that provide relevant empirical data.

Philosophy's nonempirical nature motivates what may be the only significant point of methodological consensus among the wide variety of methods in ethics. One might suppose that all of the approaches agree that a theory is rightly tested by the intuitive plausibility of its moral implications (by their resonance with our lived moral experience), yet deductivism is not committed to this criterion. Alternatively, one might presume that all of the approaches agree that the evaluation of actions is central to moral reasoning, yet proponents of virtue ethics (or at least some variants of this approach) would dissent. At the same time, all approaches must accept this requirement: The factual assumptions underlying moral reasoning must be reasonably supported by empirical evidence and observation.

Finally, there seems to be more agreement about how to write strong papers in philosophical medical ethics than there is on questions of method. Because the present chapter has focused on the latter, we here enumerate a few agreed-upon criteria of excellence for papers in philosophical medical ethics: (a) clarity of expression and organization (so that, for example, papers are not unnecessarily difficult to read); (b) rigorous argumentation, making it clear to the reader that conclusions are strongly supported by the arguments presented in their defense; (c) a firm command of leading work that has already been published on the topic; (d) novelty, so that the author is not simply duplicating work already published; and (e) an important topic, so that the work is well motivated and stands to make a contribution to the field.

Notes on Resources and Training

What sorts of training are available to those who aspire to work in ethical theory or other philosophical areas of medical ethics? Is such training necessary or merely desirable? The answers to these questions turn on an individual's specific goals.

To make significant scholarly contributions to philosophical medical ethics—in contrast to various contributions to medical ethics made by other disciplines—or to teach effectively in this area, there is no substitute for graduate training in philosophy. One possible strategy is to seek admission to a strong philosophy graduate program while planning to take several courses in medical ethics (prioritizing strength in philosophy). Another possible strategy is to apply only to philosophy graduate programs that have a medical ethics track or concentration (making medical ethics more central to one's studies). Both strategies reflect viable paths to philosophical work in medical ethics.

For those seeking basic competence (as opposed to expertise) in specific philosophical areas of medical ethics, less intensive courses of study are available. One or more courses in ethical theory—preferably, but not necessarily, at the graduate level—would be appropriate training for competence in that area. Ideally, such courses would be taken as part of a more extensive graduate training—in a master's program in medical ethics, for example—but they could also prove invaluable to the professional who is auditing courses.

In addition to courses at colleges and universities, other opportunities for education in philosophical medical ethics include intensive "short courses" taken over several days, workshops, conferences, and self-education through reading. Such educational experiences can enrich one's reasoning and discourse about philosophical issues in medical ethics. They can also enable one to learn more from scholarly writings.

There are several leading scholarly resources to which one may turn for information about or work in philosophical contributions to medical ethics. First, one may search journals for articles of particular interest. Leading journals from the standpoint of philosophical medical ethics include *American Journal of Bioethics, Bioethics, Cambridge Quarterly of Health Care Ethics, Ethics, The Journal of Medical Ethics, The Kennedy Institute of Ethics Journal, Philosophy and Public Affairs,* and *Theoretical Medicine and Bioethics.* Sometimes one can find valuable articles in strong philosophy journals that do not focus on medical ethics or ethical theory.

One systematic approach to searching for helpful journal articles is to consult *The Philosopher's Index,* which is published quarterly and lists published articles and books arranged by author and by subject; this source is now also available online at www.philinfo.org/electronic.htm. Two encyclopedias offer valuable short articles and bibliographies: *The Encyclopedia of Bioethics,* third edition (Post 2004), and *The Routledge Encyclopedia of Philosophy* (Craig 1998). Longer articles on a number of subjects can be found in *The Stanford Encyclopedia of Philosophy* (Zalta, continuously updated and still adding new articles in bioethics, at http://plato.stanford.edu/). Some comprehensive textbooks that provide both detailed discussions and leads for further research can also be a useful general resource. In addition, valuable resources, including the unique bioethics database ETHXWeb, are located at the Bioethics Research Library at Georgetown University in Washington, DC. Those cannot visit the library may call 202-687-3885, e-mail bioethics@georgetown.edu, or visit the website, http://bioethics.georgetown.edu. Finally, a new reference-database system is now available: EthicShare, a discovery and collaboration environment for ethics scholars and students, can be accessed at www.ethicshare.org. For more information or assistance, visit the website, e-mail help@ethicshare.org, or call 612-626-4357.

❧ Notes

1. Philosophy makes other contributions to medical ethics, although we cannot canvass all of them here. Examples include the contributions of action theory to a theory of informed consent and of personal identity theory to views about the definition of death and the authority of advance directives.

2. An increasingly influential variant of the human rights approach appeals to human capabilities (see, for example, Nussbaum 2000, 2006).

3. Appeals to the common morality as the source of universal norms are not intended to suggest that moral reasoning should always lead to widely accepted conclusions. Common moral experience provides the starting point of moral discourse, but critical reflection on specific ethical issues may ultimately vindicate moral judgments that are not widely shared (for example, regarding our obligations to the developing world or regarding the moral status of animals). See, for example, Beauchamp (2003), DeGrazia (2003), and Lindsay (2005).

4. For discussions of this method in bioethics, see DeGrazia (1992), Beauchamp (1994, 2007), and Beauchamp and Childress (2009). For discussions of what is now sometimes called specified principlism, see DeGrazia (1992), Davis (1995, esp. 95–102), Levi (1996, esp. 13–19, 24–26), and Strong (2000).

5. Efforts to analyze the idea of justification by coherence include Daniels (1996), DeGrazia (1996, ch. 2), and Arras (2007).

6. Their views are further developed in later writings. See Green, Gert, and Clouser (1993); Clouser and Gert (1994); Clouser (1995); Gert, Culver, and Clouser (2006); and Gert (2007).

7. Several types of ethical theory have been employed in addressing practical problems, including utilitarianism, Kantianism, rights theory, contract theory, communitarianism, virtue ethics, the ethics of care, feminist ethics, and pragmatism. Many proponents of these theories would argue, however, that specific policy and practical guidelines cannot be simply derived from these ethical theories and that some additional moral reasoning is required. Indeed, several of these theories—at least virtue ethics, the ethics of care, and feminist ethics—are often said to resist articulation in a set of principles (which is not to say that principles are rejected altogether). See Carse (1998) and Callahan (2000).

8. Rawls (1971 and, as revised, 1999) has developed a theory of justice, but not a full ethical theory, that features such a hierarchy of principles.

9. The most classic deontological theory featuring a supreme principle is that of Kant (1959). For twentieth-century representatives of this approach, see Donagan (1977), a book stressing respect for persons, and Gewirth (1978), which stresses individual rights.

10. For a variety of utilitarian theories, see Frey (1980), Hare (1981), Griffin (1986), Sumner (1987), Kagan (1989), Brandt (1992), Singer (1993), and Hooker (2000).

11. For a classic discussion of this divide among utilitarians, see Smart (1956). A rule-utilitarian may favor quite nuanced rules. For example, rather than "do not lie," she may favor a rule that incorporates one or more exceptions such as "do not lie unless lying is the only means to preventing substantial harm" or perhaps a rule building in further exceptions. However, it is extremely difficult, and often impossible, to build all nuances or exceptions into any rule.

12. For prominent contemporary representatives of Kantian ethics, see O'Neill (1989), Herman (1993), and Korsgaard (1996).

13. For a landmark work in the history of the type of reasoning described here, see Jonsen and Toulmin (1988). For additional features of the method, see Jonsen (1996, 1991, and 2000).

℘ References

Arras, J. D. 1988. AIDS and the duty to treat. *Hastings Center Report* 18 (2) (Special Supplement): 10–18.

———. 2007. The way we reason now: Reflective equilibrium in bioethics. In *The Oxford handbook of bioethics*, ed. Bonnie Steinbock, 46–71. New York: Oxford University Press.

Beauchamp, T. L. 1994. Principles and other emerging paradigms for bioethics. *Indiana Law Journal* 69:1–17.

———. 2003. A defense of the common morality. *Kennedy Institute of Ethics Journal* 13 (3): 219–30.

———. 2007. The four principles approach to health care ethics. In *Principles of health care ethics*, ed. R. E. Ashcroft, A. Dawson, H. Draper, and J. R. McMillan, 3–10. Chichester, UK: John Wiley & Sons.

Beauchamp, T. L., and J. F. Childress. 2009. *Principles of biomedical ethics*. 6th ed. New York: Oxford University Press.

Brandt, R. B. 1992. *Morality, utilitarianism, and rights*. Cambridge: Cambridge University Press.

Callahan, D. 2000. Universalism & particularism: Fighting to a Draw. *Hastings Center Report* 30: 37–44.

Carse, A. 1998. Impartial principle and moral context: Securing a place for the particular in ethical theory. *Journal of Medicine and Philosophy* 23:153–69.

Clouser, D. K. 1995. Common morality as an alternative to principlism. *The Kennedy Institute of Ethics Journal* 5:219–36.

Clouser, D. K., and B. Gert. 1990. A critique of principlism. *The Journal of Medicine and Philosophy* 15:219–36.

———. 1994. Morality vs. principlism. In *Principles of health care ethics*, ed. R. Gillon and A. Lloyd, 251–66. London: John Wiley & Sons.

Craig, E., ed. 1998. *Routledge encyclopedia of philosophy*. 10 vols. London: Routledge.

Daniels, N. 1979. Wide reflective equilibrium and theory acceptance in ethics. *Journal of Philosophy* 76:256–82.

———. 1996. Wide reflective equilibrium in practice. In *Philosophical perspectives on bioethics*, ed. L. W. Sumner and J. Boyle, 96–114. Toronto: University of Toronto Press.

———. Reflective equilibrium, *Stanford encyclopedia of philosophy* (Online, first published, April 28, 2003; accessed October 16, 2008).

Davis, R. B. 1995. The principlism debate: A critical overview. *The Journal of Medicine and Philosophy* 20:85–105.

DeGrazia, D. 1992. Moving forward in bioethical theory: Theories, cases, and specified principlism. *The Journal of Medicine and Philosophy* 17:511–39.

———. 1996. *Taking animals seriously*. Cambridge: Cambridge University Press.

———. 2003. Common morality, coherence, and the principles of biomedical ethics. *Kennedy Institute of Ethics Journal* 13 (3): 219–30.

Donagan, A. 1977. *The theory of morality*. Chicago: University of Chicago Press.

Dworkin, R. 1977. *Taking rights seriously*. Cambridge, MA: Harvard University Press.

Frey, R. G. 1980. *Interests and rights*. Oxford: Clarendon Press.

Gert, B. 2005. *Morality: Its nature and justification*. 2nd rev. ed. New York: Oxford University Press.

———. 2007. *Common morality: Deciding what to do*. New York: Oxford University Press.

Gert, B., C. M. Culver, and K. D. Clouser. 2006. *Bioethics: A systematic approach*. New York: Oxford University Press.

Gewirth, A. 1978. *Reason and morality*. Chicago: University of Chicago Press.

Green, R. M., B. Gert, and K. D. Clouser. 1993. The method of public morality versus the method of principlism. *The Journal of Medicine and Philosophy* 18:477–90.

Griffin, J. 1986. *Well-being*. Oxford: Clarendon Press.

Hare, R. M. 1981. *Moral thinking*. Oxford: Clarendon Press.

Herman, B. 1993. *The practice of moral judgment*. Cambridge, MA: Harvard University Press.

Herissone-Kelly, P. 2003. The principlist approach to bioethics, and its stormy journey overseas. In *Scratching the surface of bioethics*, ed. Matti Hayry and Tuija Takala, 65–77. Amsterdam: Rodopi.

Holmgren, M. 1989. The wide and narrow of reflective equilibrium. *Canadian Journal of Philosophy* 19:43–60.

Hooker, B. 2000. *Ideal code, real world: A rule-consequentialist theory of morality*. Oxford: Oxford University Press.

Jonsen, A. R. 1991. Casuistry as methodology in clinical ethics. *Theoretical Medicine* 12:299–302.

———. 1995. Casuistry: An alternative or complement to principles? *The Kennedy Institute of Ethics Journal* 5:246–47.

———. 1996. Morally appreciated circumstances: A theoretical problem for casuistry. In *Philosophical perspectives on bioethics*, ed. L. W. Sumner and J. Boyle, 37–49. Toronto: University of Toronto Press.

———. 2000. Strong on specification. *Journal of Medicine and Philosophy* 25:348–60.

Jonsen, A. R., and S. Toulmin. 1988. *The abuse of casuistry*. Berkeley: University of California Press.

Kagan, S. 1989. *The Limits of morality*. Oxford: Clarendon Press.

Kant, I. 1785 (1959). *Foundations of the metaphysics of morals*, trans. L. W. Beck. Indianapolis: Bobbs-Merrill.

Korsgaard, C. M. 1996. *Creating the kingdom of ends*. Cambridge: Cambridge University Press.

Levi, B. H. 1996. Four approaches to doing ethics. *The Journal of Medicine and Philosophy* 21:7–39.

Lindsay, R. A. 2005. Slaves, embryos, and nonhuman animals: Moral status and the limitations of common morality theory. *Kennedy Institute of Ethics Journal* 15:323–46.

Macklin, R. 1992. Universality of the Nuremberg code. In *The Nazi doctors and the Nuremberg code*, ed. G. J. Annas and M. Grodin, 240–57. New York: Oxford University Press.

Nielsen, K. 1991. *After the demise of the tradition.* Boulder, CO: Westview.

Nussbaum, M. C. 2000. *Women and human development.* Cambridge: Cambridge University Press.

———. 2006. *Frontiers of justice: Disability, nationality, species membership.* Cambridge, MA: Harvard University Press.

O'Neill, Onora. 1989. *Constructions of reason: Explorations of Kant's practical philosophy.* Cambridge: Cambridge University Press.

Pellegrino, E. D. 1985. The virtuous physician and the ethics of medicine. In *Virtue and medicine,* ed. Earl E. Shelp, 248–53. Dordrecht, The Netherlands: D. Reidel.

———. 1987. Altruism, self-interest, and medical ethics. *Journal of the American Medical Association* 258:1939–40.

———. 1999. The goals and ends of medicine: How are they to be defined? In *The goals of medicine,* ed. M. J. Hanson and D. Callahan. Washington, DC: Georgetown University Press.

———. 2001. The internal morality of clinical medicine: A paradigm for the ethics of the helping and healing professions. *Journal of Medicine and Philosophy* 26:559–79.

Philosopher's index. Bowling Green, OH: Philosophy Documentation Center.

Post, S., ed. 2004. *The encyclopedia of bioethics.* 3rd ed. New York: Macmillan.

Rawls, J. 1971/1999. *A theory of justice.* Cambridge, MA: Harvard University Press.

Richardson, H. S. 1990. Specifying norms as a way to resolve concrete ethical problems. *Philosophy and Public Affairs* 19:279–310.

———. 2005 Specifying, balancing, and interpreting bioethical principles. In *Belmont revisited: Ethical principles for research with human subjects,* ed. J. F. Childress, E. M. Meslin, and H. T. Shapiro, 205–27. Washington, DC: Georgetown University Press.

Singer, P. 1993. *Practical ethics.* 2nd ed. Cambridge: Cambridge University Press.

Smart, J. J. C. 1956. Extreme and restricted utilitarianism. *Philosophical Quarterly* 6 (25): 344–54.

Strong, C. 2000. Specified principlism. *Journal of Medicine and Philosophy* 25:285–307.

Sumner, L. W. 1987. *The moral foundations of rights.* Oxford: Clarendon Press.

Tarasoff v. Regents of the University of California. 1976. 17 Cal. 3d 425.

Thomson, J. J. 1990. *The realm of rights.* Cambridge, MA: Harvard University Press.

Zalta, E. N., ed. Updated and augmented continuously. *The Stanford encyclopedia of philosophy.* Stanford, CA: Stanford University Center for the Study of Language and Information. http://plato.stanford.edu/.

CHAPTER 4

Philosophy: Ancient and Contemporary Approaches

DIEGO GRACIA

Phenomenology, hermeneutics, existentialism, care ethics, gender ethics, virtue ethics, communitarianism, discourse ethics, and deliberative ethics have all been used to examine and explore questions in medical ethics. Although examining each method in detail is beyond the scope of this chapter, understanding a bit about them is important since many authors in medical ethics employ these philosophical approaches. Of special relevance is knowing not only how these methods differ from one another but also what they have in common, and this requires historical context.

Overview

In this chapter I sketch how these methods evolved in reaction to a way of thinking about ethics that became entrenched in Western philosophical thought. Next, I describe these methods and then offer a critique of them. Finally, I provide some notes on resources and training in these methods.

FIRST THINGS FIRST: ELENCHUS AND MAIEUTICS

Socrates, who founded ethics as a way of thinking in the West, seemed to identify ethics with philosophy. In his *Apology* Plato puts into the mouth of Socrates these words: "The god has commanded me that I should live philosophizing, examining myself and others" (*Apology* 28e). Philosophizing means here a way of analyzing oneself and discerning good from evil, in order to reach as much moral excellence, perfection, and happiness as possible. All must find their moral truth, examining their own moral beliefs: "The unexamined life is not worth living by man" (*Apology* 38a). The method for doing this is called "elenchus," understood as the process of refuting one's own logical inconsistencies, in view, as Aristotle said, of "the answer's own beliefs" (*De Sophisticis Elenchis* 165 b3–5). In the *Theaetetus* Socrates compared his art with midwifery. As in any analogy, there are similarities but also differences. The most relevant difference is that the Socratic art is focused on spiritual or intellectual rather than corporal labor: "The triumph of my art is in thoroughly examining whether the thought which the mind of the young man brings forth is a false idol or a noble and true birth" (*Theaetetus* 150b–c). He can ask others questions he lacks the wit to answer: "And therefore I am not myself at all wise, nor have I anything to show which is the invention or birth of my own soul, but those who converse with me profit" (*Theaetetus* 150c–d).

This was the first method of ethics in Western culture. After Socrates it was interpreted in two different ways, each one representative of the two main types of thinking on ethics in Western culture. The first is best described as idealist, and the second as constructivist. Plato and Aristotle, two disciples of Socrates, initiated these two different ways of reasoning in ethics.

LOOKING FOR AN ETHICA ORDINE GEOMETRICO DEMONSTRATA

From Plato's *Phaedo* and *Republic* to the Kantian *Critique of Practical Reason*, the history of Western ethics has been characterized by a continuous yet unsuccessful attempt at finding a way of creating a definite, universal, and immutable system of morality. This background makes it easier to understand the new developments that happened during the nineteenth and twentieth.

Plato and Stoicism

The methods that can be called Platonic, or idealist, always seek the same goal: to make ethics a scientific discipline, understood in the old meaning of this word, that is, as certain, universal, and immutable knowledge. The idea behind this assumption is that ethical principles and norms are so important for human beings that they must necessarily be absolute, invariable, and apodictic. All these theories assume that the human mind has the capacity to know universal moral principles, although how this is accomplished diverges according to the accounts of different philosophical schools. For instance, Plato thought that the idea of the good can be captured by our minds through a process of reminiscence, remembering the time in which we were in direct touch with the world of pure ideas. These ideas have not only ontic reality but also deontological power, as paradigms of human conduct. Ethics and politics, therefore, can be constructed as pure sciences, the same as mathematics. We could infer this directly from the place Plato gives to mathematics in the studies he prescribes for the rulers-to-be of his ideal polis (Plato, *Republic* 518b–531b, 537b–d; Vlastos 1991, 108).

Platonism was not, in any case, the most influential moral theory in the constitution and development of Western culture. Stoicism was the more successful moral doctrine. Stoicism was another dogmatic system that identified God with reason (*logos*) and thought that all the things of nature were governed by an internal *logos* disseminated throughout all of them (*logos spermatikos*). Nature, therefore, is the rule of morality, the only way to reach wisdom and happiness. This is the origin of the concept of natural law, which was pervasive in Western culture from Stoicism until now. Zeno, the father of the Stoic movement, established as one of his main theses that virtue is knowledge or understanding (Diogenes *Vitae Philosophorum*, VII 202;

Galen *De Placitis Hippocratis et Platonis*, VII 2). This knowledge must be absolute and apodictic, in accordance with his idea of reason as a faculty of "consistent and firm and unchangeable" products (Plutarch *De Virtute Morali*, 441c). This is the origin of the Stoic dogmatism in morals and the reason for the Stoics' rejection of emotions as interfering with reason, disturbing the *apatheia* ("indifference") that they held to be indispensable for seeing true virtue clearly and reaching it. All passions, then, should be blotted out. They should be completely eradicated in the wise man, whose state of mind will be marked by lack of passions (*apatheia*).

Medieval Natural Law

Natural law theory was assumed by theologians, who interpreted it as expression of the divine will and therefore as the law of God. This way natural law became the core of moral theology. Greek philosophers described a mental faculty that is capable of receiving the first and immutable speculative principles as the logical principles of identity, contradiction, and causality, calling this faculty *nous* or *intellectus*. But they did not describe a similar faculty in the field of practical reason. Medieval theologians tried to repair this mistake by identifying a special faculty capable of knowing intuitively and without any doubt the first moral principles, with a similar role to that played by *nous* when engaging in speculative reasoning. This was conceived as the logical setting of the principles of natural law. The first of them was that good is to be done and evil is to be avoided. Next, they included the ten Mosaic commandments, followed by all other natural duties, or *officia*. The name coined for this peculiar mental faculty was *synderesis*. This way, medieval theologians ensured the objectivity of natural law and its epistemic accessibility to human beings. This is what Somme (2006) has called "the infallibility, impeccability and indestructibility of synderesis." This concept would have seemed strange to Aristotle. Medieval moralists thought that ethics should provide for the practical part of our lives the same certainty as mathematics for the theoretical part. Moral mathematics would be a reasonable characterization of the role of ethics according to this dogmatic and idealistic tradition.

Descartes, Spinoza, Leibniz, Kant

Modern philosophy followed this trajectory. Two paradigmatic examples of this dogmatic and quasi-mathematical moral tradition were Descartes and Spinoza. Descartes thought ethics should be an exact science, like mathematics and mechanics: "If I always saw clearly what was true and good, I should never have to deliberate about the right judgment or choice" (*Discourse on Method*, VII 58). In his *Discourse on Method* Descartes presented what he called his provisional morality. Throughout his life, however, he tried to construct a more scientific system—his definitive morality. This was conceived as "the highest and most perfect moral system, which presupposes a complete knowledge of the other sciences and is the ultimate level of wisdom" (*Discourse on Method*, IX B, 15).

Spinoza, a follower of Descartes, titled his only major work of ethics *Ethica Ordine Geometrico Demonstrata*. It is evident that Spinoza was thinking of the structure of Euclid's *Elements* when he titled his book and ordered its content: "The form of the work evokes the rationalist ideal of a mind capable of taking in, in one mental gaze, a deductive network of propositions" (Lloyd 1996, 21). For him, as for Descartes, the definitive morality should be completely deductive and rational. The big difference between mathematics and ethics is that the latter deals with the real nature of human beings, including affections and emotions, and not with pure formal entities, such as numbers, points, or lines. But the goals are exactly the same: the construction of a rational and definite system, in this case of conduct (Spinoza 1927, 105).

Leibniz also tried to construct ethics as a branch of science, with the same level of demonstrative rigor as in arithmetic and geometry. In the preface to his *New Essays on Human Understanding*, Leibniz (1981, 50) wrote: "It appears that necessary truths, such as we find in pure mathematics and particularly in arithmetic and geometry, must have principles whose proof does not depend on instances nor, consequently, on the testimony of the senses, even though without the senses it would never occur to us to think of them. This distinction must be thoroughly observed, and Euclid understood that so well that he demonstrates by reason things that experience and sense-images make very evident. Logic also abounds in such products, and also metaphysics and ethics."

The last example I offer of this dogmatic and apodictic way of thinking about moral questions is Kant. At the beginning of the preface to the second edition of his *Critique of Pure Reason* (Ak B, vii), Kant defined his philosophical goal as to introduce metaphysics and ethics in the "secure path of a science," following the example of logic, mathematics, and physics. And in the conclusion of the *Critique of Practical Reason*, Kant, undoubtedly thinking of Newton, wrote, "The fall of a stone, the motion of a sling, resolved into their elements and the forces that are manifested in them, and treated mathematically, produced at last that clear and henceforward unchangeable insight into the system of the world which, as observation is continued, may hope always to extend itself, but need never fear to be compelled to retreat. This example may suggest to us to enter on the same path in treating of the moral capacities of our nature, and may give us hope of a like good result" (Ak, 163).

THE LONG RUN FROM DEMONSTRATION TO DELIBERATION

The historical analysis I have just presented demonstrates how ethics came to be constructed, from antiquity to the nineteenth century, according to a mathematical model, looking for an exact, precise, and universal system of principles and laws with which to control the behavior of human beings. Using the terminology coined by Aristotle in his treatises on logic, we can say that they understood moral reasoning as apodictic, or demonstrative. The demonstrative science par excellence is mathematics, and no less exactitude and accuracy should be demanded, they thought, of the science of human conduct.

Aristotle

The problem is that the real Aristotle did not hold this point of view. In fact, at the very beginning of the *Nicomachean ethics*, he said exactly the opposite: "Our discussion will be adequate if its degree of clarity reflects the subject-matter; for we should not seek the same degree of exactness in all sorts of arguments alike" (*Nicomachean Ethics*,

1094 b 12–14; 1094 b 19–22). It follows that moral arguments are not apodictic or scientific but of another type, which Aristotle called dialectic. They are not based on demonstrations but on what he called opinions and on the interchange of opinions through dialogue. Its end is not to capture the truth but to reach practical wisdom and to make wise or prudent decisions. Moral reasoning is, according to Aristotle, dialectical. This means that there is no room in ethics for apodictic demonstrations, only dialectical deliberations.

Aristotle made a full study of deliberation as the principal method of practical reason. First, deliberation deals with things in which demonstration is not possible: "There is no deliberation about the sciences that are exact and self-evident" (*Nicomachean Ethics*, 1112 b 1). Second, deliberation is an intellectual skill: "All deliberation is inquiry, though not all inquiry, e.g. in mathematics, is deliberation" (*Nicomachean Ethics*, 1112 b 22–23). Third, deliberation is an intellectual process that is ordered to making the right decisions in specific situations: "We deliberate about what is up to us, i.e. about the actions we can do" (*Nicomachean Ethics*, 1112 a 32–34). Decision, then, is the end of deliberation. Fourth, Aristotle notes, "What we deliberate about is the same as what we decide to do, except that by the time we decide to do it, it is definite, for what we decide to do is what we have judged to be right as a result of deliberation" (*Nicomachean Ethics*, 1113 a 3–5). Fifth and finally, because we cannot take into account all the circumstances that can determine the success or failure of a decision, when things are difficult, deliberation should include other points of view, becoming collective and not only individual. "We enlist partners in deliberation on large issues when we distrust our own ability to discern [the situation and come to the correct answer]" (*Nicomachean Ethics*, 1112 b 9–10).

It is astonishing that this method, so meticulously analyzed and described by Aristotle, and so important in the field of practical reasoning, did not have more historical success. From the Stoics onward, deliberation practically disappeared as the main method of ethics. I would argue that this was due to its incompatibility with the idea of ethics as an apodictic science, rather than as a dialectical process leading to wisdom. The Greek word for deliberation, *bouleusis*, sometimes was translated to Latin as *deliberatio*, but generally as *consilium* (counsel). Medieval theologians considered the spirit of counsel one of the gifts of the Holy Spirit, rendering the individual docile and receptive to the counsel of God. More than a moral skill, it came to be seen as a religious gift related to sanctification and salvation. Moral fault was transformed into religious sin, and deliberation became a grace reserved for religious ministers. The primary moral virtue of common people was not deliberation, but obedience.

Hume

Things did not change in the era of modernity, especially in continental Europe. Deliberation did not play any important role in the moral systems of Descartes, Spinoza, Leibniz, or Kant. They all considered deliberation a weak and insecure method, unsuitable for a matter as important and sensitive as ethics. David Hume called this antideliberative approach "dogmatism." Throughout most of its history in the West, ethics has been a dogmatic discipline, constructed as *more apodictico* and not as *more deliberativo*.

Things began to change only in the eighteenth century. The main figure was probably Hume, who wrote:

> It seems to me, that the only objects of the abstract sciences or of demonstration are quantity and number, and that all attempts to extend this more perfect species of knowledge beyond these bounds are mere sophistry and illusion.... The existence, therefore, of any being can only be proved by arguments from its cause or its effect; and these arguments are founded entirely on experience.... Such is the foundation of moral reasoning, which forms the greater part of human knowledge, and is the source of all human action and behavior. Moral reasonings are either concerning particular or general facts. All deliberations in life regard the former. (1882, 134–35)

For Hume, like Aristotle, deliberation appears as the opposite of demonstration. There is no demonstrative reasoning regarding empirical facts, including those that are the concern of morality. The reasoning concerning quantity and number is demonstrative, while the reasoning proper of empirical inquiry is deliberation. How can one construct an ethics with these tools? This was the great question facing the late nineteenth and early twentieth centuries.

Utilitarianism and Pragmatism

Different intellectual movements tried diverse ways. Two of them were utilitarianism and pragmatism. Both were developed quite exclusively in the English-speaking world, Britain and the United States. If one takes J. S. Mill's *Utilitarianism* as representative of the first branch, one notes immediately that he rejects all speculative traditions and is aware of the novelty of his own proposal (1864, 1). Speculative thinking, he argues in the same work, has been sterile in the moral setting, incapable of dealing with real problems or finding true solutions. We must, then, Mill argues, return to the beginning, when Socrates began to think about these questions. The speculative way of thinking is no longer valid.

Mill's views were typical of the thinkers of this period. Something new was needed. Mill proposed a shift from a reliance on speculative and a priori principles to considering specific and a posteriori consequences. Utilitarianism was a new way of grounding morality, avoiding and overcoming the previous speculative and apodictic approaches.

No less innovative was the point of view of pragmatists. Both intellectual movements were strongly linked with the rapid scientific developments that occurred during this period: Utilitarianism was closely related to the growth of economics as a scientific discipline and the importance of the principle of efficiency, and Pragmatism to the new biological and evolutionary data. Every day seemed to bring more evidence that the human species is but one among others in the set of all animals, sharing with them basic mechanisms, such as the need to fight for survival. In this view what we call the human mind is but a biological trait enabling the human species to adapt more readily to the environment, increasing the odds of the species's survival. Therefore, the objective of this new and peculiar trait is not primarily theoretical but practical and pragmatic, and the traditional devaluation of the pragmatic goal of our intellectual skill is, say pragmatists, completely wrong (Dewey 1997, 2). Rather than true or false, practical decisions are best described as wise or unwise. And in order to make wise decisions, two elements are necessary: evaluation and deliberation. That is why values and deliberation were two important topics in the work of pragmatist philosophers. It is not surprising, then, that just when philosophers rediscovered what Aristotle called "practical reasoning," at the turn of the nineteenth to twentieth century, deliberation reappeared as a viable method in ethics.

In Continental Europe utilitarianism and pragmatism did not have the same influence as in the English-speaking world. Continental Europe overcame the dogmatic approach to ethical thinking with its own secular traditions, which had its own pros and cons. The twentieth century, in fact, has witnessed a continuous effort to think about moral problems in a new way. All the intellectual movements of this period share several features, such as the critique of speculative reason, the importance of the idea of responsibility, and the rediscovery of deliberation as the proper method of thinking in ethics. But these common features are compatible with an enormous diversity of styles of thinking, crystallized in movements such as phenomenology, hermeneutics, existentialism, care ethics, gender ethics, virtue ethics, communitarianism, discourse ethics, and deliberative ethics. After analyzing the pivotal role of responsibility ethics in many contemporary approaches to ethics, the remainder of this chapter describes some of these movements, which have been especially important in European bioethics, in more detail.

Responsibility Ethics

At the beginning of the twentieth century, Max Weber greeted Europeans with a forceful repudiation of the old and pervasive dogmatic way of thinking in ethics, which he called conviction ethics (*Gesinnungsethik*), recalling one important concept of the Kantian tradition. Against it, Weber stressed the importance of thinking about moral problems in another way, which he called ethics of responsibility (*Verantwortungsethik*). The difference between them is crucial, because the sense of responsibility obliges one to take into account not only the values at stake but also the circumstances and consequences of the decision to be made. In ethics dogmatic and narrow-minded approaches lead necessarily either to fanaticism, typical of conviction ethics, or to the other extreme, the ethics of one's own individual success (*Erfolgsethik*). Weber thought that these two were the origin of World War I and that only an ethics of responsibility could be capable of avoiding a disaster in the future.

❧ Description of Philosophical Methods

The idea of responsibility has been one of the most important contributions of European ethics in the twentieth century. In fact, its influence pervaded the work of nearly all philosophers during this period. It also has been the background for many different developments, among them, environmental ethics, feminist ethics, and ethics of care. Carol Gilligan's studies showed that responsibility is not only a legal term but principally a way of thinking and making moral decisions. She showed that the male way of thinking is more prone to absolute decisions and that women are more contextual and have greater sensitivity to the consequences of decisions. The relevance of context, a typical note sounded in every opus marked by the idea of responsibility, is essential in the ethics of care. The ethics of responsibility has been critical to the development of bioethics in the European context. Two examples of this are the new developments in nursing ethics and in palliative care ethics.

PHENOMENOLOGY, HERMENEUTICS, EXISTENTIALISM

In the year in which the twentieth century began, a German philosopher, Edmund Husserl, published his now-famous book, *Logical Investigations*, with which another philosophical method appeared—phenomenology. Husserl came to philosophy from mathematics, his first subject of interest, and therefore came to it looking for apodictic, universal, and immutable philosophical knowledge. Through a method called "categorical intuition," he thought he was able to discover the essence of phenomena, understood in a way quite similar to the Platonic notion of Forms, as objective, ideal entities. Therefore, he concluded, there is a world, the world of pure phenomena, in which truth appears as an absolute fact. After the relativism of some movements of the nineteenth century, Husserl thought he had made possible a new foundation for philosophy on the basis of an absolute and immutable truth, which was, for him, the inalienable premise of an authentic philosophy.

The importance of this method to the development of twentieth-century European philosophy is undeniable. It did not take a long time, however, for problems to appear. One fundamental reason, among others, was the insurmountable distance between the categorical intuition and its description with words. Words are not completely adequate to ideas; they have been constructed by human beings and are therefore imperfect. Moreover, words are always polysemous, changing their meanings continuously through history. The understanding of a text is always an open question; it is much more the understanding of a human being. Our representantive thinking can be appropriate to the analysis of the "ontic" things of the world, but human beings are in touch with another level, called by Heiddeger ontologic, and here our thinking cannot be representative but hermeneutic (Richardson 1974, 630–36; Hodge 1995, 184). This discipline, developed during the nineteenth century, from Schleiermacher to Dilthey, now acquired a new interest and converted hermeneutics into one of the most useful methods of philosophical inquiry during the twentieth century.

After Dilthey and Heidegger the influence of hermeneutics on European philosophy and ethics has been progressive. In 1960 one of Heidegger's students, H.-G. Gadamer, published an influential work titled *Truth and Method*, in which hermeneutics became the method not only of social and human sciences, or of philosophy and ethics, but of all human thinking. Gadamer was completely aware that in doing this, he was connecting with the Aristotelian tradition and, more specifically, with Aristotle's theories about practical reasoning, deliberation, and *phronesis*. One of the consequences of this approach for ethics is that moral imperatives are now conceived of as imperatives of discretion and cleverness, hardly the Kantian categorical imperatives. Gadamer in an 1989 essay titled "Aristotle and Imperative Ethics," stresses the importance of the Aristotelian approach today (1999, 142). Aristotle was the father of practical reasoning, recognizing that it is impossible in the field of practical thinking for the mind to be fitted totally to reality, particularly in medicine, inasmuch as our practical statements are marked by uncertainty and probability (Svenaeus 2003).

The core idea of hermeneutics as a method of thinking is that human situations, like written texts, can be interpreted in many different ways, depending on the point of view of the observer. Between this and the question at stake, there is always a dynamic and two-way interaction. This is the origin of the hermeneutic circle. It is an indefinite circle, because no one can exhaust completely the meaning of a text or a situation. Therefore, no one can claim to possess the total truth about an event. Everyone is biased by his or her own prejudices (in the positive sense of the term, as used by Gadamer) and limitations; thus the importance of dialogue and deliberation, especially when dealing with the life and death of human beings, as in medicine (Gadamer 1996).

Hermeneutics, like all other methodologies dealing with uncertainty, is unpleasant, because humans like security, and uncertainty is always insecure. This is why in medical ethics, as in all other fields, the methodologies most frequently used are those in which certainty can be reached in a quite mechanical way or at least uncertainty is reduced to the minimum. People do not like complexity: "Therein we often find a canonical set of terms, theories, and principles explained in introductory sections and instantiated in the articles or case discussions judged worthy of inclusion" (Leder 1994, 252). Dealing with uncertainty and complexity demands a very mature personality, aware of its autonomy (in its etymological meaning of inner-directed), and capable of managing it. Apodictic systems of ethics are generally heteronomous (that is, Other-directed).

Hermeneutics is one of the various expressions throughout the twentieth century of the phenomenological tradition. Several thinkers tied to the phenomenological tradition developed another type of ethics, however, that they frequently designated as responsibility. This is a pervasive expression in nearly all the existentialists. The founder of the phenomenological school, Edmund Husserl, from time to time used this expression. It is also the best way of characterizing the ethics of Heidegger (Hodge 1995). But thinkers for whom it acquired a more coherent and developed meaning were the French phenomenologists, in particular Jean-Paul Sartre and Emmanuel Levinas. Toombs (2001) has produced an excellent study of the application of the work of these thinkers to medical ethics.

Existentialists coined the phrase "the 'essence' of human-being lies in its existence" (Heidegger 1972, 42). This is more than a witty phrase. Traditionally human beings were defined as realities with a specific essence (composed of body and soul), whose development through life was called existence. Essence, therefore, was conceived as prior to life and immutable. On the contrary, existentialists thought that the most specific characteristic of human beings is that they live in a world of possibilities and not of pure realities. As Sartre (1973) put it:

> Man is, indeed, a project which possesses a subjective life, instead of being a kind of moss, or a fungus or a cauliflower. . . . If, however, it is true that existence is prior to essence, man is responsible for what he is. Thus, the first effect of existentialism is that it puts every man in possession of himself as he is, and places the entire responsibility for his existence responsible squarely upon his

own shoulders. And, when we say that man is responsible for himself, we do not mean that he is responsible only for his own individuality, but that he is responsible for all men.

That is why "responsibility" is the proper word to designate the existentialist ethics. Its most mature and developed expression has been the ethics of Emmanuel Levinas. All these theories have been applied to medicine and medical ethics frequently during the last decades (Svenaeus 2001, 2007, 2009; Clifton-Soderstrom 2003).

For Levinas (1978) existence is anonymous and impersonal, whereas existents are subjects, persons (1969, 33–34). The Existent par excellence is the Other, which appears immediately in one's subjectivity as different from one's self, and also different from all other things. The Other is an absolute, irreducible to one's ontological grasp, which compels one to respond to him. Here one discovers that being human is being-for-the-Other. This demand is called by Levinas responsibility. Therefore, a person is responsible for the Other, and this responsibility is absolute and unavoidable. One cannot transfer this responsibility to anyone else. This is the origin of what Levinas calls first ethics, or ethics as first philosophy (1985, 98). This theory of Levinas has been frequently applied to the analysis of the clinical encounter (Tiemersma 1987).

CARE, NURSING, AND GENDER ETHICS

Care lies just a few short steps beyond responsibility. If one is responsible for the other, one must take care of him. The ethics of responsibility leads this way to the ethics of care. The being-in-the-world of Heidegger and the being-for-the-Other of Levinas both suggest that the main category of ethics is care. This is the origin of the care ethics theory, widely developed during the second half of the last century. According to Gilligan, "In this conception, the moral problem arises from conflicting responsibilities rather than from competing rights and requires for its resolution a mode of thinking that is contextual and narrative rather than formal and abstract. The conception of morality as concerned with the activity of care centers moral development around the understanding of responsibility and relationships, just as the conception of morality as fairness ties moral development to the understanding of rights and duties" (1982, 19).

The male conception of ethics is a consequence of a way of thinking characterized by the use of apodictic logic and an absolutist conception of rules and duties. That is why care and responsibility have been the two major categories in the new gender ethics. "Yet in the different voice of women lies the truth of an ethic of care, the tie between relationship and responsibility" (Gilligan 1982, 173). Peta Bowden (1997) characterized this gender-sensitive ethics of care as having four characteristics: mothering, friendship, nursing, and citizenship. It has been the main concept in modern nursing ethics (Kuhse 1997), and it is also the way in which new gender ethics has revolutionized many other fields of ethics and human life, such as politics, socioeconomic relationships, and ecology. As Gottlieb (1994) puts it, "The culturally male ego is predominantly formed through a process of separation, toward an ideal of autonomy, and results in a bounded, competitive, and dominating self. By contrast, the female ego is shaped through affiliation, toward an ideal of what is termed 'self-in-relation,' and results in an empathic, nurturing, and connected self. Women's selfhood stems from women's role as primary caretakers of infants and their responsibility for emotionality and nurturing in adult relationships" (222–40).

Although the idea of care was essential to the development of the new gender ethics, the field today has taken a direction far beyond the original Noddings-Gilligan approach to care (Gilligan 1982; Noddings 1984). Feminist ethics now strongly criticizes the strict identification of women with care. This is neither the only, nor the essential, role for women. Women have been excluded for millennia from active social life, and also from the moral life. Their moral life was reduced to obedience. One example of this is their passive role in health care (Sherwin 1996). Demanding an active and protagonistic role in social life, women are leading a full revolution and promoting the emancipation of other groups rejected or rendered submissive to the patriarchal male society. Bioethics becomes, in this way, biopolitics (Morgan 1986). Restoring the excluded "feminine," women are reversing the patriarchal construction of reality (Gudorf 1994, 166). This is not only a social or human revolution but also an ethical one. They advocate a new ethics—fairer, more embodied and contextualized, more compassionate, and more sensitive and appreciative of the role of care. Without these changes, a true ethics seems impossible. Only an ethic in which the emancipation of women could be assumed without restriction can be a true ethics (Purdy 1996).

VIRTUE ETHICS

Close to the ethics of care is another rooted in the classical tradition, especially in Aristotle, commonly called virtue ethics. Aristotle ordered moral life around the idea of virtue, *arête*, understood as the capacity of doing things well. There are moral virtues, but also virtues of a technical character. For example, justice is a moral virtue, while proficiency in performing right surgical interventions is a technical virtue (*Nichomachean Ethics*, 1106 a 17–24). The Greek word *arête* has been translated to English by two different words, "virtue" and "excellence." Today, this last translation has become more common because the word *virtue* has lost its primitive meaning, having been reduced to naming the moral but not the technical virtues.

Pellegrino and Thomasma have been two of the major defenders of the virtue approach to medical ethics. They thought that the classical four bioethical principles—autonomy, beneficence, nonmaleficence, and justice—should be taken not only as abstract and theoretical principles but also as practical virtues and that the intrinsic virtue that defines the internal morality of medicine is beneficence (Pellegrino and Thomasma 1981, 1988). Another representative book attempting to apply virtue ethics to medicine was published by James F. Drane, *Becoming a Good Doctor: The Place of Virtue and Character in Medical Ethics* (1988). His thesis, which follows ideas developed previously by Laín Entralgo (1969), is that the clinical encounter needs the exercise of many moral virtues, such as benevolence, truthfulness, respect, friendliness, justice, and religion. Drane's idea is that American medical ethics has underestimated this important element of human conduct (Drane 1988, 137). This way, Drane tried to develop this sentence of Aristotle: "We cannot be fully good without intelligence, or intelligent without virtue of character" (*Nichomachean Ethics*, 1144 b 31–32).

COMMUNITARIANISM

The tension between the ethics of principles and norms and the ethics of care, virtue, and character has also become evident in another debate—this time between the universalistic and the communitarian ways of thinking about moral problems. Universalistic theories of practical reason try to find a consistent normative standpoint external and superior to every particular society and tradition, that is, to every community. They are all, to some extent, Kantian, due to the fact that Kant was the most important promoter of the principle of universalization in ethics. But between Kant and the new universalists there is an important difference. Kant thought that human reason, used correctly, is capable of establishing universal moral principles by itself, without any other external help. These principles are, therefore, universal in a "substantive" way. The new universalists, by contrast, do not believe that the human mind is capable of reaching absolute principles; they argue that only those principles that can be assumed without coercion by all affected by them can be called universal. This way of legitimizing principles and norms is called procedural. The new universalists are proceduralists because they share with the other ethical movements of the twentieth century the belief in the weak power of human reason (Rawls 1999, 1–19). Universal principles cannot be established in a completely objective way, but only in another they call intersubjective.

John Rawls's theory of justice is one of the most important works of this new universalism. Rawls argues that in an original position, one in which participants ignore their particular, real situations, positive or negative, due to what he calls the veil of ignorance, all human beings would come to unanimous agreement regarding certain principles that are good for all, after a rational dialogue between them. Rawls takes for granted the existence of a common, rational self-interest by which the citizens, acting as free and equal moral persons, can agree and ground principles of justice, provided that religious and philosophical questions are "bracketed." Rawls calls this process deliberation but, as has been pointed out, "in that case, the process of deliberation is supererogatory" (Mouffe 1995). The Rawlsian consensus is based upon self-interest. Rawls thinks that by putting religious and philosophical questions into the background of private life, things can be decided following the model of the decision-making theory. As Mouffe (1995) wryly observes, "This is the perfect liberal utopia." Moreover, Mouffe argues, ethics ought not be reduced to a set of universal agreements about justice.

If Rawls is the American face of the new universalism, Apel and Habermas are the main figures in Europe. They are Kantians but, like Rawls, procedural Kantians. This means that both are thinking of legitimizing norms in a procedural and intersubjective way. Their procedure, like that of Rawls, is ideal, pursued through the so-called ideal community of communication. The difference between the theories is that for Rawls, the principles of justice are carried out monologically, such that one person (Rawls himself) thinks up the rules all people would agree upon if placed in an original position, whereas Apel and Habermas think that these norms can be tested only discursively, in a public deliberation with all those affected by the norm as active participants (Habermas 1990, 67).

In contrast with the continuing effort to found morality upon universal norms, other contemporary theorists have attempted to ground morality upon a more natural foundation, that is, in communities. In fact, we all develop our moral lives inside communities, assuming the values of our communities and promoting their enhancement or change. We do not develop morally thinking of ourselves as inhabitants of ideal and decontextualized utopian worlds. All these universalistic constructions are dependent on the idea of individuals as isolated entities, typical of the modern world. This was the critique argued by Charles Taylor in his book *Sources of the Self: The Making of the Modern Identity* (1989). The formal Kantian criterion of universalization purchased a radical autonomy, but at the price of emptiness. This was Hegel's critique of Kant. Opposite the Kantian *Moralität*, understood as the formal set of obligations held as an individual rational will, Hegel opposed *Sittlichkeit*, that is, the moral obligations one has to an ongoing community of which one is part (Taylor 1979, 83). The latter is the way in which ethics began in Western culture, and that is the reason why Greek philosophers conceived ethics as a part of a wider discipline, called politics (Aristotle, *Politics*, 1252 a 1–2).

DELIBERATIVE ETHICS

During the twentieth century deliberation has become more and more important. Forgotten when ethics was conceived as an apodictic discipline, it has increased its importance as thinkers have become more skeptical about the truth of moral claims. Deliberation is compatible with all the theories described in this part of the chapter. We must deliberate in order to know the set of principles or rules that would prevail in a well-ordered society, following the suggestions of Rawls, Apel, Habermas, and the proponents of principlist bioethics. But the language of values is more basic than the language of rules and norms. Among other reasons, this is because rules depend on values. The primary place for deliberation is the world of values, especially when two or more of them are in conflict. Values are not completely subjective and erratic, as philosophers used to think in the nineteenth century. The twentieth century began with the publication of G. E. Moore's *Principia Ethica* (in 1994), in which he consecrates the expression "intrinsic value." Values are the more specific human characteristics, and they cannot be dismissed as completely irrational. Certainly values are not strictly rational, but they must be reasonable. And the way of reaching this reasonability or reasonableness is what is called deliberation.

Intrinsic values constitute the argument of human lives; they structure and govern social relationships. This means that they are necessary in a well-ordered human society, so that when they are lacking we perceive an important loss. To know which values are intrinsic, G. E. Moore proposes the following rule: "It is necessary to consider what things are such that, if they existed *by themselves*, in absolute isolation, we should yet judge their existence to be good" (1994, 236). Intrinsic values are valuable for themselves, so that their lack is perceived like an important loss. Could we think of a perfect human world without peace? The answer is necessarily negative. And the same happens for justice, solidarity, love, friendship, beauty, life, health, wellbeing, and so on. Values are the matter of our duties. Our moral duty is always the same, to fulfill values, making them actual in our real world. That is not an easy task because this world is full of various constraints we must take into account to make wise and reasonable decisions. Moral decisions must be undertaken by looking to the ideal values and by including the specific circumstances of the situation in which the decision has to be made and the foreseen consequences. The way of doing that is moral deliberation, a procedure first proposed by Aristotle, forgotten during the entire period of the hegemony of apodictic thinking in ethics, only rediscovered in the twentieth century, and fruitfully applied to medical ethics (Gracia 2001, 2003, 2005).

ᝢ Critique

Taken in its broader sense, deliberation is the opposite of demonstration, covering all the movements and theories described in the last part of this chapter. A debate, more logical and metaphysical than moral, persists, however, about which approach is correct. The fundamental question is whether there are immutable principles in human reasoning about ethic, or whether, on the contrary, they all are constructed by human beings, either individually or socially. There are important reasons to think that our mind has no capacity to formulate universal and immutable moral principles, but these reasons aren't absolute either. Thus, absolutists accuse deliberationists of relativism, and deliberationists accuse absolutists of naïve idealism. The core questions of debate are two. First, whether we reach values and principles by intuition or some similar way, or by construction. Second, whether circumstances and consequences should play a substantial role in moral reasoning or not. Absolutists stress that principles, such as those of the natural law, cannot be given up for contingent reasons. Therefore, they hold that the specific circumstances of each case can modify features of the application of the rule but do not change it substantially (Finnis 1980, 1991; Spaemann 1982; Grisez 1988).

There is also another way to think about deliberation that differs from the family of philosophical approaches discussed above. Deliberation can be understood as a structured method of reasoning about facts, values, and duties, taking into account not only the abstract principles but also the specific circumstances and the predictable consequences, in order to make wise and thorough decisions. In this second meaning deliberation is different from dialogue, discussion, negotiation, and consensus. In particular it is different from the way of making decisions that is presented in decision science (see chapter 16). It is a rational process, but one that takes into account not only reasons but also feelings, values, beliefs, hopes, traditions, and expectations because human beings introduce all these things into their moral decisions. Deliberation is a rational process dealing with things that are not completely rational but that should be reasonable, wise, and prudent. This methodology has been already discussed in the political and legal settings (Habermas 1996; Bohman 1996; Gutmann and Thompson 2004), but there have been clinical ethical applications as well (Emanuel 1991; Emanuel and Emanuel 1992; Gutmann and Thompson 1997; Gracia 2009).

ᝢ Notes on Resources and Training

Moral decisions, as I have argued, are always specific and concrete and therefore dependent upon time and place. Phenomena that are not strictly rational, such as beliefs, values, and traditions, play a very important role in them. One consequence is that decisions made in some places, for instance, in the United States, are not necessarily correct in other places, such as in Europe or Latin America. For that reason the bibliographical resources that the professional must take into account in order to do research are not only those written in English and published in journals of highest impact factor but also the literature written in every particular cultural area. The National Library of Medicine database, *Bioethicsline*, later included in *Medline*, covers only literature written in English. *Medline* indexes also ethical papers published in other languages but only in medical journals. Taken as a whole this database is the most important resource available in the field of medical ethics. Scholars can make use of other, complementary resources, however, especially when working in languages other than English and their associated cultures. The European Union has promoted the construction of a European database on medical ethics called *Euroethics* (www.euroethics.de), which includes bibliographic records from fifteen partners in fourteen European countries. Other collaborative European enterprises have been the European Society for Philosophy of Medicine and Health Care (www.espmh.cm-uj.krakow.pl/) and its official organ, *Medicine, Health Care, and Philosophy: A European Journal*. There are also manuals of bioethics written in a European perspective (Have and Gordijn 2001; Lie and Schotsmans 2002). The literature of the Spanish- and the Portuguese-speaking worlds is available through BIREME (with the databases LILACS and SciELO).

Special training in medical ethics is offered by many master's degree and doctorate programs. In Western Europe there are also international collaborative courses. One example of them is the European master in bioethics, supported partially by the European Union through its Erasmus Mundus program. There are also doctoral programs in medical ethics supported by different universities.

❧ References

Aristotle. 1831. *Aristotelis opera*. Berlin: Reimer.

———. 1984. *The Complete Works of Aristotle*. Princeton: Princeton University Press.

Bohman, J. 1996. *Public deliberation: Pluralism, complexity, and democracy*. Cambridge, MA: MIT Press.

Bowden, P. 1997. *Caring: Gender-sensitive ethics*. London: Routledge.

Brickhouse, Th. C., and N. D. Smith. 1994. *Plato's Socrates*. New York: Oxford University Press.

Clifton-Soderstrom, M. 2003. Levinas and the patient as Other: The ethical foundation of medicine. *Journal of Medicine and Philosophy* 28 (4): 447–60.

Descartes, R. 1964–74. Discours de la méthode. *Oeuvres de Descartes*, 12 vols. Paris: Vrin.

Dewey, J. 1997. *The influence of Darwin on philosophy, and other essays*. New York: Prometheus Books.

Diogenes Laertius. 1964. *Vitae philosophorum*. Oxford: Oxford University Press.

Drane, J. F. 1988. *Becoming a good doctor: The place of virtue and character in medical ethics*. Kansas City: Sheed and Ward.

Emanuel, E. J. 1991. *The ends of human life: Medical ethics in a liberal polity*. Cambridge, MA: Harvard University Press.

Emanuel, E. J., and L. Emanuel. 1992. Four models of the physician-patient relationship. *Journal of the American Medical Association* 267 (16): 2221–26.

Finnis, J. 1980. *Natural law and natural rights*. Oxford: Clarendon Press.

———. 1991. *Moral absolutes: Tradition, revision, and truth*. Washington, DC: The Catholic University of America Press.

Gadamer, H.-G. 1960. *Wahrheit und methode.* Tübingen, Germany: Mohr.

———. 1996. *The enigma of health: The art of healing in a scientific age.* Cambridge, UK: Polity Press.

———. 1999. *Hermeneutics, religion, & ethics.* New Haven, CT: Yale University Press.

Galen. 1978–84. *De Placitis Hippocratis et Platonis.* Berlin: Akademie-Verlag.

Gilligan, C. 1982. *In a different voice: Psychological theory and women's development.* Cambridge, MA: Harvard University Press.

Gottlieb, R. S. 1994. Ethics and trauma: Levinas, feminism, and deep ecology. *Cross Currents* 44 (2): 222–40

Gracia D. 2001. Moral deliberation: The role of methodologies in clinical ethics. *Medicine, Health Care and Philosophy* 4:223–32.

———. 2003. Ethical case deliberation and decision making. *Medicine, Health Care and Philosophy* 6:227–33.

———. 2005. The foundation of medical ethics in the democratic evolution of modern society. In *Clinical bioethics: A Search for the foundations,* ed. C. Viafora, 33–40. Dordrecht: Springer.

———. 2010. Deliberation and consensus. In *Handbook of health care ethics in an era of globalisation,* ed. R. Chadwick and H. ten Have. London: Sage (in press).

Grisez, G. 1988. *Beyond the new morality: The responsibilities of freedom.* Notre Dame, IN: University of Notre Dame Press.

Gudorf, C. E. 1994. A feminist critique of biomedical principlism. In *A matter of principles?* ed. E. R. DuBose, R. Hamel, and L. J. O'Connell, 164–81. Valley Forge, PA: Trinity Press International.

Gutmann, A., and D. Thompson. 1997. Deliberating about bioethics. *Hastings Center Report* 27:38–41.

———. 2004. *Why deliberative democracy?* Princeton, NJ: Princeton University Press.

Habermas, J. 1990. *Moral consciousness and communicative action.* Cambridge, MA: MIT Press.

———. 1996. *Between facts and norms: Contributions to a discourse theory of law and democracy.* Cambridge, MA: MIT Press.

Have, H. T., and B. Gordijn, eds. 2001. *Bioethics in a European perspective.* Dordrecht, The Netherlands: Kluwer.

Heidegger, M. 1972. *Sein und Zeit.* Tübingen: Max Niemeyer.

Hodge, J. 1995. *Heidegger and ethics.* London: Routledge.

Hume, D. 1882. *An enquiry concerning human understanding.* London: Green and Grose.

Inwood, B., ed. 2003. *The Cambridge companion to the Stoics.* Cambridge: Cambridge University Press.

Kant, I. 1855. *Critique of pure reason.* London: Henry G. Bohn.

———. 1997. *Critique of practical reason.* Cambridge: Cambridge University Press.

Kuhse, H. 1997. *Caring: Nurses, women and ethics.* Oxford: Blackwell.

Laín Entralgo, P. 1969. *Doctor and patient.* New York: McGraw-Hill.

Leder, D. 1994. Towards a hermeneutical bioethics. In *A matter of principles?* ed. E. R. DuBose, R. Hamel, and L. J. O'Connell, 240–59. Valley Forge, PA: Trinity Press International.

Leibniz, G. 1981. *New essays on human understanding.* Cambridge: Cambridge University Press.

Levinas, E. 1969. *Totality and infinity.* Pittsburgh: Duquesne University Press.

———. 1978. *Existence and existents.* The Hague: Kluwer.

———. 1985. *Ethics and infinity: Conversations with Philippe Nemo.* Pittsburgh: Duquesne University Press.

Lie, R. K., and P. T. Schotsmans, eds. 2002. *Healthy thoughts: European perspectives on health care ethics.* Leuven, Belgium: Peeters.

Lloyd, G. 1996. *Spinoza and ethics.* London: Routledge.

Mill, J. S. 1864. *Utilitarianism.* London: Longman.

Moore, G. E. 1994. *Principia ethica.* Cambridge: Cambridge University Press.

Morgan, K. P. 1986. Gender rites and rights: The biopolitics of beauty and fertility. In *Philosophical perspectives on bioethics,* ed. L. W. Sumner and J. Boyle, 210–43. Toronto: University of Toronto Press.

Mouffe, C. 1995. Rawls: Political philosophy without politics. In *Universalism vs. communitarianism: Contemporary debates in ethics*, ed. D. Rasmussen. Cambridge, MA: MIT Press.

Noddings, N. 1984. *Caring: A feminine approach to ethics and moral education*. Berkeley: University of California Press.

Pellegrino, E. D., and D. C. Thomasma. 1981. *A philosophical basis for medical practice: Toward a philosophy and ethic of the healing professions*. New York: Oxford University Press.

———. 1988. *For the patient's good: The restoration of beneficence in health care*. New York: Oxford University Press.

Plato. 1997. *Complete works*. Indianapolis and Cambridge: Hackett.

Plutarch. 1929. *De virtute morali*. Leipzig, Germany: Teubner.

Purdy, L. M. 1996. Good bioethics must be feminist bioethics. In *Philosophical perspectives on bioethics*, ed. L. W. Sumner and J. Boyle, 143–62. Toronto: University of Toronto Press.

Rawls, J. 1999. *Collected papers*. Cambridge, MA: Harvard University Press.

Richardson, W. J. 1974. *Heidegger: Through phenomenology to thought*. The Hague: Martinus Nijhoff.

Sartre, J. P. 1973. *Existentialism & humanism*. London: Methuen.

Sherwin, S. 1996. Theory versus practice in ethics: A feminist perspective on justice in health care. In *Philosophical perspectives on bioethics*, ed. L. W. Sumner and J. Boyle, 187–209. Toronto: University of Toronto Press.

Somme, L.-Th. 2006. The infallibility, impeccability and indestructibility of synderesis. *Studies in Christian ethics* 19:403–16.

Spaemann, R. 1982. *Moralische Grundbegriffe*. Munich, Germany: Beck.

Spinoza, B. 1927. *Ethic: Demonstrated in geometrical order and divided into five parts*. Oxford: Blackwell.

Svenaeus, F. 2001. *The hermeneutics of medicine and the phenomenology of health: Steps towards a philosophy of medical practice*. Dordrecht, The Netherlands: Kluwer.

———. 2003. Hermeneutics of medicine in the wake of Gadamer: The issue of phronesis. *Theoretical Medicine and Bioethics* 24:407–31.

———. 2007. A Heideggerian defense of (and caution against) therapeutic cloning. *Theoretical Medicine and Bioethics* 28:31–62.

———. 2009. The phenomenology of falling ill: An explanation, critique and improvement of Sartre's theory of embodiment and alienation. *Human Studies* 32:53–66.

Taylor, C. 1979. *Hegel and modern society*. Cambridge: Cambridge University Press.

———. 1989. *Sources of the self: The making of the modern identity*. Cambridge: Cambridge University Press.

Tiemersma, D. 1987. Ontology and ethics in the foundation of medicine and the relevance of Levinas' view. *Theoretical Medicine* 8:127–33.

Toombs, K., ed. 2001. *Handbook of phenomenology and medicine*. Dordrecht, The Netherlands: Kluwer.

Vander Waerdt, P. A., ed. 1994. *The Socratic movement*. Ithaca, NY: Cornell University Press.

Vlastos, G. 1991. *Socrates: Ironist and moral philosopher*. Ithaca, NY: Cornell University Press.

CHAPTER 5

Religion and Theology

LISA SOWLE CAHILL

In the evolution of modern medical ethics, religious traditions and theology have interacted extensively with moral philosophy, science, public policy, health care initiatives, and global health needs. This chapter focuses on Western Christianity. Yet literature in other traditions is substantial (Sullivan 1989; *Journal of Religious Ethics* 2008). In Judaism it is abundant (Bleich and Rosner 1979; Bleich 1981; Feldman 1986; Green 1986; Novak 1990; Davis 1991; Newman 1992; Gellman 1993; Pellegrino and Faden 1999). A major new direction concerns theology, global health, and justice.

Overview

Theological medical ethics grounds arguments in religious claims and in the history and theological traditions of a religious community. For example, Jewish and Christian medical ethics originate from the conviction that humans are creatures in a created and interdependent natural world; that the Creator is good, just, and powerful; that humanity is sinful, as well as responsible for good moral behavior; and that God offers human beings healing or salvation from moral and spiritual wrongdoing.

One key set of differences has to do with the certainty and stability of theologically based moral norms. Another concerns the similarity of religious and nonreligious views. Cloning is an example. Some theologians seek clear norms to apply in a reliable, constant manner, consistent with tradition. They might propose that since humanity is finite and only God is the Creator, for humans to create children from only one parent is tantamount to playing God and is sinful. Some defending clear, stable, theologically grounded norms also appeal to a historical tradition of authoritative interpretation. Prominent examples are the Catholic Church's teaching office (*magisterium*) and the Jewish tradition of law (*halakha*) supplemented by the responsa literature, which is a collection of questions about the law submitted to individual rabbis. This kind of approach can be creative and innovative by way of its interpretation of theological tradition or religious law, but the innovations are presented as extrapolations, not departures, from teachings of the past.

Other theological ethicists take issue with the idea that theology provides specific norms that can be applied consistently and comprehensively to new or complex situations. They agree that beliefs about creation, responsibility, sin, and salvation supply parameters and establish directions. However, concrete applications must be adaptive to circumstances and emerging developments. Thus, for example, some theologians portray humans as created cocreators, arguing that human freedom and responsibility demand flexibility and even changes in ethical judgments. (For examples in genetic technology, see Peters [1996]; Chapman [1999]; and Cole-Turner [2008]).

An even more important point of difference between theological methods is whether agreement on norms and commitments requires membership in a specific religious community. All theological ethicists agree that religious identity results in a set of moral commitments but where they disagree is in relating a religiously and theologically based morality to the larger world. For example, Orthodox Jewish interpreters of the law are not interested in whether society at large accepts the norms they produce but in how Jews can live faithfully within their tradition today (Jakobovitz 1975). Some Christians write out of a story, or narrative, that claims to provide a distinctive identity not acceptable or even intelligible to outsiders (Hauerwas 1986a). It is more important to be faithful to religious and theological ideals than to have a big impact on public medical ethics and policy.

A contrasting approach accepts such premises as creation, sin, and redemption but assumes that other reasonable people can arrive at similar judgments since philosophical arguments and information from the natural and social sciences are shared. One example is Roman Catholic moral theology. Catholic medical ethicists assume a common human nature and a generally acceptable ideal of the good society. Shared human experiences and basic values provide common ground to discern whether to permit, prohibit, or limit the use of cloning, other reproductive technologies, abortion, physician-assisted suicide, or germ-line therapy. Mainline Protestants are similar, although their primary foundations are the general moral values found in scripture. Catholicism sometimes falls into the earlier category of a community-relative medical ethics, as when disputed issues are referred to Church authority and settled in a manner that avoids philosophical and scientific counterevidence. (For a discussion of the relative merits of the community-oriented and the public-oriented forms of theological medical ethics, see Verhey [1996].)

The ethical methods of theology are neither separate and insulated from one another nor detached from the realities and dilemmas of particular historical contexts. It is difficult to identify certain methods strictly with corresponding religious traditions, institutions of higher learning, or even followers and students collected around certain leading thinkers. Both the recognizable unity of theological medical ethics and some striking dissimilarities exist because of a confluence of factors that brought theologians into the growing field of medical ethics approximately four decades ago. Certain key thinkers were important in this process. How each of them envisioned theological medical ethics was heavily influenced by how they understood religious identity, interpreted new scientific and social challenges, and collaborated with nontheologians, for example, in formulating public policy.[1]

HISTORY OF THEOLOGY IN MEDICAL ETHICS

In the 1960s theologians were influential players in defining questions for the emerging field. Theologians and philosophers who created the field of modern medical ethics, and health professionals who flagged sensitive issues, were motivated by the proliferation of new biomedical technologies and a new consciousness of patients' rights and responsibilities, especially in light of well-publicized research abuses. They recognized that the ethics of medicine could no longer be contained within an individualist patient–physician model. They were aware that moral responsibility in medicine might require creativity and an orientation to future possibilities, at least as much as respect for norms and prohibitions of the past.

Protestant theologians such as Joseph Fletcher, Paul Ramsey, and James Gustafson drew on touchstones such as self-sacrificial love, covenant, creation, and image of God. They relied on information from the social and natural sciences to understand better the changing practical context. Catholic theologians like Richard McCormick, Charles Curran, and Germain Grisez looked for ways to link long-standing traditions of authoritative teaching and moral law to new developments. This was also true of such Jewish thinkers as Immanuel Jakobovitz and Fred Rosner and the Orthodox ethicist Stanley Harakas (Harakas 1980, 1999).

Theologians such as Ramsey (1970), Gustafson (1975), McCormick (1981), and Karen Lebacqz (1983) served on important policy bodies, such as the National Commission on the Protection of Human Subjects of Biomedical and Behavioral Research (1974) and the President's Commission for the Study of Ethical Problems in Medicine and Biomedical and Behavioral Research (1979). They were major players in the formation of the field—helping to create bioethics institutes such as the Institute of Religion at the Texas Medical Center in Houston (1954); the Institute of Society, Ethics, and the Life Sciences, later to become the Hastings Center (1969); and the Kennedy Institute of Ethics at Georgetown University (1971). The first edition of the *Encyclopedia of Bioethics*, whose very existence and title lent substance to the new field, was filled with entries by theologians and other articles written from religious perspectives (Reich 1978; 1996, 90). Theologians were particularly well equipped because religious communities had cultivated long-standing traditions of reflection on life, death, and suffering and had given more guidance on the specifics of moral conduct than had moral philosophy at that time (Shelp 1986; Walters 1986; Reich 1996).

Some believe this influence came at a high price (Callahan 1990; Lammers 1996). To be heard in pluralistic debates, some theologians began to operate like moral philosophers. In the 1980s as aspiring medical ethicists, even those pursuing theological degrees, were educated specifically for the new field and assumed roles in clinical settings, some paid more attention to crises and dilemmas than to theological or even philosophical foundations. Theologians soon became marginalized in a field that increasingly relied on universal, rational, and secular principles, and they sought decision-making and policy resolutions that could be squared with U.S. legal traditions and command public support. The preeminent statement of such principles (autonomy, justice, beneficence, and nonmaleficence) was made by Tom Beauchamp and James F. Childress, the latter a theologian who studied with Gustafson at Yale (Beauchamp and Childress 1979/2001).

Theologians today seek to reassert their religious identity while not giving up public credibility. This is not just about a theological identity crisis. It is also about dissatisfaction with the recent tradition of principled, secular medical ethics that prizes autonomy (and its structural protection, informed consent). Theology's search for a new model corresponds to a simultaneous philosophical development—postmodernism—and its insight that even abstract and supposedly universal principles are formulated in historical communities. Maybe such principles do express something universal but it will no longer do to view them as simple, straightforward products of rational thinking (as recognized by Childress 1994). Theological methods in medical ethics cannot be understood apart from the conditions and individuals that create and use them. They are not intellectual products to be deployed scientifically but tradition-based and contextual strategies for uniting and making concrete a number of concerns and goals having to do with biomedical trends and practices. Morality as seen from different communal standpoints may not be wholly translatable into a neutral, secular sphere. To some observers this makes communal moralities, including religious moralities and theological ethics, seem like tribal preferences, inappropriate and even dangerous candidates for public consumption (Engelhardt 1996).

To others marginality is a value, and religious and theological voices should be wary of diluting their traditions in a supposedly public square (Callahan 1990; Campbell 1990; Hauerwas 1986a, 1996; Marty 1992). Theology should be more concerned about faithfulness to its foundational texts, symbols, traditions, and moral practices than about influencing biomedical practice and policy. Its role in social ethics and policy should be primarily prophetic. Only by speaking in an authentically religious voice can theology reach practical conclusions that are truly theological.

Meanwhile, several theologians have sought a middle path (Smith 1996; Gustafson 1996a, 1996b; Reich with dell'Oro 1996; McCormick 1984; Cahill 1992; a collection of several approaches to a religious, public bioethics is Guinn 2006). The commitment to make religiously grounded ideals effective in a public setting has been particularly strong in Roman Catholicism (Hehir 1992; McCormick 1995). Protestant scholars also reinvigorate biblical roots while turning outward to a broader community of discourse (Townes 1998; Smith and Cohen 2003; Verhey 2003; Meilaender 2005). For many, religious identity, spirituality, and liturgy are very important but so is health care policy, just access to care, and global justice in health care (Guroian 1996; Sulmasy 1997; Townes 1998; Smith 2000; Hanson 2001; Ryan 2001; Christie 2003; Vogt 2004; Cahill 2005a; Ashley, deBlois, and O'Rourke 2006; Parsi and Sheehan 2006; Vigen 2006; McCarthy and Lysaught 2007; McDonough 2007). The AIDS crisis has prompted many religious responses that aim for wide social impact (Keenan 2000; Messer 2004; Cimperman 2005; Overberg 2006; Iozzo 2008).

This chapter uses a paradigm of Gustafson to sort theological methods into three categories (Gustafson 1996a, 1996b). Theology is autonomous, continuous, or in a dialectical relationship with other modes of moral knowledge. After introducing Gustafson's paradigm, I consider three of the major players in the early development of theological medical ethics: Paul Ramsey, Richard McCormick, and James

Gustafson. Then I turn to medical ethicists who have carried forward the theological interests of these greats while adapting their agendas. Important contributors today are far too numerous to treat comprehensively. Selections will illustrate major differences according to Gustafson's paradigm. Finally, I suggest contributions theology currently makes to medical ethics, including feminist and global dimensions.

❧ Description of Three Types of Theological Medical Ethics: Autonomous, Continuous, and Dialectical

Some theologians want religion to remain an autonomous sphere with its own integrity, for secular thinking amounts simply to another, competing, and ultimately hostile ideology. Still others believe that different disciplines do, in fact, offer reliable ways of understanding human behavior and human goods, so the insights generated by a religious community can be continuous with such knowledge. For others, religion and additional resources are mutually interactive. Moral discernment depends on a dialectic between religion and other sources. They may correct one another.

Different warrants for the autonomy model of theological ethics include a postmodern epistemology that relativizes the claims of religious traditions, a strong doctrine of revelation (through sacred texts, traditions, and practices), and respect for institutional authority that guards revelation and tradition. Under this model Gustafson mentions the halakhic reasoning of Orthodox Judaism; Eastern Orthodoxy's focus on the cosmological significance of Christ; forms of Christianity, Judaism, and Islam that focus on the sacred text; Catholic moral theologies that keep change within the parameters of the tradition; and churches where formal or informal structures of authority enforce compliance with revealed or traditional morality. In all cases "alteration of the religious ethic by the findings of science, medicine, and other disciplines is resisted" (Gustafson 1996b, 86).

In direct contrast to this model, the model of theological continuity holds that religious or theological ethics is not only intelligible beyond the religious community but perhaps even persuasive. The themes of religious morality can add depth and scope to other views. What is religious, then, about religiously backed medical ethics might be its source in revelation, its authorization by a sacred text, its place in a larger theological framework, or its special obligatory force for religious believers. The action-guiding rules or principles, however, are intelligible, understandable, and, even convincing outside the belief community (Gustafson 1996b, 87–88) as long as outsiders share the same moral anthropology, or basic view of humans. Gustafson mentions religious ethics informed by Aquinas's natural law or the moral anthropology of Kant. On the continuity model, "moral or ethical visions or doctrines of the human are continuous with views of the human articulated for other purposes. . . . Religious morality and ethics [is] in continuity with other ethics" (Gustafson 1996b, 91) and therefore can communicate with and transform them.

For the model that is dialectical and interactive, however, religious and theological ethics can itself be changed by other communities and fields of knowledge (Gustafson 1996b, 91). Gustafson seems to prefer this model; it certainly best describes his own theological ethics. A symbol such as "image of God" has disclosive power. Yet, while its meaning of respect for persons may be justified on other grounds, it is not completely reducible to its nonreligious equivalents. Hence the dialectical relationship. Sometimes sources turn out to be mutually compatible or complementary, and sometimes they clash. When this happens, one or the other is revised (Gustafson 1996b, 92–93). Sometimes religious backings, symbols, and moralities must be reformulated because nonreligious sources have qualified the truth claims and undermined the credibility of traditional religious interpretations of the human in relation to the divine, and of morality (Gustafson 1984, 7–8).

These models are ideal types, not strict means of classification. They have heuristic value in illuminating tendencies and divergences in the literature (Gustafson 1996b, 82). Perhaps most of the literature and methods in theological medical ethics fit into a broad dialectical category, in that they are nuanced to innovations in science and medicine. These developments change the very meaning of the human reality, including embodiment, freedom, relation to nature, and social relationships. The moral meaning of religious beliefs and symbols adapts in response. No theological medical ethics is insulated or autonomous in the full sense of the word. Due to the contextual and historical nature of religious communities and their theological reflection, no community or discipline can develop a morality that is simply continuous and fully convergent with other viewpoints.

THEOLOGY AND OTHER VOICES

Gustafson's paradigm illumines the primary worries and priorities with which theological medical ethics enters the dialectic with other discourses. In the 1960s the duty and prerogative of religious spokesmen (such as Reinhold Niebuhr, Martin Luther King, and Pope John XXIII) to exercise leadership on important social issues were less questioned than they are today. Theologians moved into the medical ethics arena perhaps more confidently, more acceptably, and more warranted in their expectation that their influence could be significant. Therefore, interpreting, "translating" so to speak, or finding functional equivalents for their religious ideals seemed to be both socially important and of little danger to their essential religious identity.

In the 1990s growing secularism in U.S. public life was accompanied by the privatization of mainstream religious morality and the growing power of a religious right that quite deliberately criticized and countered reasonable and consensus-oriented discourse on medical ethics and other social issues. Theologians found considerably less opportunity to voice their ethical views with seriousness in the public forum and less general receptivity when they did do so. In the first decade of the twenty-first century, religion was a potent force in national politics and national elections but was now paired more often and visibly with a progressive politics of social reform. From 2008 until 2010 many religious people and organizations supported President Barack Obama's advocacy for universal health care in the United States. These included the evangelical organization Sojourners; Catholics in Alliance for the Common Good; and the ecumenical Matthew 25 Network.[2] Theologians who think it is important and possible to influence social values now often try to locate points of continuity with proposals coming from secular sources or other religious traditions.

The first theological luminaries of medical ethics energetically participated in public debate. Yet they differed, like thinkers of today, in the relative priority they gave to religious identity or to general moral consensus. Ramsey was passionately interested in proclaiming the biblical foundations of ethics, including medical ethics. McCormick wanted to advance the agenda of the Catholic Church's Second Vatican Council and to engage the modern world about the nature of the person and the common good. Gustafson saw expressions of Christian morality as historically relative products of culture as well as culture's critic.

Paul Ramsey

Methodist theologian Paul Ramsey best exemplifies the concerns of the autonomy model. In his first book, *Basic Christian Ethics*, Ramsey states his purpose as "to stand within the way the Bible views morality" (1951, xi). Nevertheless, Ramsey was no apolitical Christian idealist. He summed up the relation between Christian love and existing institutions as "the constant criticism and reshaping" of the latter and the "bending" of social policies (349–50).

In later writings Ramsey adopted a mixed form of a love-based ethic, relying on reason as well as revelation (1967, 29, 122). Since Christ died for "all men," he said, including all persons in the covenant established by God in Christ, recognition of the value of altruistic love has become part of "our common humanity" (1967, 43). Thus, Ramsey protects the autonomy of Christian ethics, at least in theory, while warranting the avid participation in the practical medical and policy ethics that characterized his life and work.

Two decades after *Basic Christian Ethics*, Ramsey published his key statement of Christian medical ethics, *The Patient as Person*, addressed to, as he puts it, "the widest possible audience" (Ramsey 1970, xi). He says the governing theological categories are covenant and covenant fidelity (xii–xiii). Ramsey takes up informed consent to experimentation, brain death, care for the dying, organ donation, and the allocation of scarce resources. He translates Christian values into medical ethics primarily in terms of absolute respect for the inviolability of the individual, protected by personal consent (39). Thus all experimentation on children, however benign, is ruled out. Ramsey explicitly rejects the Roman Catholic argument that organ donation can be justified by the donor's own moral identity and holiness; the only possible Christian justification for such an act is charitable sacrifice for another (176). Concerning the allocation of kidney dialysis, one of the first crises of modern technology, Ramsey proposes that only a lottery system, and not any estimation of social worth, respects equal dignity (256).

Ramsey's covenant fidelity is designed to protect individuals from technological rationality fixed on good results. This reflects the philosophical and cultural individualism of early medical ethics. Yet Ramsey's theological perspective is operative in his refusal to define the duty to care in the vocabulary of individual rights (Smith 1993). Ramsey's stress falls much more heavily on duty and obedience: the duty, in obedience to God's saving act in Jesus Christ, to assume the burden of care for the vulnerable. His focus is not on the entitlements of individuals but on the covenantal obligations of caregivers.

Richard McCormick

Like Paul Ramsey, Richard McCormick sees theological medical ethics as reflection within a tradition, concerned "with what we, as believers in Jesus Christ, ought to be and do (or not do)" (1984, 3). However, unlike Ramsey, McCormick thinks morality consists in living up to the goods and ideals apparent in ordinary human experiences and purposes. This is so not only because the saving actions of Christ apply to all but also because the goodness of human nature survives sin sufficiently to permit discernment of basic morality and of the requirements of human well-being and the common good. (Similarly, see Curran [1973].)

McCormick elaborates six themes of medical ethics that are not exclusive to religious people: the value of life as a basic, but not absolute, good; the inclusion of the unborn in the good of human life; the definition of the highest good of human life not as physical life itself but as moral and religious experiences; the essential sociality of persons; the unity of the spheres of life-giving and lovemaking; and the normative value of heterosexual, permanent marriage (1984, 51–57). McCormick affirms that the basis for discourse between Christianity and other traditions is the essential human capacity to know good and evil and to come to reasonable (if necessarily imperfect and revisable) conclusions about what is good or evil in practice. Good morality seeks human well-being, while evil conduct undermines and destroys it.

McCormick views the dialectical relation to culture that characterized Catholic morality after Vatican II as a positive, beneficent, and necessary development. Unlike those who see the authoritative teaching of the Church as a closed system, McCormick believes Catholic moral theology is, or should be, inductive, exploratory, sometimes tentative, and "always in flux." It "takes seriously the findings of human experience and human sciences," purifying and modifying past formulations in light of basic Christian and human concerns (1984, 4).

Ethics in health and medicine is not tied to certain prescriptions and proscriptions derived from static human physical faculties and functions. It is based on "the total good of the person," or, to quote Vatican II, "the human person integrally and adequately considered" (McCormick 1984, 15). This implies that human freedom, conscience, and relationships, as well as social interrelatedness, are essential to human nature and human well-being. McCormick interprets the natural law dynamically, without losing sight of objective standards of what it means to be human and of how morality corresponds to a shared human reality (1984, 15, 17; 1989, 1–208).

McCormick addressed virtually every one of the major issues of medical ethics, carrying forward a long tradition. For example, the distinction between ordinary and extraordinary means of life support permits withdrawing or forgoing life supports, while forbidding direct euthanasia (Sacred Congregation for the Doctrine of the Faith 1980). McCormick affirms this as making sense of the human condition, valuing patient self-determination, placing choice against the horizon of objective and reasonable best interests and humanity's transcendent destiny (1984, 107–23). McCormick responds to U.S. court cases; the development of life-prolonging technology; cultural attitudes toward life, death, and medicine; and the drive toward physician-assisted suicide. He takes up the questions of access to adequate health care for all members of society that Paul Ramsey was unable to explore—and that were less publicly visible—before Ramsey's death in 1988.

McCormick interprets physician-assisted suicide as a symptom of a society in which mindless, even violent, technology has become a substitute for compassion and care (1995, 460–61). If people were assured of care and pain control, as well as the ability to refuse treatments that violate their quality of life (including artificial nutrition and hydration [1995, 461; 1989, 369–87]), they might not define suicide as a necessary option. The failure to meet health care needs of the poor reveals ultimate disrespect for life (1995, 463).

Over the years Richard McCormick and Paul Ramsey came into occasional direct conflict yet they remained colleagues and conversation partners. Ramsey's basis was absolute covenant fidelity, translated as a deontological, or duty-oriented, ethic, oriented by the inviolability of the concrete Other or "neighbor." McCormick represents a teleological ethic of human goods and purposes, in which individual good is always related to the common good. The common good is not a utilitarian concept in which the good of the many overrides individual rights but a social ethic of the participation of all in a larger enterprise from which each benefits. (For a more extensive discussion of these contrasts, with references, see Cahill [1979].)

James M. Gustafson

Gustafson sees the relation between theology and other discourses as dialectical. From the Reformed tradition in theology, he brings a central commitment to God's sovereignty. Ethics and theology should be theocentric, not anthropocentric (1981, 1984). Humans are part of the created universe; they are not its peak or center; and the world does not work so that human beings can, or should, expect all their desires and purposes to be fulfilled.

The natural and social sciences shape Gustafson's view that God's purposes are not to be confused with human purposes. They contribute to his conclusion that the moral life is full of ambiguity and conflict. The natural sciences and other experiences of the world are pathways, he says, to a human sense of the divine. Parallel to the sometimes incompatible needs of creatures in the natural environment, the resolution of a moral dilemma may lie in tragic denial or sacrifice. But human beings can keep company with one another in the midst of suffering, and sometimes experience God as friend and sustainer. (For a concise and personal presentation of these themes, see Gustafson [1994].)

Gustafson's writings in medical ethics generally stay clear of definitive pronouncements on right and wrong conduct. He introduces and explicates key theological themes and orientations (1975); outlines models, modes, and parameters for engagement with science and medicine (1988, 1996a); and incisively sorts out the consequences of certain presuppositions or approaches (1974, 273–86). Gustafson can criticize the Christian tradition, for example, by seeing suicide as a conscientious decision in cases of irremediable suffering and despair (1984, 215). He is one of the first to take global and environmental contexts of medicine and research seriously, surveying the ethics of population and nutrition (1984, 219–50). Gustafson is sensitive to Western cultural imperialism (political, ethical, or theological). He asserts that

God does not so much establish a moral order in creation (or redemption) as establish different patterns of well-being that emerge over time (1975, 39). The Christian theologian approaches medical ethics with attitudes not only of respect for life but of openness to the new, flavored with appropriate humility and self-criticism, due to finitude and sinfulness (1975, 54–75).

DEVELOPMENTS AND COMPLICATIONS

The writings of other authors, some of whom have appeared on the theological medical ethics scene more recently, may be assessed in relation to Gustafson's models; many are influenced by Ramsey, McCormick, and Gustafson.

Autonomy model

First, let us revisit the autonomy model of theological bioethics. A prominent example is Stanley Hauerwas, a student of Gustafson. Hauerwas combines a biblical vocabulary with a strong sense of historical relativity to launch a critique of cultural and theological liberalism that is almost sectarian in tone compared to the dialectical method of his mentor. Hauerwas would reject the label sectarian, although his interest in being a public spokesperson on bioethical and political issues (especially war and violence) prevents any sort of isolation from general social concerns. However, Hauerwas does use categories of narrative, story, character, and virtue to define Christian ethics as very much a community-based enterprise that may seem foolish or even senseless to those using secular standards. The theologian approaching medical ethics has the obligation, above all, to form Christian character within a narrative-based community that is true to its own identity. Christians cannot control science and technology, heal all disease, or end all suffering. What Christians can do is bear Christ's cross by keeping faithful company with those who suffer. In every suffering person, and in suffering itself, the Christian encounters God (Hauerwas 1986a, 1986b, 1990). This is a radical view insofar as Hauerwas, in effect, counsels theologians to stay away from secular philosophy and policy debates, where they can make little impact and where they are likely to be seduced by the temptation to be "relevant."

Less iconoclastic examples of the idea that Christian ethics is autonomous from alien value systems are Allen Verhey and Gilbert Meilaender. Both explicitly engage medical policy and cultural discourses through writing and professional roles. Distinctive commitments are also important. Verhey, an evangelical by background, uses biblical resources more extensively than does Hauerwas and with more attention to exegesis and biblical criticism. Verhey often interjects a biblical reference or refrain into a discussion directed ultimately toward a public or policy outcome, anticipating that religious imagery will evoke some convergence among positions that do not align on every point (Verhey 2003). Meilaender, a Lutheran, is resistant to liberalism and utilitarianism, appealing to a Barthian sense of God's ownership of human life. The Christian vision of the world defines an attitude toward life and death, in which life is understood as a trust from God and the direct causation of death remains beyond the proper limit of human powers. Similar to Ramsey, Meilaender (2005) borrows philosophical distinctions developed primarily in Catholic moral theology to define the exact limits of medical interventions; an example is the distinction between direct and indirect intention and action. (For another example of this approach, see McKenny [1997].)

Quite a different sort of autonomist is the Catholic author Germain Grisez. His theological ethics has much in common with the continuity model in that, for Grisez, ethics is based on seven basic goods that are shared and knowable by all human beings. These are self-integration; practical reasonableness; justice and friendship; life, including health and the handing on of life; knowledge of truth and appreciation of beauty; work; and play (1983, 124; 1993, 567–78). An eighth, marriage, is later added (1993, 568). However, Grisez draws conclusions about the practical import of these goods that are not so widely shared. For example, killing in abortion, euthanasia, and war are all wrong (1970; Grisez and Boyle 1975; Finnis, Boyle, and Grisez 1987); withdrawal of artificial nutrition and hydration from a comatose patient is wrong (Dennehy and Grisez 1986); and contraception is wrong (Ford et al. 1988). To defend these positions as conclusive and absolute, Grisez appeals to the Christian way of life and to the authoritative teaching of the Roman Catholic Church about what the so-called natural law is and demands. Unlike those such as McCormick who interpret the natural law in a more dialectical mode, Grisez is not open to challenge of certain specific absolutes in Catholic moral theology, mostly having to do with sexual behavior and the direct killing of innocent persons (from conception to death).

Continuity model

Moving on to the continuity model of ethics, one finds both Catholic and Protestant representatives. First consider the Catholic version. Even a Vatican document like the *Declaration on Euthanasia* (Sacred Congregation for the Doctrine of the Faith 1980), while very committed to preserving authoritative teaching, makes overtures to members of other religions and to the public at large to agree that the good of life is fundamental and that mercy killing is not acceptable social policy. This document is somewhat irenic toward those who believe that euthanasia is a form of compassion or necessary in the face of human suffering. A similar pro-public stance characterizes statements authored by the U.S. Catholic bishops and directed toward national legal or policy matters, such as health care reform (National Conference of Catholic Bishops 1993; Ashley, deBlois, and O'Rourke 2006). While adhering to official Catholic teaching on such matters as abortion, stem cell research, and euthanasia, they sometimes put the emphasis on social responsibilities for science, research, health, and equitable access to medical care.

Other Catholic authors carry this trajectory further, opening the door, as does McCormick, to revisions of specific teachings about individual "forbidden" behavior. Revisions may be based on interpretations of the human condition as evolving or changing, or on the new moral insights provided by contemporary experience. Proponents typically defend these changes, however, in terms of what they take to be the key or fundamental moral commitments that have always been honored by the tradition itself. For example, John T. Noonan argues that contraception could be accepted in changed circumstances on the basis of improved knowledge of the reproductive system and out of continuing respect for the importance of parenthood, its relation to sexual love and commitment, the protection of the unborn, the dignity of women, and the responsibility of parents to nurture children (1986). Many Catholics have made the case that quality of life is a legitimate criterion for deciding to forgo certain medical treatments and that this does not violate the traditional sanctity-of-life principle (Walter and Shannon 1990). Others have proposed that the embryo is not fully a person from conception, based on new information about early embryonic development (Shannon and Wolter 1990) or that acceptance of new genetic and reproductive technologies should be expanded (Ryan 2001; Snow 2003; Cahill 2005b).

A Protestant representative of a dialectically open continuity model of ethics is William F. May, a Methodist like Ramsey and Hauerwas. Like Ramsey, May is interested in covenantal imagery, though he too rarely takes up intensive exegesis of specific biblical texts. May's long-standing use of the covenantal metaphor to understand the physician–patient role and the place of health care and healing within community assumes that the covenant is a type of moral relationship that can be generally recognized and enacted (1996, 4, 13–14; 1983, 1991). May is not focused on concrete distinctions and rules. For example, direct euthanasia and physician-assisted suicide are not proper covenantal responses to suffering patients, but May admits a gray area for euthanasia in the rare, exceptional instance (1996, 47–48). May places life-and-death issues in a larger picture, in which a health care system that abandons the uninsured is part of the push toward legalized euthanasia (1996, 99, 103).

Dialectical model

Most theological medical ethicists today are dialectical to some degree. Some believe that the dialectical relation of theology and culture cuts both ways. This is certainly true of feminist theologians, including Barbara Hilkert Andolsen, Sidney Callahan, Dena Davis (who is Jewish), Margaret A. Farley, Christine Gudorf, Beverly Harrison, Karen Lebacqz, and Maura A. Ryan.

Margaret Farley, a senior and exemplary figure, defines feminist theological medical ethics as the unmasking of beliefs, symbols, and religious practices that foster patriarchal discrimination (1985, 166). She invokes relationality, embodiment, and the world of nature to establish the feminist perspective, and she measures the Bible and tradition according to whether, in the words of Rosemary Radford Ruether, they affirm "the full humanity of women" (Farley 1985, 175). Illustrating the new global horizon of feminist bioethics, Farley is concerned with the AIDS crisis, linking it to poverty (2002, 17) and to the status of women (2006, 230, 238). The activist, justice-oriented stance of theological bioethicists is captured in a project initiated by Farley and other Sisters of Mercy, with support from USAID, Catholic Relief Services, CAFOD in the UK, Trocaire in Ireland, and the African Jesuit AIDS Network. The project "All-Africa Conference, Sister to Sister" spearheaded three conferences (2003–04) that brought African women together with supporters from other continents to share insights and develop responses to the AIDS crisis as it affects women.[3] Globally, growing numbers of women advocate for women's health from religious and theological standpoints (Phiri and Nadar 2006).

‰ Concluding Comments

The practice of medicine in the United States has become more a scientific than a humanistic venture. It is largely directed by marketplace values. Because they deal in the elemental human experiences of birth, life, death, and suffering, however, the biomedical arts provide an opening for larger questions of meaning and even of transcendence. Religious themes and imagery can be helpful in articulating these concerns and addressing them in an imaginative, provocative, and perhaps ultimately transformative way (Thistlethwaite 2003). Religious symbolism can mediate a sense of transcendence and ultimacy that is achingly latent in the ethical conflicts, tragedies, and triumphs that are unavoidable in biomedicine. The immense current interest in the spiritual dimensions of health care exemplifies this trend.

Religion and theology stress that justice in medicine and access to care require community, solidarity, and equity, not just autonomy, individual rights, and liberty. This makes theological medical ethics more resistant to market forces controlling what research is funded, where it is conducted and on whom, who has access to the benefits, who profits from new knowledge and its implementation, and how health care is organized within a society as a whole (Chapman 1999; Hanson 2001; Cahill 2005a, 2005b; McDonough 2007; Fox and Swazey 2008). In religious traditions of practice, care of the sick has been a work of devotion and self-offering to the divine, in a communal context. In today's world, the community is increasingly international and global (Ryan 2004). Theological medical ethics is agreed that compassionate and just solidarity are essential to personal and social virtue.

‰ Notes on Resources and Training

Theological medical ethics is a national (and increasingly international) enterprise, where cross-fertilization occurs through publication, conferences, institutes that gather scholars around special projects or foci, and professional societies where numerous seminars and groups are devoted to bioethics (American Academy of Religion, Catholic Theological Society of America, College Theology Society, Society of Christian Ethics, International Association of Bioethics, World Congress of Bioethics).

Two axes along which differences in educational opportunities arise are denominational–ecumenical and academic–clinical. Identifiably Catholic faculties exist both in universities, including graduate professional schools in health and medicine, and in seminaries. Protestant faculties are more likely to exist in smaller, religiously affiliated colleges or in seminaries. This is true of Jewish education in medical ethics as well (Hebrew Union College, Jewish Theological Seminary of America, American Jewish University). Seminary faculties, Catholic or Protestant, are dedicated to work in a particular theological tradition, as are rabbinical colleges. Other Catholic, Protestant, and Jewish theologians teach and engage in scholarly research on interdenominational faculties, and those in church-related institutions often partake in the ecumenical exchange. In addition religious and theological voices are present in institutions with no specific orientation to religion, many with interdisciplinary religious studies departments (University of Virginia, Indiana University, and Yale University) as well as in departments, centers, or institutes whose mission is not specifically religious (Yale University's Interdisciplinary Center for Bioethics, Loyola Marymount University's Bioethics Institute, Indiana University Purdue at Indianapolis's Center for Bioethics).

Theological education in medical ethics that occurs in universities, as well as in many seminaries and colleges, has an academic, theoretical, scholarly, research-oriented, and properly theological orientation. Universities with a medical school, nursing school, or health care facility have programs in clinical ethics that focus more on practical decision making and holistic patient care (for example, Georgetown, Duquesne, Creighton, Saint Louis University, Loyola University of Chicago, University of Virginia, and Loma Linda University).

✎ Notes

1. For essays on and by several of the early key contributors to theological medical ethics, see Verhey and Lammers (1993) and Walter and Klein (2003). For multiple approaches to the role of religion in public bioethics, see Guinn (2006).
2. See the websites www.sojo.net/, http://matthew25.org, and www.catholicsinalliance.org/; accessed August 19, 2009.
3. See www.allafrica-sistertosister.org/; accessed August 12, 2009.

✎ References

Ashley, B. M., J. K. deBlois, and K. O'Rourke. 2006. *Health care ethics: A Catholic theological analysis.* 5th ed. Washington, DC: Georgetown University Press.

Beauchamp, T. L., and J. F. Childress. [1979] 2001. *Principles of biomedical ethics.* 5th ed. New York: Oxford University Press.

Bleich, J. D. 1981. *Judaism and healing: Halakhic perspectives.* New York: Ktav.

Bleich, J. D., and F. Rosner, eds. 1979. *Jewish bioethics.* New York: Sanhedrin Press.

Cahill, L. S. 1979. Within shouting distance: Paul Ramsey and Richard McCormick on method and morality. *Journal of Medicine and Philosophy* 4:398–417.

———. 1992. Theology and bioethics: Should religious traditions have a public voice? *Journal of Medicine and Philosophy* 17:263–72.

———. 2005a. *Theological bioethics: Participation, justice, and change.* Washington, DC: Georgetown University Press.

———, ed. 2005b. *Genetics, theology and ethics: An interdisciplinary conversation.* New York: Herder and Herder.

Callahan, D. 1990. Religion and the secularization of bioethics. *Hastings Center Report* 20:2–10.

Campbell, C. S. 1990. Religion and moral meaning in bioethics. *Hastings Center Report* 20:4–10.

Chapman, A. R. 1999. *Unprecedented choices: Religious ethics at the frontiers of genetic science.* Minneapolis: Fortress Press.

Childress, J. F. 1994. Principles-oriented bioethics: An analysis and assessment from within. In *The foundations of bioethics,* ed. E. R. DuBose, R. P. Hamel, and L. J. O'Connell, 72–98. Valley Forge, PA: Trinity Press International.

Christie, D. L. 2003. *Last rights: A Catholic perspective on end-of-life decisions.* Lanham and Boulder: Rowman & Littlefield.

Cimperman, M. 2005. *When God's people have HIV/AIDS: An approach to ethics.* Maryknoll, NY: Orbis.

Cole-Turner, R. 2008. *Design and destiny: Jewish and Christian perspectives on human germline modification.* Cambridge, MA: MIT Press.

Curran, C. E. 1973. *Politics, medicine and Christian ethics: A dialogue with Paul Ramsey*. Philadelphia: Fortress Press.

Davis, D. 1991. Beyond Rabbi Hiyya's wife: Women's voices in Jewish bioethics. *Second Opinion* 16:10–30.

Dennehy, R., and G. Grisez. 1986. *Bioethical issues*. Cromwell, CT: John Paul II Bioethics Center.

Engelhardt, H. T. 1996. *The foundations of bioethics*. New York and Oxford: Oxford University Press.

Farley, M. A. 1985. Feminist theology and bioethics. In *Theology and bioethics: Exploring the foundations and frontiers*, ed. E. E. Shelp, 163–85. Dordrecht, the Netherlands: Kluwer Academic Publishers.

———. 2002. *Compassionate respect: A feminist approach to medical questions and other questions*. New York/Mahwah, NJ: Paulist Press.

———. 2006. *Just love: A framework for Christian sexual ethics*. New York and London: Continuum.

Feldman, D. M. 1986. *Health and medicine in the Jewish tradition*. New York: Crossroad.

Finnis, J., J. Boyle, and G. Grisez. 1987. *Nuclear deterrence, morality and realism*. Oxford: Clarendon Press.

Ford, J. C., G. Grisez, J. Boyle, J. Finnis, and W. E. May. 1988. *The teaching of* Humanae vitae: *A defense*. San Francisco: Ignatius Press.

Fox, R. C., and J. P. Swazey. 2008. *Observing bioethics*. Oxford and New York: Oxford University Press.

Gellman, M. A. 1993. On Immanuel Jakobovits: Bringing the ancient word to the modern world. In *Theological voices in medical ethics*, ed. A. Verhey and S. E. Lammers, 178–208. Grand Rapids, MI: William B. Eerdmans Publishing Co.

Green, R. M. 1986. Contemporary Jewish bioethics: A critical assessment. In *Theology and bioethics: Exploring the foundations and frontiers*, ed. E. E. Shelp, 245–65. Dordrecht, The Netherlands: Kluwer Academic Publishers.

Grisez, G. 1970. *Abortion: The myths, the realities, the arguments*. New York and Cleveland: Corpus Books.

———. 1983. *The way of the Lord Jesus*. Vol. 1: *Christian Moral Principles*. Chicago: Franciscan Herald Press.

———. 1993. *The way of the Lord Jesus*. Vol. 2: *Living a Christian Life*. Quincy, IL: Franciscan Herald Press.

Grisez, G., and J. Boyle. 1975. *Life and death with liberty and justice: A contribution to the euthanasia debate*. Notre Dame, IN: University of Notre Dame Press.

Guinn, D. E. 2006. *Handbook of bioethics and religion*. Oxford and New York: Oxford University Press.

Guroian, V. 1996. *Life's living toward dying*. Grand Rapids, MI, and Cambridge, UK: William B. Eerdmans Publishing Co.

Gustafson, J. M. 1974. *Theology and Christian ethics*. Cleveland: The Pilgrim Press.

———. 1975. *The contributions of theology to medical ethics*. Milwaukee, WI: Marquette University Theology Department.

———. 1981. *Ethics from a theocentric perspective*, Vol. 1: *Theology and ethics*. Chicago: University of Chicago Press.

———. 1984. *Ethics from a theocentric perspective*, Vol. 2: *Ethics and theology*. Chicago: University of Chicago Press.

———. 1988. *Varieties of moral discourse: Prophetic, narrative, ethical, and policy*. Grand Rapids, MI: Calvin College and Seminary.

———. 1994. *A sense of the divine: The natural environment from a theocentric perspective*. Cleveland: Pilgrim Press.

———. 1996a. *Intersections: Science, theology, and ethics*. Cleveland: Pilgrim Press.

———. 1996b. Styles of religious reflection in medical ethics. In *Religion and medical ethics: Looking back, looking forward*, ed. A. Verhey, 81–95. Grand Rapids, MI: William B. Eerdmans Publishing Co.

Hanson, M. J., ed. 2001. *Claiming power over life: Religion and biotechnology policy*. Washington, DC: Georgetown University Press.

Harakas, S. S. 1980. *For the health of body and soul: An introduction to Eastern Orthodox bioethics.* Brookline, MA: Holy Cross Orthodox Press.

———. 1999. *Wholeness of faith and life: Orthodox Christian ethics, part three: Orthodox social ethics.* Brookline, MA: Holy Cross Orthodox Press.

Hauerwas, S. 1986a. *Suffering presence.* Notre Dame, IN: University of Notre Dame Press.

———. 1986b. Salvation and health: Why medicine needs the church. In *Theology and bioethics: Exploring the foundations and frontiers*, ed. E. E. Shelp, 205–24. Dordrecht, The Netherlands: Kluwer Academic Publishers.

———. 1990. *Naming the silences: God, medicine and the problem of suffering.* Grand Rapids, MI: William B. Eerdmans Publishing Co.

———. 1996. How Christian ethics became medical ethics: The case of Paul Ramsey. In *Religion and medical ethics: Looking back, looking forward*, ed. A. Verhey, 61–80. Grand Rapids, MI: William B. Eerdmans Publishing Co.

Hehir, J. B. 1992. Policy Arguments in a public church: Catholic social ethics and bioethics. *Journal of Medicine and Philosophy* 17:347–64.

Iozzo, M. J., with M. R. Doyle and E. M. Miranda, eds. 2008. *Calling for justice throughout the world: Catholic women theologians on the HIV/AIDS pandemic.* New York and London: Continuum Publishers.

Jakobovitz, I. 1975. *Jewish medical ethics: A comparative and historical study of the Jewish religious attitudes to medicine and its practice.* 4th ed. New York: Bloch Publishing.

Journal of Religious Ethics. 2008. Focus Issue on Islam and Bioethics 36 (1).

Keenan, J. F., ed. 2000. *Catholic ethicists on HIV/AIDS prevention.* New York: Continuum.

Kelly, D. F. 2004. *Contemporary Catholic health care ethics.* Washington, DC: Georgetown University Press.

Lammers, S. E. 1996. The marginalization of religious voices in bioethics. In *Religion and medical ethics: Looking back, looking forward*, ed. A. Verhey, 19–43. Grand Rapids, MI: William B. Eerdmans Publishing Co.

Lebacqz, K., ed. 1983. *Genetics, ethics, and parenthood.* New York: The Pilgrim Press.

Marty, M. E. 1992. Religion, theology, church, and bioethics. *Journal of Medicine and Philosophy* 17:273–89.

May, W. F. 1983. *The physician's covenant: Images of the healer in medical ethics.* Philadelphia: Westminster/John Knox Press.

———. 1991. *The patient's ordeal.* Bloomington: Indiana University Press.

———. 1996. *Testing the medical covenant: Active euthanasia and health care reform.* Grand Rapids, MI: William B. Eerdmans Publishing Co.

McCarthy, D. M., and M. T. Lysaught, eds. 2007. *Gathered for the journey: Moral theology in Catholic perspective.* Grand Rapids, MI: William B. Eerdmans Publishing Co.

McCormick, R. A. 1981. *Notes on moral theology: 1965 through 1980.* Washington, DC: University Press of America.

———. 1984. *Health and medicine in the Catholic tradition: Tradition in transition.* New York: Crossroad.

———. 1989. *The critical calling: Reflections on moral dilemmas since Vatican I.* Washington, DC: Georgetown University Press.

———. 1995. Technology, the consistent ethic and assisted suicide. *Origins* 25:459–64.

McDonough, M. J. 2007. *Can a health care market be moral? A Catholic vision.* Washington, DC: Georgetown University Press.

McKenny, G. P. 1997. *To relieve the human condition: Bioethics, technology and the body.* Albany: State University of New York Press.

Meilaender, G. 2005. *Bioethics: A primer for Christians.* 2nd ed. Grand Rapids, MI: William B. Eerdmans Publishing Co.

Messer, D. E. *Breaking the conspiracy of silence: Christian churches and the global AIDS Crisis.* Minneapolis: Fortress Press, 2004.

National Conference of Catholic Bishops. 1993. Resolution on health care reform. *Origins* 23:97, 99–102.

Newman, L. E. 1992. Jewish theology and bioethics. *Journal of Medicine and Philosophy* 17:309–27.

Noonan, J. T. 1986. *Contraception: A history of its treatment by the Catholic theologians and canonists.* Enlarged edition. Cambridge, MA: Harvard University Press.

Novak, D. 1990. Bioethics and the contemporary Jewish community. *Hastings Center Report* 20:14–17.

Overberg, K. R. 2006. *Ethics and AIDS: Compassion and justice in global crisis.* Lanham, MD: Rowman & Littlefield.

Parsi, K., and M. N. Sheehan. 2006. *Healing as vocation: A medical professional primer.* Lanham, MD: Rowman & Littlefield.

Pellegrino, E. D., and A. I. Faden, eds. 1999. *Jewish and Catholic bioethics: An ecumenical dialogue.* Washington, DC: Georgetown University Press.

Peters, T. 1996. *For the love of children: Genetic technology and the future of the family.* Louisville, KY: Westminster/John Knox Press.

Phiri, I. A., and S. Nadar, eds. 2006. *African women, religion and health: Essays in honor of Mercy Amba Oduyoye.* Maryknoll, NY: Orbis.

Ramsey, P. 1951. *Basic Christian ethics.* New York: Charles Scribner's Sons.

———. 1967. *Deeds and rules in Christian ethics.* New York: Charles Scribner's Sons.

———. 1970. *The patient as person.* New Haven and London: Yale University Press.

Reich, W. T. 1978. *Encyclopedia of bioethics.* New York: Macmillan Free Press.

———. 1996. Bioethics in the United States. In *Bioethics: A history,* ed. C. Viafora, 83–118. Bethesda, MD: International Scholars Publications.

Reich, W. T., with the assistance of R. dell'Oro. 1996. A new era for bioethics: The search for meaning in moral experience. In *Religion and medical ethics: Looking back, looking forward,* ed. A. Verhey, 96–115. Grand Rapids, MI: William B. Eerdmans Publishing Co.

Ryan, M. A. 2001. *Ethics and economics of assisted reproduction: The cost of longing.* Washington, DC: Georgetown University Press.

———. 2004. Beyond a Western bioethics? *Theological Studies* 65 (1): 174–76.

Sacred Congregation for the Doctrine of the Faith (Vatican). 1980. *Declaration on euthanasia.* Boston: St. Paul Editions.

Shannon, T. A., and A. B. Wolter. 1990. Reflections on the moral status of the pre-embryo. *Theological Studies* 51:603–26.

Shelp, E. E., ed. 1986. *Theology and bioethics: Exploring the foundations and frontiers.* Dordrecht, The Netherlands: Kluwer Academic Publishers.

Smith, D. H. 1993. On Paul Ramsey: A covenant-centered ethic for medicine. In *Theological voices in medical ethics,* ed. A. Verhey and S. E. Lammers, 7–29. Grand Rapids, MI: William B. Eerdmans Publishing Co.

———. 1996. Religion and the roots of the bioethics revival. In *Religion and medical ethics: looking back, looking forward,* ed. A. Verhey, 2–18. Grand Rapids, MI: William B. Eerdmans Publishing Co.

———, ed. 2000. *Caring well: Religion, narrative and health care ethics.* Louisville: Westminser John Knox Press.

Smith, D. H., and C. B. Cohen, eds. 2003. *A Christian response to the new genetics: Religious, ethical and social issues.* Lanham, MD: Rowman & Littlefield.

Snow, N. E., ed. 2003. *Stem cell research: New frontiers in science and ethics.* Notre Dame, IN: University of Notre Dame.

Sullivan, L. E., ed. 1989. *Healing and restoring: Health and medicine in the world's religious traditions.* New York and London: Macmillan.

Sulmasy, D. P. 1997. *The healer's calling: A spirituality for physicians and other health care professionals.* New York/Mahwah, NJ: Paulist Press.

Thistlethwaite, S. B., ed. 2003. *Adam, Eve, and the genome: The Human Genome Project and theology.* Minneapolis: Fortress Press.

Townes, E. M. 1998. *Breaking the fine rain of death: African American health issues and a womanist ethic of care*. New York: Continuum.

Verhey, A., ed. 1996. *Religion and medical ethics: Looking back, looking forward*. Grand Rapids, MI: William B. Eerdmans Publishing Co.

_____. 2003. *Reading the Bible in the strange world of medicine*. Grand Rapids, MI: William B. Eerdmans Publishing Co.

Verhey, A., and S. E. Lammers, eds. 1993. *Theological voices in medical ethics*. Grand Rapids, MI: William B. Eerdmans Publishing Co.

Vigen, A. M. 2006. *Women, ethics, and inequality in U.S. healthcare: "To count among the living."* New York: Macmillan.

Vogt, C. P. 2004. *Patience, compassion, hope and the Christian art of dying well*. Lanham, MD: Rowman & Littlefield Publishers.

Walter, J. J., and T. A. Shannon. 1990. *Quality of life: The new medical dilemma*. New York/Mahwah, NJ: Paulist Press.

Walter, K., and E. P. Klein, eds. 2003. *The story of bioethics: From seminal works to contemporary explorations*. Washington, DC: Georgetown University Press.

Walters, L. 1986. Religion and the renaissance of medical ethics in the United States. In *Theology and bioethics: Exploring the foundations and frontiers*, ed. E. E. Shelp, 3–16. Dordrecht, The Netherlands: Kluwer Academic Publishers.

CHAPTER 6

Codes, Virtue, and Professionalism

EDMUND D. PELLEGRINO

Until very recently, in both Eastern and Western medicine, codes of ethical conduct provided the only source of judgment of good and bad, right and wrong, professional conduct. They were, therefore, the only method of ethical argumentation. However, from the beginning of the contemporary era of medical ethics, ethical codes have been challenged by a wide variety of alternate modes of argumentation, as the other chapters in this book attest. Nonetheless, in most of the world, among professionals and laypersons, codes continue to set standards for ethical conduct, to define new ethical issues, and to support one position or another in ethical discourse.

The purpose of this chapter is to examine the use of codes in medical ethical discourse, to define their sources of moral authority, and to relate them to virtues and professionalism. Properly employed, professional codes still have an important place in medical practice, provided their limitations are taken into account and their moral precepts are grounded more securely in a moral philosophy of the professions. The delimitation of such a philosophy has been a long-term project of the author of this chapter and his colleague, David C. Thomasma (Pellegrino 2008).

ᴗ Description of Codes, Virtue, and Professionalism

The discussion of codes, virtue, and professionalism proceeds as follows: an overview of the historical presence and ubiquity of ethical codes in medicine; the use of codes in argumentation; challenges to the moral authority of codes; proposed sources of their moral authority, including an argument relating codes to virtue and professionalism based on a moral philosophy of medicine; and the abuse of codes.

THE PERSISTENCE AND UBIQUITY OF CODES

It is important at the outset to distinguish codes from oaths, with which they are frequently confused. Sulmasy has made this distinction quite explicit (Sulmasy 1999). He understands an oath to be a formal, solemn, publicly proclaimed commitment to conduct oneself in certain morally specified ways. Codes, on the other hand, are simply enumerations, codifications, or collations of a set of moral precepts. One may or may not swear fidelity to a code. When one does swear solemnly to abide by a specific codification of moral precepts, then code and oath coincide but do not lose their separate identities. This chapter refers to the codification, and not necessarily the oath to abide by that codification.

No attempt is made here to summarize the history, variable content, or provenance of the wide variety of ethical codes now extant in the medical and other health professions (Etziony 1973; Konold 1978; Veatch 1978; Gorlin 1995; Spicer 1995). Rather, the focus here will be on the Hippocratic ethic, that is, the Hippocratic Oath and the other so-called deontological books: *Precepts, Decorum, Law, The Physician,* and *Aphorisms* (Hippocrates 1972, vol. 1; Hippocrates 1981, vol. 2; Hippocrates 1979, vol. 4). The multitudinous medical oaths and codes of the modern era reflect, in significant degree, the prescriptions and proscriptions of these books of the Hippocratic ethic. For this reason the Hippocratic Oath will be used as a paradigm for this inquiry into the use of codes in ethical argumentation.

Today, the popularity of codes is not limited to medicine. One of the most active areas is in business and corporate ethics. In recent decades U.S. businesses have sought to combat public distrust by institutionalizing ethics (Sims 1994). For example, in 1990, of the Fortune 500 companies that responded to a survey, 94 percent had ethics codes, 32 percent had ethics committees, and 15 percent employed full-time ethicists (Petry 1993). Many of the issues addressed in this chapter with regard to medical codes, their use in argumentation, and their moral authority can be found in the expanding literature relative to business codes.

Despite the criticisms and doubts about the moral authority of professional codes, they continue to proliferate. The second edition of the *Encyclopedia of Bioethics* takes 243 pages simply to reproduce the texts of codes related to the health professions (Spicer 1995). Veatch lists forty-one health professions with codes (1978). Gorlin presents fifty-one codes in business, health, and law (1995). The Hippocratic Oath is simply an orally verbalized code. Recitation of the Hippocratic Oath, or some variation of it, is regaining popularity in American medical schools after a lapse some years ago (Orr et al. 1997). Clearly there is a latent attraction to codes as a mark of serious professionalism, even though the degree to which they are observed or felt to be binding is in considerable doubt.

In medicine professional codes go back at least to the ancient Code of Hammurabi (1792–1750 BCE), which, itself, was probably derived from earlier Sumerian sources dating to 3000 BCE (*Encyclopedia Britannica* 1979; Hamarneh 1993). Since then, every era and all the major cultures have produced codifications of right and wrong professional behavior (Muthu 1930; Bar-Sela and Hoft 1962; Etziony 1973; Levey 1977; Temkin 1991; Baker, Porter, and Porter 1993; Baker 1994). In the West the dominant code of oldest provenance is the Hippocratic Oath and elements drawn from the deontologic books of the Hippocratic corpus. The oath and its ethic, revised to conform to theological presuppositions, were given added moral authority during late antiquity and the Middle Ages by the major monotheistic religions (Temkin 1991; Amundsen 1996).

All these codes and their variations describe in some detail what was expected in the way of moral conduct, as well as personal decorum of those who professed to be physicians. Taken together, their prescriptions and proscriptions constitute the Hippocratic ethos and ethic or, more simply, the Hippocratic tradition. They survive, with suitable modification, in the multiplicity of codifications adapted for virtually all the health professions.

To be sure, the Hippocratic ethic has undergone changes in language, interpretation, and emphasis over the centuries (Baker 1993). It was never fully embraced by all physicians in any era. It was frequently violated by individual physicians, or modified or reshaped to suit contemporary mores—just as it is being reshaped today. Some historians have taken those uncertainties of provenance and interpretation as reasons to deny or doubt that the Hippocratic code was ever a universal, unchanging set of moral principles (Baker 1993; Nutton 1995).

Those ambiguities are significant, but they must not obscure the fact that despite changes and variations in interpretation, codes have persisted for 2,500 years in Western and Eastern medicine. There is still substantial agreement across historical eras and cultures on many of the core precepts of these codes (Pellegrino 1999). Until the past several decades, the Hippocratic ethos and its variants have carried significant moral authority for many physicians. However, in the last few decades the widespread deconstruction of the Hippocratic Oath and ethics has made it mandatory to develop a moral philosophy for medicine on which the normative authority of the code can be based (Pellegrino and Thomasma 1981; Pellegrino 2001; Jotterand 2005).

CODES AS AN ARGUMENT FROM AUTHORITY

Strictly speaking the use of professional codes in moral discourse and argumentation does not fit precisely under the rubric of "methodology" as that term is used to define other modes of argumentation represented in this book. Codes are not modes of analysis, like the application of prima facie principles or the use of paradigm cases, as in casuistry. Neither are they elements of a robust moral philosophy external to medicine, such as Kantian deontology, Millian utilitarianism, Thomistic natural law, or Aristotelian virtue theory. Rather, the Hippocratic code and its historical congeners are assertions of moral precepts presented as self-evident and self-justifying prima facie obligations.

Nonetheless, codes are the reference point for a long-standing method when they are used in argumentation. Their method is the rhetorical method of the argument from authority. In classical logic as well as in scientific reasoning, arguments from authority have often been judged to be the weakest sort of argument. Yet arguments from authority are used universally—in court cases, in everyday discourse, in scholarly papers, and even in scientific investigations. Moreover, argument from authority has been recognized in classical rhetoric as a valid form of argumentation under certain specified conditions that define its valid use (St. Aubyn 1985; Perelman 1982; Weston 1992; Scriven 1976; Mackin 1969).

In classical logic the argument from authority was known as *argumentum ad verecundiam*; that is, an argument accepted out of deference for the prestige, stature, or presumed expertise of a person, institution, or office holder. This argument gained a bad reputation because of its frequent misuse and because it was used in the wrong context (e.g., in matters where demonstrable truth was possible) or without proper qualification (e.g., when Nobel laureates in physics or chemistry expatiate on theological or moral matters or on clinical medicine). The strength and validity of any argument from authority vary directly with the strength of the proof of that authority's qualification to command respect.

Thus, in theology, for those who believe in God, argument from authority, as with the Ten Commandments, is the strongest possible argument. It is absolute, and given that premise, it overrides every other argument. Believers may differ in their interpretation of precisely what these divine commands require but not with their authority as binding obligations. For nonbelievers, on the other hand, the Decalogue is, at best, a social construction and subject to challenge and doubt just as the Hippocratic ethic is today.

A related mode of argument is the *argumentum ad populum*, which appeals to general opinion, to categories of people who hold a certain view, or to a cultural or ethnic tradition. This argument has understandable appeal in democratic societies. Like the argument from authority, great dissonance can result from differences in interpretation of what is popular opinion. *Argumentation ad populum* is classically understood to be a weaker argument than argument from authority—to be used sparingly and only when demonstrable proof, valid expertise, or other arguments are not available (Weston 1992).

The moral authority of a professional act cannot be based, therefore, on the fact that it is sanctioned by a majority of physicians, the law, or the general public. This would give moral status to social or public opinion, which per se is not a source of moral justification. In the recent past pathological communities and societies, for example, have completely subverted medical ethics to political or social ideologies. This is the danger in all forms of social constructions of morals. While more sophisticated than a simple argument by public opinion, social construction suffers the same limitations. Such arguments surface whenever the possibility of objective moral truth is abandoned. When this occurs the validity of the moral authority of a professional code can be established only by first establishing the moral validity of the community giving it its consensus.

To be valid and effective, any argument from authority must establish the qualifications of the authority, whether that authority is vested in a person, institution, or tradition (Dauber 1996). The authority must be free of conflicts of interest and use expertise in the right circumstances and the right field of inquiry. Genuine qualification and appropriate context are the two essentials of the valid use of authority in argument.

The use of codes in medical ethics argumentation clearly is dependent, therefore, upon the legitimacy of the moral authority of the code in question. Today the authenticity of the moral authority of any code is under significant attack. An essential step, therefore, in a consideration of codes as a method of argumentation is to examine the criticisms of the paradigm medical ethical code, the Hippocratic Oath, and then to establish its moral authority as clearly as possible. Only then can we proceed to delineate the proper and improper ways of employing codes to define or settle an ethical issue or question.

CHALLENGES TO THE MORAL AUTHORITY OF CODES

In recent years, as a result of intensive historical and social scrutiny, the moral authenticity and authority of the Hippocratic Oath and ethic are suspect. Some critics interpret it as a self-serving creed, created by a self-appointed guild to monopolize the healing arts (Berlant 1975). Others reject it as unilaterally proclaimed, rather then being a contract negotiated between individual patients, society, and physicians (Veatch 1991). Still others see physician– and nurse–patient relationships as matters of character: virtuous persons have no need for codes; those who need them are unlikely to respect them (Lebacqz 1985; Warren 1993). Rules may impede the exercise of virtue, displace accountability from persons to codes, and foster "cookbook" ethics (Sanders 1993).

Still further, some see codes as impediments to teaching ethics since they encourage the simplistic reading of codes as duties to be accepted on authority alone (Kluge 1992). In addition they are thought to stifle individual expression (Downey and Calman 1994). Others, however, argue that the use of codes may, in fact, require heightened ethical sophistication (Hussey 1996).

An increasingly widespread criticism is that the inherent anachronism of any unchanging code cannot carry moral authority in our times, which are characterized by changes in gender, power, and societal mores and the commercialization and bureaucratization of medicine. The admixture of ethics and etiquette in the Hippocratic ethic bespeaks an outdated elitism, insincerity of motive, and obsession with personal comportment (Foot 1972; Goodfield 1973; Newton 1978; Sugarman 1994).

The more pragmatic critics point out that codes have historically been ineffective in making physicians virtuous. This is clear from the many times ethical imperatives have had to be imposed on the profession—for example, the code of Hammurabi (1792–1750 BCE); in Babylonian times, the *Lex Aquilia*; in Roman times, the *Lex Cornelia*; the German "medical police" (Castiglioni 1941; Frank 1976; *Encyclopedia Britannica* 1979) in the nineteenth century; and the medical licensing authorities in the United States today. Moreover, some critics argue that codes cannot be effective without better support systems for whistleblowers, without which, as Tadd writes, self-regulation of the profession becomes a mockery (1994). Nutton (1995) has recently summarized many of the common criticisms of the Hippocratic Oath and casts doubt as well on the current resurgence of interest in the oath, attributing it to a desire for ceremony as a substitute for religious belief and exclusivity.

More recently Miles (2004) has offered a series of criticisms of the Hippocratic ethic from a sociohistorical perspective. He faults it for its insensitivity to matters of social justice in the distribution of health care resources, to the difficulties of defining right and wrong in a changing, morally pluralist society, and to the deprofessionalization of the doctor by the societal mechanisms within which he or she must function today.

In a comprehensive article Jotterand (2005) reviews these and other criticisms of the Hippocratic ethic. To remedy them, he makes a strong case for a moral philosophy of medicine to undergird its ethics. This is the same proposal that Thomasma and I (1988, 1997; Pellegrino 2008) have made for many years. Indeed, we have suggested a moral philosophy derived from the nature of medicine as a special kind of human relationship that entails certain ethical obligations on the part of those who profess it. For us this is an ethic of medicine, an internal morality of medicine, based on the existential realities of being ill, needing healing and helping, and the act of profession of the physician as a promise to help and heal.

This is not the place to attempt to evaluate or respond to each of those criticisms. Obviously, anyone who intends to adhere to the precepts of the Hippocratic code or any professional codes must be aware that there is some measure of truth in many of them. One must decide whether a code is simply a social construct without any intrinsic claim to moral authority, whether it has a claim to authority that is only transient and subject to change in response to social preferences, or whether the moral authority of medical codes rests in their being stable reflections of moral obligations rooted in the nature of medicine itself.

SOURCES OF MORAL AUTHORITY

It becomes important, therefore, to examine the possible sources of moral authority of professional codes. These sources of moral authority may be derived externally—that is, from moral theories outside medicine—or internally, from the nature and ends of medicine itself.

External sources of moral authority

One possible means of justifying medico-moral codes is by applying general moral theories to the practice of medicine. The code that results is derived from each moral theory.

Social construction. A widely accepted source for the moral authority of codes (and the one inherent in most of the criticisms cited above) is some form of social construction. In this view the ends of medicine are grounded in societal consensus about the uses and goals that medicine should pursue. Here, codes are instruments designed to attain certain predefined social ends of medicine. The ethics of medicine derives from whatever values, guidelines, beliefs, or principles a society chooses to impose upon its practitioners at a particular time.

The requisite consensus can be derived in several ways. One way is by plebiscite or referendum, where a majority vote of the polity would be decisive. This is, in effect, to equate the major tenets of democratic political philosophy with moral discourse. Another way that the precepts of a code could be determined would be by their fitting into a coherence theory; that is, by the fit or misfit of the precepts within a context of other beliefs already socially accepted. Still another method of social construction is reflective equilibrium, whereby judgments about particular theories or precepts are tested systematically for congruence or incompatibility with particular judgments and vice versa. The socially preferred or accepted precepts are those that come closest to equilibrium between a theory and particular judgments.

Another form of social construction is the social contract—as construed by Hobbes, Locke, and Rousseau. In this view the relationship of a profession with society is in the form of a mutually constructed contract. Society affords certain privileges to a profession in order to gain, in return, the special services that the profession can provide. Here the moral authority of a code resides in the bilateral obligations of the contracting parties. As a result the obligations incurred are social constructions whose authority depends on societal concurrence.

The moral authority of a socially constructed code is defined by particular social forces in particular historic settings. It is subject, therefore, to continuing processes of change. Today, such codes must accommodate the prevalent mores of moral pluralism and moral skepticism. In this setting, linkages between physicians and patients of different cultures or nations would be morally insecure. The notion of a moral tradition would be suspect.

Deontology. Another external source of moral authority would be Kantian deontology. L'tang (1992) argues that professional codes are codifications of Kantian perfect duties; that is, duties that are obligatory because they derive from the categorical imperative. According to this view, to generate valid duties, codes must be voluntary and must shape the will of the participants, irrespective of personal inclination. The difficulty here is that codes are intended to articulate specific precepts to guide professional action whereas the categorical imperative is the standard by which every potential precept ought to be evaluated. L'tang recognizes this limitation but justifies the Kantian approach by what it can contribute to policy formulation and decision procedures and by its insistence on the participation of rational, autonomous human beings (1992).

Utilitarianism. Starr justifies the moral authority of codes on grounds of their socially useful consequences, such as the stability of society and the establishment of a set of expectations to guide law and policies (1982). Professional codes also yield social benefits for all by encouraging physician compliance.

Utility as a source of moral authority encounters the usual problems of any utilitarian theory: defining what precisely is in the public interest, quantifying and calculating utility, and paying inadequate attention to intentionality. Moreover, the way utility itself is to be defined is problematic. As totalitarian regimes have repeatedly demonstrated, professional ethics are susceptible to subversion and compromise with nonmoral or immoral societal purposes (Pellegrino 1995).

Prima facie justification. W. D. Ross's notion of prima facie obligations has enjoyed wide popularity as a basis for biomedical ethics (1988; Beauchamp and Childress 1994). It appeals to many professionals as a justification of professional codes as well. According to this view some set of rules or precepts could gain universal approbation as reflections of a common morality. These rules become prima facie obligations to be respected ipso facto unless some overriding justification could be offered for violating them.

The problem with prima facie principles as the basis of moral authority is that they require agreement on a common morality. This is more and more difficult to attain in today's pluralistic, multicultural, morally divided societies. Also, there remains the problem of reconciling prima facie rules when they conflict with each other.

Postmodern ethics. Postmodernism is a multifaceted philosophical and cultural move-ment with many ramifications for codes of ethics. Postmodernists deny the validity of any foundational theory for moral authority and, thus, any stable codification of moral precepts. They would read a professional code of ethics as a text susceptible, like any other text, to deconstruction and individual interpretation.

The only possible basis for moral authentication would be praxis (Toulmin 1997). If a code worked—for example, in the sense of achieving some measurable differ-ence in conduct—it would be authenticated. The problem, of course, is that what works may not be moral. In any case one would have to define both terms: "works" and "moral." This would press us to find some other justification for moral author-ity. Some suggest that the normative dimension can be reintroduced by the fact that everyone is a game-player and moral norms are the rules of the game (Nuyen 1998). This is a far cry from the ideal of a code. It reduces ultimately to another form of social construction.

Internal sources of moral authority

Two internal sources of moral authority rest in the practitioners of the profession in question and the activity peculiar to the profession they practice. One source consists in practitioners' discerning, through moral reflection, something special in their art that imposes moral obligations upon them. A second source is found in a more for-mal analysis of the peculiar nature of the practice, its ends, purposes, and phenomena, from which a set of duties is derived if the defined goals are to be achieved.

Moral reflections of practitioners. In its origins the Hippocratic Oath was developed as a statement of freely asserted moral precepts without argumentation. A group of physicians in ancient Greece saw their art intuitively as a moral enterprise that required a high degree of moral commitment. By their collective oath, they commit-ted themselves publicly to beneficence, confidentiality, competence, and fidelity to promises, while abjuring maleficence, abortion, euthanasia, and sexual congress with patients. Their profession of this oath carried with it the penalty of reproach for its infraction. By their collective oath, they recognized that commitment and thus estab-lished themselves as a moral community distinct from the main body of practitioners of their day (Edelstein 1943; Carrick 1985).

The validity of those moral commitments should rest on their merit, not on the way in which they were derived or proclaimed. The voluntary taking of the oath is a freely made promise and, as such, is binding, like all promises, on those who make the promise in good faith. This was the case with those physicians, few or many, who took the Hippocratic Oath in centuries past and those who take it today, and it serves as one source of the Hippocratic Oath's moral authority. But the moral validity of the oath transcends communal or societal acceptance.

A teleological account of moral authority. I contend that what the Hippocratic physi-cians grasped intuitively as the moral basis for their oath was the moral imperative embedded in the nature of their art. They took the end of that art to be relief of pain and suffering, lessening what they called the violence of the disease—thus, healing.

Moreover, the first moral precept of the oath (its first codification in ethics) is the promise to use medical knowledge for the good of the patient and to refrain from harm—deemed to be that which distinguished medicine from other arts (Hippocrates 1981). Plato discerns this more explicitly, setting medicine apart from carpentry or navigation or money making by its end and function (*Cratylus; The Republic*). For both Plato and Aristotle medicine was the paradigm of an art, or *tekné*, practiced within a moral framework.

In its classical Platonic, Aristotelian, and Thomistic sense, the term "teleology" refers to the study of ends. This differs from the modern Benthamite or Millian ethical teleology with emphasis on consequences or outcomes. Classically, the *telos* of a thing is intrinsic to its nature, to what it is, what it is intended for, and what its purpose is. The essence of an act and its *telos* are connected in such a way that an act is a good act of its kind if it attains its proper end or purpose, its *telos*.

In this way the end or purpose is linked with the good. To know the end is to know the particular excellence that can enable one to attain it with perfection (Guthrie 1971). In moral terms this idea of the *telos* incorporates an "ought" dimension. Any trait or disposition that enables an agent to achieve the end is a virtue; that is, it confers a power (*virtus*) to attain that end with perfection.

Aristotle incorporated this notion of *telos* in his definition of final causes and his definition of a definition (*Metaphysics; Posterior Analytics*). It was further refined by Thomas Aquinas, who defined both the good and the end as being "that for the sake of which other things are done" (1960). Aquinas is quite specific about teleology as the basis for ethics "so the subject matter of moral philosophy is human action as ordered to an end or even man as he is acting voluntarily for the sake of an end" (1960).

This concept of teleology, classically defined, is not consistent with current consequentialist preferences for social constructions of the goals of medicine. Indeed, the use of goals as opposed to ends in a new treatment of this subject is indicative of the contemporary preference (Hanson and Callahan 1999). Goals are human societal constructs and can be changed at will. Ends, on the other hand, have an ontological status that is not susceptible to manipulation even for ostensibly good reasons. Those objections notwithstanding, it is important to compare and contrast a teleological account of the moral basis of codes with contemporary theories.

Let us now apply this notion of *telos* and its accompanying ethic of the good to medicine. Such an account provides the elements of an internal morality of medicine and, thus, a moral philosophy for medical practice. Medicine exists because humans become ill and want to heal, ameliorate, cure, or prevent this universal human frailty. These are the ends of medicine, those things that define it for what it is. These are, therefore, the good for which medicine strives and for which health professionals act.

Physicians, nurses, and other health professionals are the human agents through whom the essential ends of medicine are achieved. They effect these ends in clinical medicine through particular relationships with individual patients. The *telos*, or end, of the clinical relationship is the same as the generic *telos* of medicine as an art. This generic end is brought about clinically through a more proximate and specific end—namely, making and effecting a technically right and morally good healing decision for, and with, a particular patient (Pellegrino and Thomasma 1988). A right decision is one that is scientifically correct; that is, it is congruent with the best scientific evidence. A good decision is one that is morally good; that is, it is in the best interests of the patient and protects or preserves the good of the patient. The good of the patient is, in turn, a composite notion of four elements: the medical good; the patient's perception of his or her good; the good of the patient as a human being; and the spiritual good of the patient (Pellegrino and Thomasma 1988).

The good of the patient thus defined is the immediate end of the clinical encounter attained through making right and good decisions, and these, in turn, serve the more distant good of the restoration of the patient's health, care, cure, or amelioration of illness or disability. Medicine is judged good or bad depending on whether it facilitates those ends. Those ends are intrinsic to medicine, and those who practice this art are under a moral constraint to bring them about. The ethics of medicine arises, therefore, in the nature of medicine, in the definition of its ends, and in the possession, by the medical agent, of those traits of character that enable and empower the closest approach possible to those ends.

The ancient codes of medicine and their contemporary counterparts are public commitments to strive to attain the ends of medicine. They are implicitly proclaimed in the codes that commit doctors to the patient's good through fulfillment of duties and necessary virtues. Thus, in the Hippocratic ethic, one finds the positive duties of beneficence and nonmaleficence; fidelity to trust; preservation of confidences; and not taking sexual advantage of patients, not practicing abortion or euthanasia, and not engaging in practices beyond one's competence. Professional codes of medicine are explicit declarations of commitment to those duties that are required if the ends of medicine are to be attained and a physician is to be a good physician.

A teleological validation of moral authority yields a professional code at variance with current moral theory. Such a code is essentialist, stable at least in its core precepts, and universally binding on all who profess to be healers. It would eliminate from the codes those elements that cannot be justified on grounds of the ends and nature of medicine or the other health professions. It would hold all members of a profession who ascribed to the code morally responsible for its observance.

If a minimal core of moral commitments can be fashioned that focuses on the obligations of health professionals as professionals, there is every probability that it would eventuate in a code common to all health professions. Such an effort is under way under auspices of the Tavistock Group, which is attempting to fashion a guide to ethical decision making for all health professionals (Smith, Hiatt, and Berwick 1999). What is proposed is a set of universal principles that might apply to health care systems throughout the world. Allowance would be made for additional ethical principles peculiar to each of the separate professions. Some differences suited to national, sociopolitical, and economic preferences are contemplated as well.

If such a universal code were to succeed, its moral authority would have to be derived from something more fundamental than the interests or assertions of any one of the health professions. The moral grounding in the primacy of the welfare of those to be served will be essential. Only in this way will the differences between health care systems and health professionals be reconciled. Only in this way can a legitimate and morally defensible criterion be established to distinguish essential from nonessential or self-defeating differences in ethical guidelines.

In today's moral discourse, the objections to a teleological essentialist derivation of moral authority are many. First is the total negation of any theory of a stable foundation for moral philosophy. Second is the tendency to confuse classical teleology with theological cosmology; that is, the argument for a design built into nature in the form of unbreakable laws. Third is the antimetaphysical conviction of contemporary philosophy. Fourth is the postmodern resistance to the possibility of grasping moral truths by the use of reason. Finally, any teleological ethic based in objective reality is susceptible to the accusation of the naturalistic fallacy; namely deriving an "ought" conclusion from an "is" premise—an error in moral reasoning pointed out by David Hume and G. E. Moore.

This is not the place for a rebuttal of the arguments against the teleological foundation for the moral authority of codes. The purpose of the preceding section has been to illustrate ways moral authority can be established. Which one is chosen will condition the form of the dialogue. But without some degree of moral authority, there can be no dialogue or argumentation.

THE ABUSE OF CODES

As indicated at the beginning of this chapter, the methodology underlying the use of codes is the rhetorical methodology of the argument from authority. The use or abuse of codes is determined in terms of the criteria for a valid argument from authority. These criteria in moral argumentation reduce to: the authenticity and validity of the authority cited; the use of that authority in the proper context; and the absence of conflicts of interest.

Even if a robust interpretation of the moral authority of a code is accepted based on one of the justificatory arguments discussed above, that authority, like any authority, can be misused so that it becomes self-defeating and ineffective. Indeed, some of the current criticisms of codes speak more of their misuse than to a fundamental moral defect. There are many ways to misuse the authority of codes.

For example, the code may be cited to claim or defend some self-serving professional prerogative, such as restricting the exercise of a legitimate technical expertise by members of other health professions. Similarly, some physicians might claim that the code demands so much of them morally that they are thereby justified in assuming moral primacy in team decisions or disputes. Some doctors read the Hippocratic Oath, for example, as giving them automatic leadership of the health care team or the right to dictate what is right or wrong without challenge from their colleagues. Still others take the oath to be a unilateral license to paternalism that brooks no disagreement.

Some also misuse the code to argue against the need for teaching medical ethics or for further analysis and study of its history, meanings, and interpretation. It is said that everything can be deduced from the Hippocratic Oath or reduced to the simple phrase "Do no harm." This ignores the fact that beneficence, rather than nonmaleficence, is the first moral principle of the code and of the whole Hippocratic ethic.

It also ignores the fact that codes, however defensible their moral precepts may be, are subject to continuing analysis of their moral implications as each new clinical dilemma presents itself.

A few physicians may still quote the preamble of the Hippocratic Oath to justify their preferences for elitism, sexism, or the guild mentality. These elements of the oath may not even have been part of the original text. In any case they would not survive ethical scrutiny today. Neither were they ever ethically defensible on principled grounds.

An overemphasis on the etiquette of the so-called deontological books of the Hippocratic corpus that focuses on details of comportment, dress, manner, and style may encourage honoring professional loyalty over loyalty to the welfare of patients. This misinterpretation is especially dangerous in matters of malpractice, physicians' personal conduct, or protection of the impaired physician. To err in that way is to subvert patients' interests to those of physicians—a clear violation of the central commitment of the oath to patient welfare. It is worth bearing in mind that the intentional or unintentional misuse, abuse, or violation of a code does not vitiate the code itself.

The grossest documented abuse of the Hippocratic ethic was that of the physicians of the Third Reich. Those who were indicted for their roles in human experimentation and the Holocaust protested that they had obeyed the precepts of the oath (Pellegrino 2009; Pellegrino and Thomasma 2000). Indeed, a telling lesson of the Nuremberg trials was the fragility of the Hippocratic Oath and ethic, resting as they do on moral assertion without a moral philosophy to ground them more securely.

The fragility of the oath also has been evidenced by its more subtle deconstruction in the last several decades as its precepts have been subjected to individual interpretations. In this era of autonomy, individual preference, freedom of choice, and moral skepticism, many physicians feel free to pick and choose which precepts (if any) they will accept or reject. The variability of oaths at medical commencements attests to the growing insistence on a more secular-sounding, more inclusive oath. This variability is exacerbated by the gradual transformation of patient autonomy into patient sovereignty (Veatch 2008).

Without a moral philosophy to ground them, the Hippocratic Oath and ethic are fragile and are threatened with progressive fragmentation and, perhaps, complete dissolution.

∾ Concluding Comments

A code binds physicians not only because they have voluntarily and publicly proclaimed allegiance to it but also because its moral precepts can be individually justified and defended by sound moral argumentation. Despite the emergence of a variety of other powerful methods of doing medical ethics, codes will continue to play a prominent role in the indefinite future. They are simple, direct codifications of moral conduct to which large numbers of today's professionals commit themselves. If codes are to satisfy the rhetorical canons for the proper use of arguments from authority, the moral authority of codes will have to be continually validated. This means that scholarly study of codes remains a requisite for sound discourse in medical ethics.

Inquiry into the provenance, content, sociohistorical settings, and social evolution of the meanings of codes will require the knowledge and skills of sociology, history, and politics. Inquiry into the philosophical origins and moral validity of codes and their critical evaluation against modern ethical theory and practice will require the skills of philosophers. Relating these facets of codes to each other will demand a level of interdisciplinary study difficult to attain. In all of this the error of presentism—that is, interpreting events of the past in terms of the present—must be avoided. Equally seductive is the misuse and abuse of texts simply to score a victory in argument.

In the end the major problem is not the fragility of the code but the character of the physician. Any moral code must be translated into a moral act by a human person, and that moral act will reflect the moral values and sensitivities of that agent. In this view virtues are character traits that predispose the physician habitually to act in such a way that the intended end (which is the fundamental point of the code) is the good of the patient. To achieve that end entails certain virtues both intellectual and moral.

Thomasma and I (1988, 1993) have identified those virtues as practical wisdom (prudence), justice, temperance and courage, as well as fidelity to trust, benevolence, some suppression of self-interest, intellectual and personal honesty, humility, and compassion. In our view these virtues are entailed by the nature of the physician–patient relationship, that is, by what the physician promises and the patient is entitled to receive.

The strongest assurance of the code's survival is the fact that it speaks to realities of human existence that do not change in their essence. As long as humans are mortal, they will become ill and will face predicaments that will give rise to a need for assistance from someone who professes and practices healing and helping. The nature of the predicament of one human seeking help from another who offers to help is what prompted a small group of Greek physicians to commit themselves to moral obligations they freely assumed. That reality is today more complex and filled with more hope for comfort or cure, but it is also as central to human welfare as it has always been.

∾ Notes on Resources and Training

Those who plan research in professional codes, and especially the Hippocratic code, may do so from a wide variety of perspectives—including historical, sociological, and philosophical. Educational requirements will vary with the perspective chosen. Serious textual scholarship regarding ancient declarations requires knowledge of the languages in which they were written. What can be certain is that this is a well-tilled field of scholarship. This does not preclude further study but does require in-depth preparation if new insights are to be discovered.

The literature on professional ethics in general, and medical ethics in particular, is voluminous. The citations in the references for this chapter are a small sample, selected for their relevance to the limited question of the use and abuse of codes in bioethical argumentation. Each contains an extensive bibliography that can be used to extend the reader's studies further.

1. The article on codes in the *Encyclopedia of Bioethics* by Carol Spicer (1995) is the most comprehensive current collation of the content of professional codes.

2. For the AMA code, see American Medical Association, Council on Ethical and Judicial Affairs, *Code of Medical Ethics: Current Opinions with Annotations* (Chicago: American Medical Association, 1999).

3. Eliot Freidson's *Profession of Medicine* (New York: Dodd, Mead, 1973); Talcott Parson's "The Sick Role and the Role of the Physician Reconsidered," *Milbank Memorial Fund Quarterly* 257 (1975): 53ff.; and Renée C. Fox's *The Sociology of Medicine: A Participant Observer's View* (Englewood Cliffs, NJ: Prentice Hall, 1989) are excellent examinations of professions in general from the sociological point of view.

4. For the Hippocratic texts, the literature is enormous. For those with the requisite facility, the Greek text will be preferred. Of these I would single out the following: Loeb Classical Library, eight volumes in Greek and English, at present, with various translators (Cambridge, MA: Harvard University Press); *Hippocratic Writings*, trans. Frances Adams, in the Great Books of the Western World Series, Vol. 10 (Chicago: Encyclopedia Britannica, 1952).

5. Edelstein's *Ancient Medicine*, ed. Owsei Temkin and C. Lilian Temkin (Baltimore: Johns Hopkins University Press, 1967) represents the work of one of the most respected commentators on the Hippocratic corpus.

6. Paul Carrick's *Medical Ethics in Antiquity* (1985) is an excellent review of specific ethical issues as treated by ancient authors.

7. Owsei Temkin's *Hippocrates in a World of Pagans and Christians* (1991) is a study of the evolution of the Hippocratic ethos during the Christian era.

8. Wesley D. Smith's *The Hippocratic Tradition* (Ithaca, NY: Cornell University Press, 1979) is an essential commentary on the ways the Hippocratic tradition has been variously interpreted over the centuries and why. Robert Baker's "The History of Medical Ethics" (1993) is a concise, up-to-date history including later codes—for example, Percival, Gregory, and AMA.

9. Anthony Weston's *A Rule Book for Arguments* (1992) is a concise summation of proper and improper use of arguments in discussion.

10. The subject of codes of ethics appears periodically in almost every medical journal. Especially pertinent would be, for example: *Bulletin of the History of Medicine, Hastings Center Report, Kennedy Institute of Ethics Journal, Journal of Clinical Ethics, Journal of History of Medicine and Allied Sciences, Journal of Medicine and Philosophy*, and *Theoretical Medicine and Bioethics*.

Electronic resources include AMA Code of Medical Ethics (American Medical Association): www.ama-assn.org/ama/pub/physician-resources/medical-ethics/code-medical-ethics.shtml; Bioethics Information Resources at the U.S. National Library of Medicine: www.nlm.nih.gov/bsd/bioethics.html; Center for the Study of Ethics in the Professions at IIT (Illinois Institute of Technology): www.iit.edu/libraries/csep/; ETHXWeb database (National Reference Center for Bioethics Literature, Kennedy Institute of Ethics, Georgetown University): http://bioethics.georgetown.edu/data

bases/ETHXWeb/basice.htm; UNESCO's Global Ethics Observatory (GEObs), which includes Database #5: Codes of Conduct: www.unesco.org/shs/ethics/geobs.

ᔕ Note

The author wishes to express his gratitude to Martina Darragh, reference librarian, at the National Reference Center for Bioethics Literature, Georgetown University, for compiling this list of electronic resources. The National Reference Center may be reached at 202-687-3885 or 888-BIO-ETHX (888-246-3849); e-mail: bioethics@georgetown.edu; url: bioethics.georgetown.edu.

ᔕ References

Amundsen, D. W. 1996. *Medicine, society, and faith in the ancient and medieval worlds*. Baltimore: Johns Hopkins University Press.

Aquinas, T. 1960. *The pocket Aquinas*, ed. Vernon J. Burke, 185, 190. New York: Washington Square Books.

Aristotle. 1984a. Metaphysics. In *The complete works of Aristotle, the revised Oxford translation*, ed. Jonathan Barnes, 1646. Princeton, NJ: Princeton University Press.

———. 1984b. Posterior analytics. In *The complete works of Aristotle, the revised Oxford translation*, ed. Jonathan Barnes, 154–55. Princeton, NJ: Princeton University Press.

Aubyn, Saint G. 1985. *The art of argument*. New York: Taplinger.

Baker, R. 1993. The history of medical ethics. In *Companion encyclopedia of medical history*, ed. B. Bynum and Roy Porter. Vol. 2. London and New York: Routledge.

———. 1994. *The codification of medical morality: Historical and philosophical studies of the formalization of medical morality*. Vol. 2: *The nineteenth century*. Dordrecht, The Netherlands: Kluwer Academic Publishers.

Baker, R., D. Porter, and R. Porter, eds. 1993. *The codification of medical morality: Historical and philosophical studies of the formalization of medical morality*. Vol. 1: *The eighteenth century*. Dordrecht, The Netherlands: Kluwer Academic Publishers.

Bar-Sela, A., and H. Hoff. 1962. Isaac Israeli's fifty admonitions to physicians. *Journal of the History of Medicine and Allied Health Sciences* 17:243–54.

Beauchamp, T. L., and J. F. Childress. 1994. *Principles of biomedical ethics*. New York: Oxford University Press.

Berlant, J. 1975. *Profession and monopoly: A study of medicine in the United States and Britain*. Berkeley: University of California Press.

Carrick, P. 1985. *Medical ethics in antiquity: Philosophical perspectives on abortion and euthanasia*. Dordrecht, The Netherlands, and Boston: D. Reidel/Kluwer Academic Publishers.

Castiglioni, A. 1941. *A history of medicine*. Trans. and ed. E. B. Krumbhaar, 226–27. New York: Alfred A. Knopf.

Dauber, F. W. 1996. *Critical thinking: An introduction to reasoning*. New York: Barnes and Noble, 37–45.

Downey, R. S., and K. C. Calman. 1994. *Healthy respect*. 2nd ed. London: Faber and Faber.

Edelstein, L. 1943. The Hippocratic Oath: Text, translation, and interpretation. *Bulletin of the History of Medicine* Supp. I.

Encyclopedia Britannica. 1979. Code of Hammurabi. 15th ed. Vol. 11. Chicago: Encyclopedia Britannica Inc., 823.

Etziony, M. B. 1973. *The physician's creed*. Springfield, IL: Charles Thomas.

Foot, P. 1972. Morality as a system of hypothetical imperatives. *Philosophical review* 81:305–16.

Frank, J. P. 1976. *A system of complete medical police*. Baltimore: Johns Hopkins University Press.

Goodfield, J. 1973. Reflection on the Hippocratic Oaths. *Hastings Center Studies* 1:79–92.

Gorlin, R. A., ed. 1995. *Codes of professional responsibility*. Washington, DC: Bureau of National Affairs.

Guthrie, W. K. C. 1971. *Socrates*. Cambridge: Cambridge University Press, 146.

Hamarneh, S. K. 1993. Practical ethics in the health professions. *Hamdard Medicus* 36:11–24.

Hanson, M., and D. Callahan, eds. 1999. *The goals of medicine: The forgotten issues in health care reform*. Washington, DC: Georgetown University Press.

Hippocrates. 1972. *Hippocrates*. Loeb Classical Library 147, with an English translation by W. H. S. Jones, 291–301, 312–33. Vol. 1. Cambridge, MA: Harvard University Press.

———. 1979. *Hippocrates*. Loeb Classical Library 150, with an English translation by W. H. S. Jones. Vol. 4, 97–222. Cambridge, MA: Harvard University Press.

———. 1981. *Hippocrates*. Loeb Classical Library 148, with an English translation by W. H. S. Jones. Vol. 2, 190–217, 262–65, 278–301, 305–13. Cambridge, MA: Harvard University Press.

Hussey, T. 1996. Nursing ethics and codes of professional conduct. *Nursing Ethics* 3:250–58.

Jotterand, F. 2005. The Hippocratic Oath and contemporary medicine: Dialectics between past ideals and present reality. *Journal of Medicine and Philosophy* 30:107–28.

Kluge, E. H. 1992. Codes of ethics and other illusions. *Catholic Medical Association Journal* 146:1234–35.

Konold, D. 1978. Codes of medical ethics: History. In *Encyclopedia of bioethics*, vol. 1, ed. Warren T. Reich, 162–71. New York: MacMillan/The Free Press.

L'tang, J. 1992. A Kantian approach to codes of ethics. *Journal of Business Ethics* 11:741–43.

Lebacqz, K. 1985. *Professional ethics*. Nashville: Abingdon Press.

Levey, M. 1977. Medical deontology in ninth-century Islam. In *Legacies in ethics and medicine*, ed. Chester Burns, 129–44. New York: Science History Publications.

Mackin, J. H. 1969. *Classical rhetoric for modern discourse*. New York: Collier-MacMillan, 125–26.

Miles, S. H. 2004. *The Hippocratic Oath and the ethics of medicine*. New York: Oxford University Press.

Muthu, D. C. 1930. The antiquity of Hindu medicine and civilization. London, n.p. Cited in Will Durant. 1994. *Our Oriental heritage*. New York: Simon and Schuster, 530.

Newton, L. 1978. A professional ethic, a proposal in context. In *Matters of life and death*, ed. John Thomas, 264. Toronto: Samuel Stevens.

Nutton, V. 1995. What's in an oath? *Journal of the Royal College of Physicians of London* 29:518–24.

Nuyen, A. T. 1998. Lyotard's postmodern ethics and the normative question. *Philosophy Today* 42:411–17.

Orr, R. D., N. Pang, E. D. Pellegrino, and M. Siegler. 1997. Use of the Hippocratic Oath: A review of twentieth-century practice and a content analysis of oaths administered in the U.S. and Canada in 1993. *Journal of Clinical Ethics* (Winter): 377–88.

Pellegrino, E. D. 1995. Guarding the integrity of medical ethics: Some lessons from Soviet Russia. *Journal of the American Medical Association* 3:1622–23.

———. 1999. Traditional medical ethics: A reminder. *American Board of Internal Medicine Forum for the Future Report*. Philadelphia: American Board of Internal Medicine.

———. 2001. The internal morality of clinical medicine: A paradigm for the ethics of the helping and healing professions. *Journal of Medicine and Philosophy* 26 (6): 559–79.

———. 2008. *The philosophy of medicine reborn: A Pellegrino reader*, ed. H. T. Engelhardt and F. Jotterand. Notre Dame, IN: University of Notre Dame Press.

———. 2009. When evil was good and good evil: Remembrances of Nuremberg. In *Medicine after the Holocaust: From the master race to the human genome and beyond*, ed. S. Rubenfeld. New York: Palgrave-Macmillan.

Pellegrino, E. D., and D. C. Thomasma. 1981. *A philosophical basis of medical practice: Toward a philosophy and ethic of the healing professions*. New York: Oxford University Press.

———. 1988. *For the patient's good: The restoration of beneficence in health care*. New York: Oxford University Press.

———. 1993. *The virtues in medical practice*. New York: Oxford University Press.

———. 1997. *Helping and healing: Religious commitment in health care*. New York: Oxford University Press.

———. 2000. Dubious premises—evil conclusions: More reasoning at the Nuremberg trials. Cambridge Quarterly of Healthcare Ethics 9:261–74.

Perelman, C. 1982. *The realm of rhetoric*. Notre Dame, IN: Notre Dame University Press.

Petry, E. D. 1993. The wrong way to institutionalize ethics. *Conference proceedings, Shefield business school* (April 1990): 30. Cited in Richard C. Warren, Codes of ethics: Bricks without straw. *Business Ethics* 2:184–91.

Plato. 1982a. *Cratylus*. In *The collected dialogues of Plato including the letters*, ed. Edith Hamilton and Huntington Cairns, 389c–e, 427. Princeton, NJ: Princeton University Press.

———. 1982b. *The Republic*. In *The collected dialogues of Plato*, ed. Edith Hamilton and Huntington Cairns. Book I, 342c–e, 592. Princeton, NJ: Princeton University Press.

Ross, W. D. 1988. *The right and the good*. Indianapolis: Hackett, 18–19.

Sanders, J. T. 1993. Honor among thieves: Some reflections on professional codes of ethics. *Professional Ethics* 2:83–103.

Scriven, M. 1976. *Reasoning*. New York: McGraw-Hill, 227–28.

Sims, R. R. 1994. *Ethics and organizational decision making: A call for renewal*. Westport, CT: Quorum Books.

Smith, R., H. Hiatt, and D. Berwick. 1999. Shared ethical principles for everybody in health care: A working draft from the Tavistock Group. *British Journal of Medicine* 318 (1999): 248–51 and *Annals of Internal Medicine* 130:143–47.

Spicer, C. M., ed. 1995. Appendix: Codes, oaths, and directives related to bioethics. In *Encyclopedia of bioethics*. 2nd ed. Vol. 5., ed. Warren T. Reich, 2599–2842. New York: MacMillan/Simon & Schuster.

Starr, P. 1982. *The social transformation of American medicine*. New York: Basic Books.

Sugarman, J. 1994. Hawkeye Pierce and the questionable relevance of medical etiquette to contemporary medical ethics and practice. *Journal of Clinical Ethics* 5:22–30.

Sulmasy, D. P. 1999. What is an oath? *Theoretical Medicine and Bioethics* 20 (4): 329–46.

Tadd, V. 1994. Professional codes: An exercise in tokenism? *Nursing Ethics* 1 (1): 15–23.

Temkin, O. 1991. *Hippocrates in a world of pagans and Christians*. Baltimore: Johns Hopkins University Press.

Toulmin, S. 1997. The primacy of practice: Medicine and postmodernism. In *Philosophy of medicine and bioethics: A twenty-year retrospective*, ed. Ronald A. Carson and Chester Q. Burns, 41–54. Dordrecht, The Netherlands, and Boston: Kluwer Academic Publishers.

Veatch, R. M. 1978. Codes of medical ethics: Ethical analysis. In *Encyclopedia of bioethics*, ed. Warren T. Reich, 172–80. Vol. 1. New York: MacMillan/The Free Press.

———. 1991. *The patient as partner in the physician–patient relationship*. Bloomington: Indiana University Press.

———. 2008. *Patient, heal thyself: How the "new medicine" puts the patient in charge*. New York: Oxford University Press.

Warren, R. C. 1993. Codes of ethics: Bricks without straw. *Business Ethics: A European Review* 2 (4): 185–91.

Weston, A. 1992. *A rule book for arguments*. Indianapolis: Hackett, 28–35.

CHAPTER 7

Casuistry and Clinical Ethics

ALBERT R. JONSEN

Clinical ethics is that part of bioethics that attempts to provide a structured approach to the identification, analysis, and resolution of ethical problems in clinical medicine (Jonsen, Siegler, and Winslade 2006). Clinical medicine is always about cases. The vast science of medicine funnels down to a case: a patient in the care of doctors and nurses within the institutions of health care. However, the ethical analysis of cases, once commonly called casuistry, has been ignored by modern moral philosophy, on which bioethics relies for its principles and theories. One of the seminal books of modern moral philosophy, G. E. Moore's *Principia Ethica*, opened with the assertion that there is "a study different from Ethics and one much less respectable, the study of Casuistry . . . (although Ethics cannot be complete without it)." He goes on, "The defects of Casuistry are not defects of principle; no objection can be taken to its aim and object. It has failed because . . . the casuist had been unable to distinguish, in the cases which he treats, those elements upon which their value depends" (1903, 4–5). In subsequent ethical scholarship, Moore's statement seems to have been taken as definitive. Moral philosophers showed little interest in remedying the defects of casuistry. This chapter outlines an approach to cases that may remedy some of these defects and, thereby, make case analysis more useful to clinical ethics.

The casuistry to which Moore refers had a long history. As far back as the Roman Stoics and Cicero, philosophers aimed to give advice about how to act in particular morally charged situations (Cicero, *De Officiis*). This practice continued into the Christian Middle Ages to train priests as confessors, and in Roman Catholic and Anglican theology, scholarly consideration of cases of conscience or case divinity was a vigorous enterprise from the sixteenth to the nineteenth century. At that time, the word "casuistry" was applied to this enterprise, usually as a term of abuse. The abuse was first instigated by the brilliant French mathematician, Blaise Pascal, who, speaking as an ultradevout Catholic, excoriated the casuistry of his time, both because it led to moral relativism and laxism and for the reason mentioned by Moore, its failure to base case reasoning on sound foundations (Pascal, *Provincial Letters*). The word *casuistry* itself became a synonym for an overly clever, self-serving, totally relativistic form of moral analysis. The *Oxford English Dictionary* definition includes the quote, "Casuistry destroys by distinctions and exceptions all morality and effaces the difference between right and wrong." By the time bioethics emerged and engaged the ethics of medical cases, casuistry had faded away. Few moral philosophers knew or cared what it was. It was not only "much less respectable" than ethics, as Moore said; it was essentially unknown. Still, Moore added, parenthetically, "yet ethics cannot be complete without it."

❧ Description of Casuistry and Clinical Ethics

Jonsen and Toulmin (1987) attempted to resuscitate casuistry, that is, to breath life into casuistical reasoning by understanding the methods casuists employed and attempting to ground it more solidly within moral reasoning. Subsequently, the prominence of cases and case reasoning has given medical ethics a distinctly casuistic tone. As the previous chapters in this section show, medical ethicists have an intense interest in theory and principle, but when they get down to work, particularly as consultants in clinical medicine, they perforce become casuists. They wittingly or unwittingly follow the advice of Aristotle, who remarks, "Agents are compelled at every step to think out for themselves what the circumstances demand, just as happens in the arts of medicine and navigation.... Prudence is not concerned with universals only; it must also take cognizance of particulars, because it is concerned with conduct, and conduct has its sphere in particular circumstances" (*Nichomachean Ethics* 1104a 6–9, 1141b 15–16).

The essential steps of casuistic reasoning are three: discerning the topics under consideration, weighing the principles involved, and employing analogical reasoning. Each of these will be considered in turn. First, however, we should be clear about what case means. A case is a sphere of particular circumstances. The English word *case* is a homonym: One of its meanings is "the instance of a thing occurring, an actual state of affairs"; the other totally different meaning is "that which encloses or contains something, as box, bookcase, briefcase." The first derives from the Latin *casus*, an event, from *cadere*, to happen; the second derives from the Latin *capsa*, from *capere*, to hold, which comes into the Romance languages as *cassa*. These are very different meanings and derivations, yet for the purpose of explaining the term "case method" they are suggestive. The most colloquial use of the first meaning, for example, "well, it was the case that..." is made into technical jargon in medicine and in law, for example, "this is a case of pneumonia," or "this is a case of treason," meaning "this event is a particular instance of the general condition called pneumonia or the crime called treason."

This technical use reminds us of the second meaning of case. All human events are complex, filled with behaviors, beliefs, motivations, and emotion. Its components, so tumbled together in life, are sorted into mental compartments so that they can be seen more distinctly, that is, they are boxed. A medical text will describe pneumonia in terms of certain changes in respiration and body temperature, certain findings on the chest x-ray and in the sputum, certain physiological responses to administration of antibiotics. A legal text will describe treason as a witnessed and overt act of aiding the enemy with treasonable intent. These are general descriptions that fit many cases, each of which has certain features that presumably correspond to the general description but that present themselves in unique ways. Thus, the doctor might say, "It looks like this patient has pneumonia but there are atypical features"; the prosecutor may say, "This government scientist communicated with foreign scientists about classified material, but did this communication rise to the level of the crime of treason?"

This boxing of circumstances requires, of course, a box or boxes into which the circumstances are sorted. In the above examples, the medical box might be Pulmonary Diseases, within which there would be smaller boxes, such as Obstructive Lung Disease, Infiltrative Lung Diseases, and Infectious Lung Diseases. Some of the signs and symptoms would sort into several boxes, some into only one. What I have called boxes, the classical rhetoricians, who influenced casuistic argument, called topics (*topos* in Greek means place). They designate standard, common, invariant elements of some enterprise or activity. For example, in making an argument about "who done it?" a detective would have to refer to contiguity of cause and effect, temporal priority of one over the other, and the sufficient and necessary relationship of both. This form of argument penetrates all cases of causality. Readers of murder mysteries will recognize this as the sleuth's reasoning, and those familiar with the law will be reminded of the structure of argument about negligence.

TOPICS

The first move in casuistic reasoning is to designate the topics that constitute the structure of the activity to be examined. The ethics of politics, the ethics of business, and the ethics of medicine deal with very different forms of activity. As forms of human conduct, they will be marked by some common ethical features that identify the moral aspect of any human intercourse. Honesty, fairness, altruism, restraint from violence, and so forth are constants through all intercourse between human persons in communities. The academic field of moral philosophy has engaged in attempting to explain what these common features are, what purpose they serve, and how they fit into a general understanding of human life. But it is also necessary to discern the topics appropriate to each realm of activity. Business ethics might be boxed into form of corporate governance, finance, markets, and so on; political ethics into type of government, public welfare, system of law, and so forth.

Jonsen, Siegler, and Winslade (2006) suggest that the complex practices of clinical medicine can be reduced to four topics. These topics constitute the essential features and structure of that encounter between physician and patient that is called clinical medicine. They are the boxes that structure the cases of clinical ethics. The first topic is Medical Indications: the medical facts, the physical signs, and symptoms that initiate the encounter between patient and physician, and that suggest diagnoses and forms of treatment. The second topic is Patient Preferences: the wishes and choices that a patient has about illness and treatment and its possible results. The third topic is Quality of Life: the physical, intellectual, affective, and social states that individuals wish to attain by means of health interventions and the probability that those interventions will contribute to such states. The forth topic is Contextual Features: the social, organizational, administrative, financial, and legal structures within which health interventions take place and that enhance or limit their efficacy. Any case or particular instance of the medical relationship manifests these four topics. Into these four boxes the particular circumstances of each are sorted and arranged for evaluation.

Take a case: A man is brought to an emergency department bleeding severely. The doctors and nurses recognize that he needs a blood transfusion. He says he is a Jehovah's Witness and refuses transfusion. What should the doctors and nurses do? "Bleeding" and "needs a transfusion" are medical indications. "Says he is Jehovah's Witness and refuses the transfusion" are patient preferences. The providers know the patient's quality of life will be nil, since he will be dead; the patient believes his quality of life will be in the splendor of salvation if he dies being faithful to God's command. That the patient is the father of several young children, the mission of the hospital and its emergency department, the extant law, the possibility for malpractice claims, the distress of the Emergency Department staff, the doctrine of the Jehovah's Witness faith, and the rallying of the local congregation to support their brother are contextual features. This is, then, a case of refusal of medical care. A general philosophical response to the case might be, "The principle of respect for autonomy dictates that the patient's refusal be respected," and the philosopher might go on to provide strong arguments to justify the principle of respect for autonomy. However, those faced with the question "What shall I do?" (which includes the patient, his family, and fellow believers as well as the doctors, nurses, administrators, and legal counsel) cannot be satisfied with that response. It is generally accepted, in ethics and in law, that competent patients may refuse medical care, but in this case, should that general principle be implemented?

This question can be answered only when we examine in detail the actual features of this case. We need quite specific information about this patient's medical condition, its causes, his medical history, and his physical and psychological status at admission. We need to know how urgent is the need for transfusion and whether there are alternatives. We have to be accurately informed about the tenets of his faith and about how committed he is to these tenets. We must know the relevant policies and legal provisions that might apply. In other words each of the four topics must be filled with information specific to this case. When this is done it might be seen that, given the blood loss, the need for blood transfusion is not urgent or, conversely, that even a transfusion might be useless. We might learn that the person who brought him, rather than the patient himself, expresses this preference or that the patient expresses it only vaguely in his confusion. We might find that, although we assumed he would be expelled from his congregation if he was transfused, in fact he would be received with love as one who had been wronged. We might be astonished to learn from legal counsel that the hospital policy and the state law support the right of Jehovah's Witnesses to refuse transfusions even at risk to life. These particular features of this particular case are crucial: They allow us to move toward an ethical resolution. Thus, the first act of casuistic reasoning is to sort the particular details of the specific case into the appropriate topics.

ETHICAL PRINCIPLES

Up to this point this chapter has focused on the factual details that constitute the case. Specific cases are always a riot of detail, and it is the details that attract attention. Casuistic reasoning begins by sorting those details in an orderly way. The development of topics is the technique or method for doing such sorting. However, the conjunction of the topics and the factual details reveals not merely an empirical state of affairs, the facts of the case. It also begins to disclose the moral dimensions of the case. Human practices are shaped by more than conventional and customary understandings and ways; they have embedded in them a host of normative features that reveal not only how people engaged in that practice behave but also how they ought to behave. Morality describes human action and character in light of certain features generally called moral principles, rules, values. Moral philosophers work to give precise meaning to these principles, rules, and values, but they appear, as if spontaneously, in daily discourse. A philosophy text might read, "Truthfulness is the essential ingredient in trust." Moral arguments pivot on these principles. Thus, someone might say, "President Nixon was wrong to deceive the American people, because he forfeited their trust. After all, truth is the essential ingredient in trust." The argument may then go on to show that trust is the basis for political authority and effectiveness, using other moral principles to enforce the argument. Principles are stated in a more general fashion and are related to more general theories of moral justification. Contemporary moral philosophy has concentrated on giving theoretical explanations for the origin and certainty of moral principles. Bioethics has adopted much of this work but has generally accepted four principles as fundamental: respect for autonomy, nonmaleficence, beneficence, and justice (Beauchamp and Childress 1994).

The casuistry that G. E. Moore contrasted to ethics undertakes to relate the very specific details of particular cases to the sweeping range of an abstractly defined moral principle. Does the principle of autonomy resolve the case of the Jehovah's Witness believer arriving in this clinic at this time? In addition to the principle of autonomy, many other moral principles appear in this case, such as beneficence, nonmaleficence, and justice. Are we morally permitted to allow a person to die when he can be saved by appropriate care? Is not his death a harm for which we are responsible? Are we bound by a belief that we do not understand and share? Is it right to allow this person, who is father of a family, to leave his wife and children fatherless? Would it not be better to force a transfusion on him and let him be welcomed back to family and congregation, not as a sinner but as one whom we have sinned against? These and other principles provide the moral ambiance of the case. How do we find the route to travel between these moral principles and the facts of the case so that we might arrive at a resolution useful to those who must make decisions reflective of moral standards?

The metaphor of balancing and weighing is favored by many ethicists when explaining how principles relate to decisions in particular cases. For example, in *Principles of Biomedical Ethics*, Beauchamp and Childress reject theories such as classic utilitarianism, which rely on a single principle by which all cases are resolved. They propose what they call a composite theory, which "permits each basic principle to have weight without assigning a priority weighting or ranking. Which principle overrides in a case of conflict will depend on the particular context, which always has unique features." They then recall philosopher W. D. Ross's thesis (1930, 19–36) that when two or more obligations conflict, balancing is necessary and "we must examine the situation carefully until we form 'a considered opinion (it is never more)' that one obligation is more incumbent in the circumstances than any other." Ross invokes the metaphor of weights moving on a scale to describe how principles are balanced. Yet, even with this departure from the rigid adherence to a single theory and a univocal principle, we are left with some mystery. What does it mean to say, as Beauchamp and Childress do, "what principle overrides . . . will depend on the particular context, which always has unique features"? (1994, 33, 104–11). How do the unique features of a particular context provide weight to a principle or tip the balance toward one rather than the other?

At the most abstract level, two principles—beneficence and respect for autonomy—strive for attention in the case of the Jehovah's Witness believer. These principles are in apparent conflict. As the factual details of the case emerge, however, these abstract principles begin to take on (or lose) weight. If the details show that the patient had in fact reached hemoglobin levels too low to sustain organ perfusion and life, and also reveal that he is a truly committed believer and is (or was at the moment of admission to the Emergency Department) clear and competent in expressing his beliefs, the two competing principles remain in balance. This patient can be benefited by transfusion; he competently rejects transfusion. However, as more details about the nature of his beliefs and the doctrines of his church appear, and as possible medical alternatives are considered, weight may begin to shift.

Without pursuing the case in detail, the accumulation of details may finally weigh down the principle of autonomy to the point where its importance becomes compelling: It may become clear that the beneficence that sustains organic life by blood transfusion is not, for this patient, a benefit. It will give him not the gift of life but a burden of guilt, either for his own sin or for occasioning the sin of others. Even his continued fatherly presence may be less a benefit than an example of infidelity to divine commands. The abstract principles of beneficence and autonomy take on their respective weight as the factual details relative to the topics and maxims are filled out and amplified. Each one of the circumstances does or does not weigh down the principles: Their relevance to the weight of the principles can be judged only in the full context of the case as it presents itself to those who must decide. "Circumstances make the case" is an old adage, familiar to lawyers and doctors and beloved of casuists.

Circumstances exert a powerful pull on principles, but principles, abstract though they may be, carry some weight in themselves. Failure to appreciate the weight of principles allows good casuistry to collapse into situationism: the ethical doctrine that circumstances alone determine the moral quality of decision and action (Jonsen 1993a). Further examination of the metaphor of weighing may clarify the role of principles in casuistic reasoning. Weight, in classical physics, is the result of the pull of gravity toward a center. A moral principle is weighty when it falls to the center of consideration within the universe of moral considerations relevant to the problem under consideration. Its weight is its importance or significance in deliberation about the issue. That weight derives from several related sources. First, it comes from the way in which a society cultivates certain ideas and values, enacting and reinforcing them in its intellectual, social, and religious life. For example, in American culture, individualism is a central value, as the sociologists Robert Bellah et al. demonstrated in *Habits of the Heart*: "American cultural traditions define personality, achievement, and the purpose of human life in ways that leave the individual suspended in glorious, but terrifying, isolation" (1985, 6). This is the modern precipitate from a long historical conversation that includes biblical and republican strands. Our current American emphasis on respect for autonomy as an ethical principle is the precipitate of that tradition.

Thus, in American culture, respect for persons is a principle that has considerable weight. It outweighs other principles that are commonly accepted as worthy but that have lost weight by attrition of the social conditions in which they flourished. For example, it would be commonly accepted that family loyalty and respect for elders were good things but, given significant changes in the sociology and economics of the family in our culture, these good things are much less weighty than in earlier times. Clearly the principle of autonomy outweighs a panoply of moral notions that may serve major purposes in other cultures but are only minor in American culture. Punctilious etiquette toward individuals of various social classes, rigorous conventions of honor, and elaborate linguistic formulas are important morally in other societies but not in ours. Thus, in this sense, it not difficult to find some principles that are more weighty than others within a social tradition.

These anthropological observations do not get us far enough, however. It is not the balancing of central against marginal principles or significant against trivial ones that causes moral perplexity. It is the balancing of central and significant ones against each other. It is easy to demonstrate that individualism, with its consequent ethical principle of respect for persons, is central in American culture. However, it is also possible to demonstrate that beneficence, the duty to help others, has played a consistent place in Western culture and American life. Similarly, justice and fairness are central and significant notions. The problem of balancing arises when autonomy must be balanced against beneficence and beneficence against justice. These notions all have, in the abstract, equivalent gravity, or put less surely, it is difficult to show by theoretical argument how one should prevail over the other.

The critical reflection of scholars within the culture provides a second way in which a moral principle acquires weight. In some cultures there is a formal intellectual enterprise that is called philosophy; in other cultures, intellectual life runs in other courses but there is, nonetheless, a recognized cultural wisdom that articulates ideals and announces priorities for social and personal life. Whenever this happens, respected thinkers select certain principles, ideals, and virtues for special attention. These principles are drawn from those available in the cultural tradition; the philosophers promote them to the center of the system of reflective thought that they construct. Their gravity becomes apparent when other ideas are drawn into their orbit and circle around them as implications. Thus, the notion of the individual as autonomous subject enthralled the thinkers of the Enlightenment and gradually attained a central place in the thought of leading philosophers such as Hobbes, Locke, Rousseau, Kant, and Mill. The philosophical reflections of British liberalism and American pragmatism elaborate and refine these central ideas. In the United States, Ralph Waldo Emerson gave philosophical and rhetorical power to individualism, from which American thought has never recovered. The principle of respect for persons becomes a familiar, indeed, indispensable notion among those who read and write in the Western philosophical traditions; those who ignore it do so at peril of exclusion from philosophical society, and those who criticize it must fight an uphill battle.

This sort of weight, however, is somewhat illusory. A system of moral philosophy is not a morality. Although those who write philosophy may give great weight to a principle because it has made a system of thought coherent and convincing, that principle may not be as weighty in the life of those who live the morality of the culture. Even if they do acknowledge its importance, they may not give it the preeminence or the priority accorded to it within some systems of thought. For example, in recent years we have seen the principle of autonomy become the weightiest of bioethical principles. It is congenial to American moral tradition. However, we are beginning to hear protests from those who speak with other voices within the dominant moral tradition and who are in the process of elaborating alternative moral philosophies, emphasizing community rather than individual or a gender-balanced ethic. The scholarly authority of authors and the elegance of their argument may give weight to their notions; yet it may be years, if ever, before their voices are heard outside the scholarly world.

Weighty principles, then, acquire their gravity from tradition and culture, as well as from systems of moral reflection. Sensible casuists will admit this. When they do, they encounter one of the most common denunciations of casuistry, namely, that casuistry entails moral relativism. Relativism questions whether there are universal, unexceptionable norms of moral conduct at some level of moral reflection. It is an amorphous accusation, for it always raises the questions, "relative to what?" and "relative in what manner?" The classical casuists firmly grounded their casuistry on a philosophy of natural law, derived from Cicero and Aquinas. At the same time they engaged in moral reasoning that, as Aristotle said, "is not concerned with universals only; it must also take cognizance of particulars, because it is concerned with conduct, and conduct has its sphere in particular circumstances." Contemporary casuists may admit to relativism or reject it. If they do, they face the task of building a foundation that can support the structures of all levels of moral reasoning. Contemporary work in moral psychology may provide the materials (Sinnot-Armstrong 2008).

The metaphor of weight can be employed in a third way, briefly described above: Moral principles are given weight by being loaded with circumstances. This third way is the most characteristic of casuistic reasoning. To understand it, we might change the metaphor of weighing: The principles are the scales on which the burdens of circumstances are placed. Principles do weigh on a final decision, but the scales dip, not under the principles' weight, but under the accumulated circumstances that pull on one or the other principle. Moral judgments bear on whole cases; the principles are welded together with the circumstances. Principles, values, circumstances, and consequences must be seen as a whole. The judgment about them covers all of them. Casuists do not, in Platonic fashion, turn their eyes from a vision of moral principle down to the factual circumstances of a case. They sweep facts, values, consequences, and principles into a single vision.

Take a case (from research ethics): should children be subject to research procedures, not for their own good, but for the sake of developing new knowledge? *The Report on Children as Subjects of Research*, from the National Commission for Protection of Human Subjects (1977) argues the case. Since children generally cannot give consent (a circumstance), the principle of respect for autonomy is of less weight than the principle of nonmaleficence. However, the principle "do no harm" must be interpreted in the context of research. It is necessary to clarify what constitutes harm and how research might do harm. The commission's conclusions bear witness to the realization that there are harms of many sorts and many degrees and that most research maneuvers do not do harm but pose risks of harm and that these are of many sorts and degrees. The harm of deliberate death or maiming is unquestionably unethical; how should the harm that comes from a needle stick to draw blood be judged? Is it more harmful or risky if the child is healthy and normal than if the child is a leukemia patient for whom needle sticks are routine? Is a change of daily activities for research observation a harm or risk of harm? Would it be so if the change involved placing the child for a day in the care of strangers rather than familiar caretakers? Should it be considered a harm to be randomized into a treatment regimen that turns out at the conclusion of the study to be the less effective? These and many other variations on the theme of harm and risk are essential to any reasonable judgment that the maxim "do no harm" is being honored or violated. It is the total picture in the instant case that allows such a judgment to be made. The moral weight of "do no harm" is manifested only amid the greater and less, the probables and the possibles of quite particular circumstances. This is the task of an institutional review board (IRB) as it examines any proposal to use children as research subjects.

ANALOGICAL REASONING

I have thus far discussed the initial two steps of casuistic reasoning. The first is the designation of topics for the sorting of circumstances; the second is the weighting of principles within the sphere of those circumstances. One final step of casuistic reasoning remains: finding firm ground for the moral authority of a proposed resolution of the case. How does the casuist test his conclusions in the particular case? In casuistic reasoning conclusions in a contested case are compared to conclusions in similar cases in which the relation between principles and circumstances suggests an obvious resolution. The casuist reflects on the similarities and differences between the contested case and the uncontested cases—similarities and differences that are manifested in the actual circumstances of each case. This comparison of similar cases is called analogous reasoning. It is widely used in Anglo-American common law, in which a new case is seen against a background of similar cases. The casuist, like the jurisprudent, always notes, "This case is very like or somewhat like, the previous case of X," and then asks what it is about the instant case that might suggest a different judgment than did the prior case (in Anglo-American jurisprudence, this process is canonized in the use of precedents).

For example, the principle that parents should determine what is best for their children is, in the usual circumstances of familial life, uncontested, even though some parents may make ill-considered judgments. However, given the circumstance that the parents are devoted believers in a sect that forbids medical care for children, another principle, the protection of a vulnerable human being, grows strong enough to challenge the first principle. Cases can then be lined up in which the uncontested case stands as a paradigm and other cases stand at various removes from it. At the first remove, the parents' faith does not forbid medical care but rather recommends that prayer be the first recourse; at the second remove the belief forbids all but emergency treatment; at the third remove, it forbids all medical attention without exception. At each remove the danger to the child increases and the moral challenge to parental authority grows stronger. This simple example (which in reality might be very complex) shows how the circumstances change the case, modify moral judgment about it, and justify different practical responses to it. The paradigm case is a clear expression of principle, as instantiated in typical circumstances. The contested case is analogous to the paradigm, that is, a similar yet relevantly different instance in a series of cases in which the paradigm case is the most clear and compelling.

Reasoning by analogy is quite different than reasoning by logical deduction from premise to conclusion. Analogous reasoning does not move in a straight line between propositions, and its terms are not primarily conceptual. Rather, it moves back and forth within myriad empirical details as well as conceptual propositions. It is rather like an art critic comparing several paintings. One detail on one canvas is noticed and evaluated in view of another detail on the second canvas. The comparison highlights certain features of both paintings, and only then can the critic render a judgment about the painting as a whole. Obviously, the details compared must be similar to each other in some respect—in both paintings, the intensity of the color of the sky might be the point of comparison—sky color is the similarity; intensity is the difference. The casuist is a sort of art critic, glancing at several cases, their principles and circumstances, in order to compare one to the other and to render a judgment about the value of each (Jonsen 2000).

In casuistic reasoning, then, moral authority derives from the comparison of clear instances of morally right (or wrong) action, in which principle and circumstances are well aligned, with contested cases in which it is less and less clear how the principle can be applied within these circumstances. Resolution of these more contested cases becomes more and more probable and tentative, but sufficiently reasonable to command assent. This form of analogical reasoning is not a repudiation of ethical principles or theory: It acknowledges that principles will always appear within a mélange of circumstances within which their relevance and weight must be assessed.

ꙮ Critique of Casuistry

Casuistry hardly needs another critique. It and its practitioners have been the object of the most scathing criticisms over the centuries. One of the world's most renowned satires is Blaise Pascal's *The Provincial Letters*. This book excoriates the classical casuists. Casuists are portrayed as adept at sharp distinctions and striking comparisons, and those with such skills can make a case that almost anything can squeeze under the ethical bar. Pascal found such casuistry in which the outrageous act won casuistic approbation (an arsonist could be absolved of burning down a house because he set fire to the wrong one), and such casuistry exists even today (an act of fellatio, for example, might count as a sex act for the one performing it but not for the one on whom it was performed). Pascal's sarcastic criticism, however, does not reach to the casuistic method as such. Indeed, if it had, the human activity of moral judgment would itself be accused, since the essential methods of casuistry mirror the common, untutored process of moral judgment. Nevertheless, since Pascal's time, the word *casuistry* itself has come to mean the unscrupulous art of making groundless distinctions to defend obviously outrageous behavior (Jonsen 1993b).

The renewal of interest in casuistry that followed the publication of *The Abuse of Casuistry* stimulated criticisms quite different from those of Pascal. These modern critiques touch the important elements of casuistic reasoning: topics, principles, and paradigms. Since casuistry begins by designating the topics inherent in a particular enterprise, some critics have questioned whether any human enterprise has a structure so defined and permanent as to permit the identification of a finite number of topics. All human enterprises, from marriage to medicine and from economics to education, are fluid and shift their constituent features over time and in different settings. The casuist who wishes to hang a particular case on a permanent structure will not find that structure in the human institutions.

A second criticism also concerns topics. The purpose of designating topics is to create the boxes into which multitudes of heterogeneous circumstances can be filed. Although it is useful in any ethical discussion to get one's facts sorted out, casuistic sorting is deceptively simple: One may sort circumstances into the wrong topics, particularly when many circumstances are open to several interpretations, and, even worse, one sorts some circumstances in and others out. This latter fault arises from biases in the casuist and obviously biases the case. How can the casuist know that all the relevant circumstances have been collected and sorted? How can the casuist ensure that the right circumstances are in the right boxes? Another casuist might construct the case quite differently, using different circumstances or topics and combining them in different ways. Similarly, those presenting the case might, consciously or unconsciously, select certain details to the detriment of others (Kopelman 1994).

Classical casuistry countered these threats to good casuistic reasoning by sustaining a vigorous conversation within the community of casuists: volumes of cases, in repeated editions, cited the arguments and analyses of various casuists and opened them to challenge and criticism. They devised a sort of rating system to designate the probability that an author's opinion was sound or defective in some respect (Fleming 2007).

Critics challenge the casuist's manner of relating principles to circumstances. The principles are, in the casuist's view, embedded in the case. They convey only the most general meaning when stated in the abstract and without illustrating instances, which will always be cases. Yet the critic can ask what is the origin and nature of principles. It is not enough to assert that they are embedded in cases and need case-specificity for their meaning. Principles do appear to have at least general meaning on their own. We say without hesitation that lying is wrong or that superiors should not exploit the vulnerability of their inferiors. Also, principles are often used as the critical tool to attack a practice or an institution. Respect for persons, fairness, and equity, we might say, show that sexual harassment is immoral. Principles, then, appear to have some logical, epistemological, and ethical function apart from cases. Casuistry does not offer an account of that function. Indeed, it seems not only to ignore it but also to undermine it, since maxims and principles are always open to revision as new cases arise, and as they are revised in the light of circumstances, they lose their power as critical tools of moral discourse (Arras 1991). It is this feature of casuistic reasoning that leads some to assert that casuistry is a form of situation ethics.

This criticism raises the broader question of the relation of casuistry to ethical theory. Some casuists seem to imply that casuistry can thrive independently of ethical theory; cases and case series are, as was once said of the American Constitution, "an engine that runs by itself." This view of casuistry is historically wrong and logically incorrect. Casuistry may, indeed, run rather free from theory, but it is tethered to theory in many ways. The classical casuists honored the theory of natural law. Utilitarian moral theory involves casuistry in every determination of how the good is to be maximized. Bentham's felicific calculus sets the terms for utilitarian casuistry. Even Kantian theory draws on cases to illustrate the application of the categorical imperative. Indeed, Kant wrote a little manual of (rather clumsy) casuistry. To assert that casuistry does not depend on theory, however, may mean only that case reasoning is not deduction from theory and principles. It is not a denial that moral theory may serve as a broad background or an atmosphere for casuistic reasoning. It does not deny that certain methodological moves in moral theory might be quite relevant to casuistic thinking, such as the reflective equilibrium and specification methods mentioned in chapter 3.

Casuists are frequently accused of teaching that ethical principles and theory somehow emerge from cases; they have no independent source as grounds of morality. While some enthusiastic casuists may imply this, it is an exaggeration. Some thoughts on this question have been proposed earlier in this chapter, where we discussed the source of the weight of principles, but pursuit of this question would take us further into moral epistemology than this chapter allows. It might simply be said that moral philosophy always arises in some way from contemplation of moral experience, and moral experience is fashioned of cases. Yet the point at which principle and theory are abstracted from experience may be, and probably must be, distant from the riot of detail that makes up cases. It is intriguing to note that contemporary moral philosophers, utilizing the methods of cognitive psychology and neuroscience, discover the frameworks of deontological and teleological moral thinking in very concrete moral decisions, such as the now familiar case of having to decide whether to divert a trolley toward one person in order to avoid killing five (Appiah 2008; Sinnot-Armstrong 2008).

Finally, casuistry's reliance on paradigm cases and analogous reasoning has attracted criticism. The casuist maintains that moral reasoning moves not from theory and principle down to judgment but that it moves sideways from clear to less clear case. This leaves open what makes a case clear enough to be a paradigm. In general the casuist might say that a clear case is one in which the circumstances are such that the relevant principle can be readily realized in choice and action, and no other maxims contest for primacy. However, this still leaves many questions.

One casuist's paradigm may not be that of another casuist, since cases can be viewed under different perspectives. For example, the same facts constitute a case of assisted suicide and a case of medical manslaughter, but one casuist comes at those facts from the stance of personal autonomy and another comes at the same facts from the perspective of protection of the vulnerable. Also, paradigm cases are not Platonic ideas, free of earthly connections. They are instances found in quite real cultural settings imbued with custom and history. The moral judgment made about their paradigmatic status cannot be isolated from those earthly connections. Furthermore, in the culture of moral pluralism that we inhabit it is unlikely that everyone or even many will settle on a set of paradigms satisfactory to all. Also, paradigm cases do not appear in full dress. Often, they are cases that at first view are very perplexing. Through examination and argument, they move into the paradigm status, because the relationship between principle and circumstance comes strikingly clear. The case of Karen Ann Quinlan, for example, begins in confusion, but persistent examination reveals how the conjunction of circumstances meets the principles of respect, beneficence, and non-maleficence. It early became and still stands as a paradigm.

Finally, if paradigms are the final testing ground for moral judgments about analogous cases, the certitude of the paradigm must be guaranteed in some fashion. If casuistry declines to refer its judgments to some prior ethical theory, then the paradigms themselves must be the locus of certitude. This appears to invoke the questionable moral epistemology of intuitionism, moved from its usual place among principles to the realm of paradigm cases (Juengst 1989; Wildes 1991). Yet intuitionism is finding new support in the new moral psychology mentioned above.

Finally, DeGrazia and Beauchamp assert, in chapter 3, that "casuistry risks being unable to make progress on controversial issues . . . and overlooking very general and fundamental issues, the resolution of which may be relevant to specific cases." This is true, but it is not a problem for casuistry as such. Rather, it criticizes any casuist who claims that casuistry is the whole of moral philosophy. It is but a method of reasoning that aims to make broad generalizations about the moral life relevant to particular cases. Broad generalizations as such emerge from critical moral philosophy and social commentary, as well as from groundswells of moral indignation or aspiration in a society. A functioning casuistry will be sensitive to these as explained above in the discussion of weighting of principles. DeGrazia and Beauchamp offer treatment of animals as an example of their criticism. Casuistry would have relatively little to say on this subject if it relied on the history of moral debate, but it can enter that debate as it becomes controversial, and as various broad principles emerge, by working to elucidate the particular cases that are brought to attention, for example, treatment of animals as experimental subjects, as trained for sports, or as food for humans (Jonsen 2005). Still, it is reasonable to ask the casuist, as Stanley Hauerwas (1983) does, how do competing, critical, innovative moral notions force their way into a moral tradition?

If the casuist is more than a moral mechanic, fiddling with the machinery of cases, the questions will be taken seriously. Even the dedicated casuist must admit that the work of casuistry is, as one critic said, "only an engine of thought" (Arras 1991). It stimulates the mind to move in certain directions as it asks what ought to be done "in the occasion," as Aristotle said. It is a tactic of bringing the circumstances into the moral evaluation of the case. Techniques and tactics are never the whole story; they work within a larger context of understanding. So the techniques of casuistry, topics, principles and circumstances, paradigms and analogy, work within a broader understanding of the nature of the moral life, of moral reasoning, of the history of ethics, and of cultural and institutional values.

❧ Concluding Comments

Casuistry is not "a much less respectable" study than theoretical ethics. Professor Moore, who wrote those words, was a Cambridge don for whom respectability came from lineage and who probably left details of daily life to the college servants. The lineage of classical casuistry was, unfortunately, tainted by some of its practitioners and so must have gained Moore's disdain. However, today we can trace that lineage back to more reputable ancestors, including Aristotle, Cicero, and the Stoics.

Even more important than ancestry, we find contemporary casuists who are honest ethicists working with difficult problems. Also, the details of daily life are no longer beneath the notice of respectable people. Those details are the stuff of ethical judgment, and they come to us in the form of cases, episodes real or imagined of human action. Casuistry is ethics respecting the moral dimensions of the gritty stuff of daily life and, as such, deserves respect. The casuistic method not only respects the mundane but helps the ethicist, whether philosopher or physician, to work within the circumstances of the mundane. Its ultimate title for respect derives from the ability of its practitioners to elucidate the obscurities of particular cases so that people may be helped to make responsible decisions, that is, decisions that are responsive to the needs, desires, exigencies, and hopes that generate the case, as well as responsive to the principles and values that sustain human dignity. To the extent that casuistry achieves this end, it deserves (as Professor Moore does admit) respect as an endeavor that "ethics is not complete without."

❧ Notes on Resources and Training

The job description for a casuist is peculiar. First, there is no Department of Casuistry (although the various centers that go by the names "practical" or "applied ethics" might offer a class or a course). Also, there are no jobs for casuists as such. Professors of ethics or ethics consultants might use casuistry from time to time and even pride themselves for their skill at case analysis, but they don't inscribe "Casuist" on their name tags. Second, the training specified in the job description might contain some rather odd requirements, referring to skills rarely attained in courses. Indeed, the casuist might be defined in terms of his or her virtues. Aristotle remarks, "Prudence is not concerned with universals only; it must also take cognizance of particulars, because it is concerned with conduct, and conduct has its sphere in particular circumstances" (*Nichomachean Ethics* 1141b 15–17). Those circumstances are, he says, "the agent, the act, the object of the act, the instrument, the aim and the manner" (*Nichomachean Ethics* 1111a 1–5). The prudent person, he says, is one who can deliberate well about particulars. And again, he says, "The field of deliberation is that which happens for the most part, where the result is obscure and the right course not clearly defined; and for important decisions we call in advisors, distrusting our own ability to reach a decision" (*Nichomachean Ethics* 1112b 9–11). A casuist should be such an adviser.

The casuist should be cognizant of particulars, that is, should have a solid, even scientific understanding of the topics within the endeavor in which advice is given (thus, a medical ethicist must be reasonably familiar with medical science and clinical medicine, a business ethicist must understand economics, banking, investment, and commerce). He or she should recognize the obscurity of situations and thus depend on other involved parties to illuminate as best they can. He or she must be able to hear and hold in mind a variety of arguments appropriate to the complex situations and be aware of possible paradigm cases. He or she should be able to tolerate uncertainty about the right course and, within that uncertainty, find a reasonable course of action, that is, the course recommended by the most persuasive argument in the circumstances, with due recognition of other arguments that are plausible. A good casuist must, then, have all the intellectual virtues recommended by Aristotle: science, prudence, intuition, wisdom.

Casuistry can be taught as a skill by outlining the technique and by inviting the student to apply it to cases again and again. Persons more adept can criticize the adequacy of the application. However, the casuist must constantly argue his or her analysis with others from and outside the world of ethics. The initial framing and analysis of a case must be subject to other views and other sources of information. Casuistry should not be a solitary reflection but a vivid interchange of facts and ideas. This sort of exercise is training for casuistry. Another aspect of training is the broadening education about ethical theory, history of ethics, and the ethos of the culture (or cultures) where casuistry is being performed. Practicing casuists should regularly read and contribute to the published case studies that are now available in the literature of bioethics. In this way they can re-create something of the community of criticism that once existed within classical casuistry.

A final characteristic of a casuist is a controversial one: The casuist must be a person of probity. As Pascal brilliantly exposed, casuistry can be cleverness that makes convincing arguments in defense of reprehensible behavior. The casuist must be able to control his or her cleverness, or ethical virtuosity, and link it to serious moral intent. Aristotle recognized this, saying, "If the aim of action is noble, cleverness is praiseworthy but if the aim is ignoble, cleverness is unscrupulousness ... now since only a good person can discern the good for humans and because wickedness can distort this vision and cause serious error about the principles of conduct, it is evident that one cannot be prudent without being good" (*Nichomachean Ethics* 1144a 24–27). This is a strong proposition and unwelcome to many modern hearers, yet it is worth pondering. Even if we cannot conceive a model of virtue, or demand that every person be a paragon of all virtues, at least we can recommend honesty, truthfulness, fidelity, compassion, and responsibility, and hope that ethical advisers possess these moral characteristics. Whether these virtues come by nature or nurture remains a perennial question.

The principal resources for the study of casuistry lie hidden in rare book libraries. The casuistic books of the era of high casuistry, 1550–1650, contain the full panoply of cases and analyses that lay the foundations for the methodology proposed by contemporary commentators. A list of the major casuistic books of that era can be found as an appendix to *The Abuse of Casuistry*. Contemporary resources for the study of casuistry are both historical and analytic. An adequate understanding of casuistry and a sound criticism of its strengths and weaknesses must be informed by both its history and by the critical analyses employed by philosophers, theologians, and rhetoricians.

A collection of informative essays, *Conscience and Casuistry in Early Modern Europe* (Leites 1988), exposes the social and religious changes in the seventeenth century that radically modified the perceived relationship between personal conscience and law, and the consequent shifts in the ways in which morality was conceived and taught, stimulating the growth of casuistic thinking. The acute crisis of conscience that the English Reformation forced on many religious people was a significant source of much seventeenth-century casuistry; that story is told in detail in Elliot Rose's *Cases of Conscience: Alternatives Open to Recusants and Puritans under Elizabeth I and James I* (Rose 1975). Pascal's critique of casuistry is itself criticized by Richard Parish (1989) in *Pascal's Lettres Provinciales: A Study in Polemic*, a book that sustains in substance the critique of Pascal's attack made by Jonsen and Toulmin (1987) in *The Abuse of Casuistry*.

The contemporary literature cited previously in this essay, particularly the essays mentioned in "Critiques of Casuistry," constitute the principal resources for the current reflections on the use of the casuistic method. However, much of that literature is polemical rather than systematic. Efforts to explain the nature of casuistic reasoning more systematically are rare, but several are worthy of notice. One of these, Kenneth Kirk's *Conscience and Its Problems*, was written many years ago (1927) but a recent reedition, with introduction by David Smith, makes available a learned and literary exposition of classical casuistic ethics (1999). Kirk's remark, "The abuse of casuistry is properly directed, not against all casuistry, but only against its abuse," suggested the title for Jonsen and Toulmin's *Abuse of Casuistry* and many of Kirk's insights informed the theses of that book.

The Abuse of Casuistry surveyed rather summarily the ancient and medieval precursors to the high casuistry of the Renaissance. A volume of essays edited by James Keenan and Thomas Shannon, *The Context of Casuistry* (1995), goes more deeply into that earlier literature, particularly the writings of the nominalist theologians who immediately preceded the neo-scholasticism of the Renaissance. Several essays explore the work of the Anglican casuists and the effect of casuistry (or its abuse) in the moral theology manuals of the nineteenth century. This volume is a valuable addition to the history of casuistic thinking. Baruch Brody's *Life and Death Decision Making* (1988) is the major exposition of a form of casuistic reasoning that gives a larger place to ethical theory than does the method explained above. Carson Strong has written many essays in defense of a paradigm-based casuistry and lucidly applied his own version of casuistic method in the analysis of difficult cases in pediatrics, obstetrics, and reproductive medicine (1988, 1997, 1999, 2000).

Richard B. Miller's *Casuistry and Modern Ethics* (1996) is a book about casuistry that would be dear to any casuist's heart. He explains casuistic methodology as he works through particular cases. He moves beyond the bioethical problems that have absorbed the attention of the bioethical casuists and turns to cases raised by modern warfare, politics, and social issues. His use of casuistic method is insightful and imaginative, balanced and provocative, all virtues required in the contemporary casuist. In *Fragmentation and Consensus*, Mark Kuczewski (1999) explores the similarities and differences between two approaches to moral philosophy, casuistry and communitarianism and, in so doing, explicates several of the most difficult problems inherent in casuistic reasoning, the selection of paradigms, and the role of consensus.

Julia Fleming's book, *Defending Probabilism: The Moral Theology of Juan Caramuel* (2007), is a meticulous exposition of the system of rating moral opinions found in the classical casuists, with particular reference to the seventeenth-century theologian Caramuel, who was known as the Prince of Casuists, a prolific producer of opinions about complex moral conundrums. A recent interest in pragmatism as a method in bioethics relies heavily on one feature of casuistry, the aim toward practical resolution of cases, relying on empirical exploration (McGee 2003).

Finally, it should be mentioned that the new interest that moral philosophers, cognitive psychologists, and neuroscientists have taken in moral psychology touches casuistry at many points. Cases are regularly published in several of the major journals of bioethics and are often accompanied by critical commentary. Collections of cases and commentary can be found in many bioethics textbooks and anthologies. Among these are the cases that have appeared in the *Hastings Center Report* from its beginnings in the 1970s (Crigger 1998) and Gregory Pence's narrative of many of the major cases that have engaged bioethicists (1995).

❧ References

Appiah, Kwame Anthony. 2008. *Experiments in ethics*. Cambridge, MA: Harvard University Press.

Aristotle. 1976. Nichomachean ethics. In *The ethics of Aristotle*. Trans. and ed. J. A. K. Thomson and Hugh Tredennick. London: Penguin Books.

Arras, John. 1991. The revival of casuistry in bioethics. *Journal of Medicine and Philosophy* 16:29–51.

Beauchamp, Tom, and James Childress. 1994. *Principles of biomedical ethics*. 4th ed. New York and Oxford: Oxford University Press.

Bellah, Robert, Richard Madsen, William Sullivan, Ann Swidler, and Steven Tipton. 1985. *Habits of the heart*. New York: Harper and Row, 6.

Brody, Baruch. 1988. *Life and death decision making*. New York: Oxford University Press.

Cicero. 1975. *On duties (De officiis)*. Trans. Walter Miller. Cambridge, MA: Harvard University Press.

Crigger, Bette-Jane. 1998. *Cases in bioethics. Selections from the Hastings Center Report*. 3rd ed. New York: St. Martin's Press.

Fleming, Julia. 2007. *Defending probabilism: The moral theology of Juan Caramuel*. Washington, DC: Georgetown University Press.

Hauerwas, Stanley. 1983. Casuistry as a narrative art. *Interpretation* 37:377–88.

Jonsen, Albert R. 1993a. Casuistry, situationism and laxity. In *Joseph Fletcher: Memoir of an ex-radical. reminiscence and reappraisal*, ed. Kenneth Vaux. Louisville: John Knox Press.

———. 1993b. Platonic insults: Casuistical. *Common Knowledge* 2:48–66.

———. 2000. Strong on casuistry. *Journal of Medicine and Philosophy* 3:348–60.

———. 2005. *Bioethics beyond the headlines*. Lanham, MD: Rowman & Littlefield, ch. 14.

Jonsen, Albert, Mark Siegler, and William Winslade. 2006. *Clinical ethics. A practical approach to ethical decisions in clinical medicine*. 6th ed. New York: McGraw-Hill, 1.

Jonsen, Albert R., and Stephen Toulmin. 1987. *The abuse of casuistry. A history of moral reasoning*. Berkeley: University of California Press.

Juengst, Eric. 1989. Casuistry and the locus of certitude in ethics. *Journal of Medical Humanities* 3:19–27.

Keenan, James F., and Thomas A. Shannon. 1995. *The context of casuistry*. Washington, DC: Georgetown University Press.

Kirk, Kenneth. 1927 [1999]. *Conscience and its problems*. Introduction by David Smith. Louisville: John Knox Westminster Press, 126.

Kopelman, Loretta. 1994. Case method and casuistry: The problem of bias. *Theoretical Medicine* 15:21–37.

Kuczewski, Mark G. 1999. *Fragmentation and consensus: Communitarian and casuist bioethics.* Washington, DC: Georgetown University Press.

Leites, Edmund, ed. 1988. *Conscience and casuistry in early modern Europe.* Cambridge: Cambridge University Press.

McGee, Glen, ed. 2003. *Pragmatic bioethics.* Cambridge, MA: MIT Press.

Miller, Richard B. 1996. *Casuistry and modern ethics.* Chicago: University of Chicago Press.

Moore, G. E. 1903. *Principia ethica.* Cambridge: Cambridge University Press, 4–5.

National Commission for the Protection of Human Subjects of Biomedical and Behavioral Research. 1977. *Research involving children.* Washington, DC: Government Printing Office.

Parish, Richard. 1989. *Pascal's lettres provinciales. A study in polemic.* Oxford: The Clarendon Press.

Pascal, Blaise. 1657/1967. *The provincial letters.* Trans. A Krailsheimer. London: Penguin Classics.

Pence, Gregory. 1995. *Classical cases in medical ethics.* New York: McGraw-Hill.

Rose, Elliott. 1975. *Cases of conscience: Alternatives open to recusents and Puritans under Elizabeth I and James I.* Cambridge: Cambridge University Press.

Ross, D. W. 1930. *The right and the good.* Oxford: Clarendon Press, 19–36.

Sinnott-Armstrong, Walter, ed. 2008. *Moral psychology.* 3 vols. Cambridge, MA: MIT Press.

Strong, C. 1988. Justification in ethics. In *Moral theory and moral judgments in medical ethics,* ed. Baruch Brody, 193–211. Dordrecht, The Netherlands: Kluwer Academic Publishers.

———. 1997. *Ethics in reproductive and perinatal medicine: A new framework.* New Haven, CT: Yale University Press.

———. 1999. Critiques of casuistry and why they are mistaken. *Theoretical Medicine and Bioethics* September 20 (5): 395–411.

———. 2000. Specified principlism: What is it and does it really resolve cases better than casuistry? *Journal of Medicine and Philosophy* June 25 (3): 323–41.

Wildes, Kevin. 1991. The priesthood of bioethics and the return of casuistry. *Journal of Medicine and Philosophy* 18:33–49.

CHAPTER 8

Legal Methods

MARK A. HALL AND NANCY M. P. KING

American bioethics owes much of its existence, and derives much of its content, from the law. Biomedical ethics first gained force and prominence in the 1960s through the judicial development and application of the informed consent doctrine. In the 1970s and 1980s, legal disputes over the right to die dominated the field, culminating in the 1990s with Supreme Court decisions in the *Cruzan* (feeding tube) and *Glucksberg* (assisted suicide) cases, followed by the legal battles against Dr. Kevorkian and within the Schiavo family. The list goes on and continues to expand (Poland 1997). Much of the debate over organ transplants, genetic technologies, reproductive rights, and access to care is framed, at least initially, in terms of what the law should or does allow or prohibit (Mazzoni 1998). Legal disputes like these are the means by which medical ethics frequently comes into the public eye. In addition, medical ethics jobs can be created thanks to the law, especially after an institution suffers some legal action or public humiliation. In short, both for better and for worse, law permeates medical ethics. Therefore, those who study medical ethics need at least some understanding of how legal institutions and legal analyses function.

Because medical ethics is not itself a discipline and those who practice medical ethics come from a range of disciplines, it should not be a surprise that there are many lawyers whose work is exclusively in bioethics. Some rarely (if ever) publish in law reviews, teach law students, or contribute to legal briefs. Others divide their efforts between primarily legal and predominantly medical or medical ethics audiences. Those who work in medical ethics and wish to immerse themselves in the law can learn to read cases and statutes and learn how legal scholars analyze cases and statutes in law review articles and law–medicine casebooks, simply through exposure to these strictly legal genres. Indeed, a number of prominent medical ethics scholars without formal legal education are well known for their mastery of the law.

Many resources provide legal primers for the uninitiated so that is not this chapter's objective. Indeed, "legal methods" is a somewhat imprecise term in this context. Instead, we aim to provide an overview of law's role in medical ethics, in order to assist readers in using legal materials and understanding legal thinking well enough to grasp when and how legal methods can do ethics work. In short, this chapter bridges between law and medical ethics by increasing the ability of nonlawyers to appreciate and incorporate legal perspectives usefully into their medical ethics work. We start with a perspective on law from the view of practicing lawyers and then shift to the variety of ways that legal scholars seek to deepen understanding of the theory and impact of law.

☙ Description of Legal Methods

One can approach the law in each of three mindsets: as a practicing lawyer, as an academic theoretician, and as a social scientist. The first approach is descriptive, the second is analytic, and the third is empirical. This section discusses each in turn.

PRACTICING LAWYERS

To learn to practice law, one must go to law school. Nonetheless, while a short chapter is not a substitute for a proper legal education, we can usefully describe attributes of how practitioners approach and analyze legal problems.

First, lawyers are obsessed with jurisdictional questions (meaning the reach of legal authority in any specific situation). A common error in legal research is to focus exclusively on one source of law (e.g., federal legislation) to the exclusion of others (e.g., administrative regulations, case law, or state statutes). Even if it is determined that a piece of federal legislation is relevant, how is it interpreted by the courts or through administrative regulations? Furthermore, has Congress exceeded its own powers or violated constitutional guarantees of individual rights in enacting the law?

These are critical questions that often require some sophisticated comprehension of the law, so generally we turn to lawyers for answers. Even so, nonlawyers can fully appreciate that law emanates from many sources that are arranged hierarchically. Federal law trumps state law, and the Constitution trumps statutes, which trump regulations. The residual source of law that fills the remaining empty spaces is known as the common law—law created solely by court decisions, also often referred to as case law. In American jurisprudence the common law is a relatively powerful instrument, even though the body of statutory law (enacted by legislatures) is vast and growing all the time. A generalization that contrasts common-law jurisdictions (the United States and the United Kingdom) with civil law (or statutorily based) jurisdictions (e.g., the European Union) is this: According to civil law, everything not permitted is forbidden; according to common law, everything not forbidden is permitted. It is, in part, the creativity allowed by judge-made common law that accounts for law's considerable influence in medical ethics.

Contrary to initial appearances, there often is a rhyme and a reason for deciding which legal issues fall into which cells in this complex hierarchical matrix, but the reasons may be hard to identify. The federal Patient Self-Determination Act (PSDA) is a good example. Although the PSDA was enacted to avoid *Cruzan/Schiavo*-type scenarios by encouraging advance care planning, its authority is necessarily limited. It requires hospitals that receive federal funding to ask patients whether they have an advance directive (AD), and if they do not, then to provide an opportunity for them to complete one during their hospitalization. The requirement targets hospitals because federal authority can reach those institutions, even though everyone acknowledges that education about and completion of ADs before hospitalization is far more preferable (since this provides more time for reflection and full discussion, strengthens the patient–clinician bond, reduces emotional trauma, and helps to counter the mistaken notion that ADs are recommended only for those in dire medical situations). To allay concerns that the PSDA might be viewed as a means of pressuring patients to have ADs, or even to write ADs as a way to express cost-saving choices (as opposed to merely ensuring that the opportunity to have an AD is made available to all), the PSDA requires only that hospital personnel ask questions and provide information. Because it is an unfunded mandate, however, the PSDA alone does not ensure that any hospital provides adequate, comprehensive, or timely resources and assistance to patients.

Judicial opinions

In trying to understand other parts of the law, one frequently starts with reading judicial opinions. These fascinating texts are especially important in our legal system for two reasons: first, statutory (or codified) law is usually general and ambiguous in important respects and so can be fully understood only as interpreted and applied to particular factual scenarios by the courts; and second, judicial decisions have precedential effect, meaning that lower courts must honor the principles announced by higher, appellate courts, and courts at the same level see great value in remaining consistent with each other and with their past decisions.

Only the decisions of higher courts have value as precedent. When a higher (appellate) court makes a decision, it relies on a certain construction of the facts that have been determined, or found, by a lower court. However, seldom are two legal scenarios precisely the same. Therefore, even with clearly decided cases as precedent, lawyers must rely on some form of what might be called analogic reasoning. They compare the facts of their situation to a previous decision and analyze the extent of similarity and whether the differences are likely to affect the outcome of a hypothetical new dispute. This requires experiential professional understanding of which factors courts or administrators deem most or least relevant.

When lower courts make determinations of fact, these have no precedential value, are not reported, and are therefore invisible to legal analysts. In the medical arena, the fact that one jury may have found a doctor negligent for failing to do a test says nothing about whether the law requires the test to be done. This is only a single datum regarding the risk another physician might face—a datum that hardly is conclusive. Each case is distinct, and each jury decides based only on its own deliberation over the evidence it hears.

Clearly this is not a scientific or quantitative enterprise. The practice of law is much less evidence based than even the practice of medicine. Ultimately lawyers must make judgments about probabilities, but these judgments are highly uncertain and usually are expressed in primarily qualitative terms. Few scenarios are clearly legal or clearly illegal; rather, a variety of different legal consequences are usually arrayed over a range of very high to very low likelihoods.

These probability predictions frequently depend on factors other than a bare description of the law. We know the speed limit with precision, but the practical questions posed might be: "How likely am I to be caught?" and "What is the penalty?" How parties choose to act on these predictions depends a great deal on what the stakes are. On the one hand, no one wants to be charged with a criminal act. On the other, being found in violation of a contract might be viewed not as immoral or disreputable but as simply an honest difference of opinion or, even more pragmatically, as just a cost of doing business. Thus, to nonlawyers, the law may seem to operate with a sometimes substantial disconnect between court decisions and the real world.

Law and real world medical ethics

Another brief example helps to illustrate the difference between the law in the books and the law in action. One of the seminal decisions on end-of-life treatment is *Barber v. Superior Court*, in which the court declared that disputes about the appropriateness of withholding or withdrawing treatment at or near the end of a patient's life should not be heard in the criminal courts.[1] The clear assertion that medical decision making lacks criminal intent except in unusual circumstances was extremely important for physicians, patients and families, and medical institutions. However, after the decision exonerated the Kaiser physicians who had withdrawn life support at the family's request, the policy at Kaiser hospitals regarding end-of-life treatment abatement became highly restrictive, at least for a time. This seems paradoxical: If physicians and their institutions need not fear criminal prosecution, it should become easier for physicians, patients, and families to make appropriate decisions at the end of life. Yet it is also reasonable for hospital counsel to consider the cost of public scrutiny too high. Thus, risk managers see both the need and the legal justification for a conservative interpretation of statutory and case law—leaving it to patient advocates, practicing clinicians, and medical ethics scholars to continue to press for greater patient and family autonomy in end-of-life choices. The result is a negotiation process that remains ongoing in health care facilities nationwide.

We see, then, that another commonality between legal practice and medical ethics practice is an interest in improving and reforming real-world policies and institutions. A good example comes from the development of end-of-life decision making since the *Cruzan* case in 1990.

This literature is truly enormous, extraordinarily varied, and impossible to summarize here. However, a brief tour of provides a good sense of the ongoing role of lawyers doing medical ethics at many levels, from legislatures to client advice to hospital ethics committees. The legal trajectory of the *Cruzan* decision can be captured, albeit rather cursorily, by noting what happened in its immediate aftermath: extensive state legislative activity amending living will statutes to explicitly address artificial nutrition and hydration and permanent loss of consciousness; and enacting health care proxy statutes permitting individuals to name substitute decision makers to make treatment decisions for them should they become decisionally incapable (King 1996). Those with medical ethics training often worked with medical societies and other groups to provide analysis or advocacy regarding proposed post-*Cruzan* statutory changes. New state laws also meant amended or new AD forms, which then required extensive education and translation between legal and lay understandings. Those with medical ethics and legal expertise worked with hospital policy and forms committees to devise workable systems for capturing ADs; with hospital ethics committees to interpret and make use of ADs in the decision-making process; and with health care providers and the public to educate them in a wide variety of settings, from conferences to shopping mall information tables, often with the assistance of advocacy groups.

It was not surprising, then, that when the *Schiavo* case became national news, the first reaction of many in medical ethics was "But haven't we already *done* all that?" Nevertheless, among the many effects of Teresa Schiavo's sad story was a new round of state legislative activity, including efforts in many states to narrow the permissible scope of ADs, efforts by legal and medical ethics scholars to resist restrictive changes and improve education for legislators and public alike, and renewed attention to interpretation of state laws, including creation of new AD documents and educational materials.[2] In these ways common and statutory law provide the framework upon which medical ethics builds much of its scholarship and service.

Despite the limited view that judicial opinions give of the actual operation of the law, the law's focus on case law is especially convenient for medical ethics, which also often takes a case-based analytical approach called casuistry (see chapter 7). But perhaps the similarities have done harm to medical ethics by causing it to emulate judicial reasoning too much. Judges are called on to make authoritative and binding decisions, while medical ethics usually aspires only to better understanding of a situation or conflict. For these reasons medical ethics might borrow more profitably from academic rather than real-world legal methods.

LEGAL SCHOLARS

Practicing lawyers are concerned with the application of general legal principles to specific cases. Academic lawyers are more concerned with understanding the general principles of law. They develop descriptive or predictive theories about why law is the way it is and normative theories about how law should be. A leading, and perhaps dominant, branch of legal theory is economic analysis of law, many of whose principal scholars have been associated with the University of Chicago (e.g., Richard Epstein and Judge Richard Posner). Classical economic theory views law instrumentally— as a means to achieve greater social or personal welfare—denying that it has any intrinsic moral value. Critics charge that this reductionist view neglects both the wider range of values that law advances and the inevitably emotional and illogical dimensions of human action.

Even when law is viewed as value laden, however, moral theory does not necessarily match up well with practical legal realities. An example is the doctrine of informed consent, which, as previously noted, represents one of the earliest connections between law and medical ethics. The contemporary judicial interpretation and state statutory creation of the doctrine as a type of medical malpractice means that the failure to obtain a patient's informed consent represents negligence by the treating physician (Faden, Beauchamp, and King 1986). Thus, a complaint alleging lack of informed consent must meet a set of standards that is in large part common to all malpractice claims, including proof that the patient was injured as a result of the treatment and that a reasonable person in the patient's position, if properly informed, would have refused the treatment and therefore would not have suffered the injury. This requires proof not only that a reasonable person in the patient's position would consider the omitted information "material" to the decision whether or not to consent to treatment but also that it would have been reasonable to refuse the treatment if the omitted information had been provided.

This complex doctrine means that, in practice, the law plays out much differently in court than the way physicians are and should be taught to inform patients. The informed consent process is prospective, but the courts necessarily look backward, to what actually transpired in a case gone wrong. Physicians in training are generally taught to provide more information than that which is likely to result in liability if not provided, and ethical and professional training tends to be fairly uniform across the country even though important aspects of the legal doctrine of informed consent vary considerably from state to state.

Moreover, the informed consent doctrine's legal characterization as medical negligence ensures that litigators view it somewhat differently from legal scholars. Litigators tend to view the doctrine primarily as an invention designed to get around the problem of expert testimony in ordinary medical negligence cases. The success of a medical malpractice case depends upon the testimony of an expert that there was indeed negligence in the treatment itself, and in the 1960s and 1970s many plaintiffs' lawyers encountered what they termed a "conspiracy of silence," whereby physicians were reluctant to testify against their fellow professionals. Many of those who did provide expert testimony for plaintiffs were widely regarded as providing opinions for hire rather than highly credible testimony. Thus, many apparently meritorious medical negligence cases—and many seriously injured plaintiffs—could not get a hearing. The development of the informed consent doctrine as a theory of liability circumvented the need for expert testimony, often in those same cases, by measuring the standard for required disclosure according to the needs and interests of the reasonable patient facing treatment rather than according to the medical community's expert judgment. To plaintiffs' lawyers, then, the informed consent doctrine was primarily a new way for injured patients to prevail in court and get financial relief; to academic lawyers and medical ethics scholars, it was more important that it offered a novel legal formulation of a central principle of medical ethics (Faden, Beauchamp, and King 1986).

Is vs. Ought: How law does medical ethics

Legal scholarship resembles medical ethics scholarship in this respect: They both draw from eclectic sources. The branches of legal scholarship are as varied and numerous as the methods found in all of the humanities and social sciences. Recognizing the value of a broad theoretical armamentarium, the law professor, like the bioethics scholar, is the original "jack of all trades, master of none." Legal scholars experiment with the tools of historians, economists, sociologists, literary theorists, moral philosophers, and many others (Crump 2001). Rather than attempting to examine the methodology of legal scholarship as typified by law review articles addressing topics and issues of interest to medical ethics, we provide two key examples of how legal considerations and legal arguments can contribute to the ways in which medical ethics issues are discussed in the literature and addressed in law and policy. These examples illustrate how legal scholarship can help distinguish between what law is and what it ought to be, with respect to a medical ethics issue, by examining important dimensions of theory, policy, and practice.

Key example 1: Genetic discrimination legislation. The first example we consider is the issue of genetic discrimination, as addressed through legislation. Although family history has always provided important information regarding the heritability of a variety of disorders and conditions, it was not until the advent of genetic testing that concerns about discriminatory practices in insurance and employment, based on genetic information, became widespread. Breast cancer susceptibility test results were at the forefront of concern. States began to pass legislation prohibiting genetic discrimination in the mid-1970s and early 1980s, and continued through the 1990s.

Early legal scholarship addressing genetic discrimination fell into several categories: surveying, cataloguing, and critiquing existing legislation (e.g., Rothenberg 1995); detailed analysis of statutory terminology (e.g., Rothstein 1998); proposals for amended and new legislation (e.g., Annas 2001); and research examining whether the fear of genetic discrimination exceeded the reality of actual discriminatory denials of insurance or employment (e.g., Hall and Rich 2000).

Public concern about genetic discrimination persisted throughout the 1990s and beyond, despite a paucity of evidence of actual discrimination. Genetic testing technologies became more powerful and broader in scope (Kahn and Wolf 2007), and large-scale databases emerged combining genetic with phenotypic data from medical and other records; still, there was little evidence of discrimination. Even as more states enacted legislation, calls for comprehensive federal legislation began to mount as early as the mid-90s, spurred in part by NIH scientists, who viewed enactment of clear federal law as essential to the progress of genomic research. After extensive discussion and advocacy, the Genetic Information Nondiscrimination Act (GINA) ultimately passed in 2008. Legal scholarship played and continues to play an important role in this policy arena, from advocacy for GINA's passage to explanations of precisely what protections it affords and recommendations about improving critical aspects of laws governing the use of genetic and other health information (Hudson, Holohan, and Collins 2008; Rothstein 2008a, 2008b, 2008c).

Key example 2: Biospecimen ownership. Our second example is drawn from case law regarding the ownership of biospecimens. The realization that biospecimens can have not only research importance but also significant competitive and commercial value has generated an important policy debate about intellectual property and ownership considerations deriving from biospecimens provided to researchers. The first and still most famous court decision, *Moore v. Regents of University of California*, 793 P.2d 479 (Cal. 1990), considered whether the specimen provider could claim any financial interest from the development of a scientifically lucrative cell line derived from his successfully treated cancer. A later case, *Greenberg v. Miami Children's Hosp. Research Inst., Inc.*, 264 F. Supp. 2d 1064 (S.D. Fla. 2003), addressed the patenting of a genetic test by a university that employed a faculty member who had worked with a disease constituency to develop the test and had not anticipated that the test would be made available only at a high cost.

Most recently, the *Catalona* decision (*Wash. University v. Catalona*, 490 F.3d 667 [8th Cir. 2007]) addressed the critical question of ownership of biospecimens provided by patients to a biorepository. Briefly, Dr. Catalona is a urologist and urological surgeon and researcher, with many loyal patients whom he has treated for prostate cancer. He is the developer of the widely used prostate-specific antigen (PSA) test for prostate cancer. While he was a faculty member at Washington University–St. Louis, he collected biospecimens for his research into the genetic basis of prostate cancer and helped to establish a large repository of biospecimens for genitourinary research at Washington University. When Dr. Catalona moved to Northwestern University, he asked specimen contributors for permission to bring the specimens with him so that he could continue his research. About six thousand of those who were contacted agreed; Washington University, however, contended that it alone owned all specimens in the biorepository and that, therefore, neither Dr. Catalona nor the specimen providers had the right to determine their disposition or use. The courts agreed. The 8th Circuit Court of Appeals, looking to the language of the consent forms employed and to Washington University's financial and infrastructure support of the repository itself, reasoned that the biospecimens were gifts to the university.

A considerable body of legal scholarship addresses all these cases and their attendant ethical issues, including not only ownership of biospecimens but also informed consent, the intent of biospecimen providers (usually called donors), commodification, and the profitability of health care applications of genetic information. Much of this is familiar law review territory. However, the enormous growth of scholarly commentary on biobanking and related topics has broadened the scope of legal commentary and firmly ensconced it outside law reviews. To give just one example, in the last few years alone the *Journal of Law, Medicine and Ethics* has published symposia on international biobanking regulation (Rothstein and Knoppers 2005), group interests in genetic biospecimen collection and research (Tsosie and McGregor 2007), and incidental findings in research with human subjects, a topic of special concern in genetic research and biobanking (Wolf et al. 2008).

The *Catalona* decision exemplifies this expanded focus in some of the work of Lori Andrews (2006), a prominent health lawyer and medical ethics scholar. During this litigation Andrews published an article detailing some of the nuances of the legal, regulatory, and policy arguments raised in the case. She and other scholars filled familiar roles for legal academics in the case: advising the parties' attorneys, helping to write *amicus* ("friend of the court") briefs, even providing testimony. Her writing about the case, however, while in form an analysis of the legal arguments, ranged widely enough to place the dispute in the larger policy framework surrounding genetic research, including the role and intentions of specimen providers, the commercial value of biospecimens, the permissible scope of biospecimen research, and the researcher–subject relationship.

This critique of the applicability of state law on *inter vivos* gifts to the circumstances of the case is a useful example of medical ethics and legal scholarship that begins from but expands beyond familiar law. It is positioned for a broader audience and fits well into the scholarly literature, based in many of the disciplines that make up medical ethics, addressing the human body and examining embodiment, identity, and commodification.[3]

EMPIRICAL STUDY OF LAW

The variety and complexity of legal scholarship is so great that it is not possible or useful in this space to survey all the methods employed, so we will focus on one that is especially relevant to medical ethics: empirical content analysis. Despite legal scholars' rich interdisciplinary study of legal doctrines and institutions, they have yet to identify an empirical methodology that is uniquely their own.[4] Instead, traditional legal methods, like ethics methods, are interpretive and qualitatively analytic. The researcher of case law reads a handful of appellate opinions and comments on their themes and likely social effects. This is done in a subjective, interpretive, or advocacy mode more akin to how a literary critic might interpret poetry than to scientific observation. Although legal or ethics writing in this mode may contain many assertions about how judges think or act, these are empirical only in a casual way. These analysts report what they see in key cases and how they interpret these observations, which others may agree or disagree with as they wish, rather than making any higher ontological claims about the true reality of case law or judicial behavior.

When legal scholars choose to employ empirical methods, often these are standard applications of basic social science methods to subjects of legal interest. Treating statutory, regulatory, or case law as a dependent variable, the range of potential social and economic influences on law that might be studied empirically is limited only by the bounds of a researcher's imagination. Or empiricists can treat law as an independent variable, meaning that they ask how case law influences other social and economic conditions.[5] With its diverse "laboratory of states," the United States offers boundless opportunities to learn from the "natural experiments" created by the inevitable differences in judicial and statutory law among jurisdictions and over time (Morriss 1995; Tremper et al. 2010).

In doing this kind of work, researchers may ably step into the shoes of social scientists, but their methods are not uniquely or especially legal methods. One standard social science technique—content analysis—could, however, form the basis for an empirical methodology that is uniquely legal. On the surface, content analysis appears simple, even trivial, to some. A researcher collects a set of documents (for instance, judicial opinions on a particular subject), reads them systematically, records consistent features of each one, and then draws inferences about their use and meaning (Krippendorff 2004). This method holds the potential for bringing social science rigor to the empirical understanding of case law, and therefore for creating what is distinctively a legal form of empiricism. For instance, claims about whether and how the informed consent doctrine shapes medical practice could be tested using content analysis to identify and verify different versions of the doctrine among the states.

Content analysis is a social science alternative that seeks objective understanding of a large number of decisions. The method also helps a researcher sort out the interaction of multiple factors that all have some bearing on an outcome in the legal system. The epistemological roots of content analysis lie in legal realism, the school of jurisprudence that rejects legal formalism (Leiter 1997). Oliver Wendell Holmes Jr. (1897) famously proclaimed that "prophecies of what the courts will do in fact, and nothing more pretentious, are what I mean by the law." This realist credo's call to empirical methods is obvious, but the call was never heeded by most of the original legal realists. Content analysis can help legal realists achieve their jurisprudential aims more scientifically—by generating objective, falsifiable, and reproducible knowledge about what courts do and how and why they do it.

Content analysis has it limits. It is best used when each decision should receive equal weight, that is, when it is appropriate to regard the content of opinions as generic data. Counting cases assumes that the information from one opinion is potentially as relevant as that from any other opinion. Because content analysis tends to regard all cases, judges, courts, and jurisdictions being studied the same, it should be used only with great caution when any of these have a great deal more status or influence than the others for the question addressed. This is often true in ethically relevant legal analysis because precedent and persuasiveness depend on various qualitative judgments about the reasons given or the source of the decision. "The legal and cultural salience of *Roe v. Wade* far outruns its statistical significance" (Goldsmith and Vermeule 2002).

Taking this limitation into account, scholars have found that it is especially useful to code and count cases in studies that question or debunk conventional legal wisdom. Using content analysis to disprove widely held views about case law has been especially successful because it highlights the methodological weakness of traditional legal analysis. One example relevant to health law is work that one of us did to show that ERISA does not have the protective effect on insurance companies defending coverage denials that many doctrinal scholars had assumed (Hall et al. 1996).

Analyzing the cause-and-effect relationship between legally relevant factors and the content of judicial opinions, however, raises a serious circularity problem: the facts and reasons found in an opinion might or might not accurately describe the real-world facts or the true nature of the judge's decision process. There is no reason to expect that appellate opinions should provide complete, objective, and result-neutral statements of all the facts in each case. Indeed, there is every reason to think just the opposite. Therefore, content analysts must acknowledge that "our information comes from what the judges decide to tell us about the cases, and it comes with all the blinders and biases of the bench job. . . . The judicial opinion is the judge's story justifying the judgment. The cynical legal realist might say that the facts the judge chooses to relate are inherently selective and a biased subset of the actual facts of the case" (Mendelson 1963, 558–59). In short it is circular or tautological to predict judicial outcomes from facts that reflect rather than generate the result.

From another viewpoint, however, the presumed bias created by courts' justifying their decisions may be precisely what a researcher wishes to study. After all, the facts and reasons the judge selects are the substance of the opinion that creates law and binding precedent, so they merit careful study for this very reason. This justification calls, however, for restraint and precision in setting the goals of the study. Instead of predicting outcomes, content analysis is better suited to studying judicial reasoning itself, retrospectively. Scholars can use the method to learn more, for instance, about how opinions are constructed and how results are justified. This type of study may be less relevant to practicing lawyers trying to predict successes and failures but perhaps is more relevant to legal and ethics scholars seeking a systematic and measurable understanding of the substantive law and the legal process.

In the most common approach, researchers simply observe and document what can be found, much like a naturalist might explore a new continent or even a familiar patch of woods, by turning over stones to see what crawls out. This general approach contrasts with more focused analytic projects that use formal, statistical hypothesis testing to generate fairly definitive conclusions about cause–effect relationships. Descriptive or exploratory studies are more akin to mapping than to testing. They discover and document a relevant legal landscape, often suggesting how or why it came to be but sometimes only noting its relevant features.

The primary criticism of these descriptive/exploratory studies is that they sometimes draw conclusions about features of the legal landscape that cannot be observed fully from judicial opinions. Observing win/loss records from published opinions tells us nothing, necessarily, about the decisions that judges chose not to write or to publish. Similarly, observing general trends in litigation shows only what the parties were not able or willing to settle before the matter reached trial or appeal.

In summary, content analysis does not lead to the Holy Grail of a true legal science as early proponents claimed it might. It is not possible to scientifically analyze legal principles and precedent at the level that is relevant to practicing lawyers or doctrinal scholars. For that, subjective interpretation of key cases remains the best method. Understanding law, like ethics, is no more easily reduced to a wholly scientific method than interpreting poetry is reducible to a literary science. However, content analysis is a useful adjunct to conventional legal analysis. It enables scholars to read and analyze decisions more systematically and objectively, to complement insights gained through conventional interpretive methods.

◦❖ Critique of Law's Influence on Medical Ethics

There are probably more negative than positive things to say about law's influence on medical ethics, but we will start with what's good. Among law's redeeming features is that it is concerned principally with solving disputes. Therefore, it has developed great acuity on two fronts relevant to medical ethics: a focus on fair and effective procedures, and resort to neutral (that is, not unduly subjective, value-laden) principles. Those concepts map, roughly speaking, to the terms "procedural justice" and "substantive justice" in political philosophy.

Only those who are exceptionally devout or naïve believe there is a right answer to every important question. Most of us understand that doing what is right is often more a matter of *how* rather than *what* decisions are reached. Legal theorists have dubbed this basic insight the legal process school of analysis. Following it, law has spun out a panoply of dispute resolution mechanisms and principles, both within and outside official legal settings, that have served medical ethics well.

Second, law in modern liberal democracies strives to articulate its substantive principles in a neutral fashion that is not unduly moralistic, theological, or personally subjective. Instead, law strives to be general, universal, and fairly objective. As the gender-specific slogan goes, we strive to be a "nation of laws, not men." This strength can also be seen as a weakness, though, because it suggests that biolaw must be value neutral. Often, it is inappropriate to claim that bioethics should ignore people's religious views or idiosyncratic subjective opinions, yet an unduly legalistic outlook might lead in that direction.

The role of law in medical ethics can be critiqued on a number of other fronts, which we summarize in quick order.

One: The legal mindset tends to engender a narrow, compliance-oriented focus that can fail to keep animating purposes front and center. By analogy, health care quality improvement is often criticized as unduly focused on structure and process measures rather than on actual outcomes. Similarly, a legal compliance orientation can distract attention from moral substance with the implicit assumption that ethical behavior is best captured through a set of enforceable rules and protocols. To the contrary, one eminent law professor once quipped that "the better the society, the less law there will be. In Heaven there will be no law, and the lion will lie down with the lamb. The values of an unjust society will reflect themselves in an unjust law. The worse the society, the more law there will be. In Hell there will be nothing but law, and due process will be meticulously observed" (Gilmore 1977).

Two: Law often is too blunt an instrument to do the fine-chiseled work required by ethics. As Carl Schneider (1994) aptly explains,

> the idioms of the law . . . have arisen in response to needs for social regulation, but the systemic imperatives that shape the law are sometimes a poor pattern for bioethical discourse. For example, the law of torts is centrally a way of compensating victims of an injury. But bioethicists have wanted the law of informed consent not just to remedy specific failures to inform patients, but to fundamentally reform the relationship between doctors and patients. However, tort law ill suits this ambitious goal. For one thing, the language of torts is the language of wrongs. . . . A doctor may obey it through quite mechanical and sadly unsatisfactory routines that mock the dialogue bioethicists imagine for doctors and patients.

Ethics, in contrast to law, requires "a rich vocabulary of ethical considerations, styles, and approaches. . . . Different bioethical issues arising in different contexts may demand a regime of rules or the flexibility of discretion, a rights discourse or a language of duties, public policy analysis or private preference, the salvation of religion or the neutrality of liberalism, the profits of principles or the insights of casuistry, the uses of utilitarianism or the devices of deontology, the rigors of economics or the consolations of philosophy" (1994).

Three: The failure of law to do a better job of regulating ethics would not be as much a problem if it did not also threaten to displace more nuanced ethical reflection. Frey (1997) refers to this as a crowd-out phenomenon. He observes that people can act out of either intrinsic or extrinsic motivation. Surveying a range of social and economic settings, he shows that regulatory legal regimes tend to crowd out intrinsic ethical motivation by replacing it with extrinsic rules. Legal rules usually are meant to enforce only minimally acceptable behaviors rather than to inspire aspirational ethical goals. It is just as wrong for law to demand perfection as it is for ethics to be content with legal minima, but conflating law with ethics tends to produce both results.

Medical law is not condemned to this gloomy fate. Conscious of these various pitfalls, law is capable of attending to the nuanced, relational features of medical settings and issues (Hall 2006). In better adapting to the medical context, there is much that law can and has learned from the analytical methods of medical ethics. Similarly medical ethics necessarily draws from the tools and concepts of law to advance its disciplinary aims. In doing so ethicists will become more conversant in the law and adept at its methods, but ethicists should resist displacing ethics with law.

ᴥ Notes on Resources and Training

Studying the legal dimensions of medical ethics requires an understanding not only of various bodies of legal doctrine (constitutional, tort, criminal, and so on) but also of how courts, legislatures, and administrative agencies function and interact at both the federal and state levels. Law-related courses in various parts of the university, including schools of public health, management, and public policy, can provide useful introduction and orientation, but there is no substitute for a formal legal educational and experience acquired through legal practice. Law libraries have rich repositories of primary and secondary legal resources, but many of these require significant training to be used effectively. This is also true for electronic legal databases, including Westlaw® and LexisNexis®, and many other web-based legal resources.

Still, useful sources abound for introductions and summaries of the law. The following are online sources accessible to nonlawyers:

> American Law Sources On-Line, www.lawsource.com/also/. A comprehensive and uniform compilation of links to freely accessible online sources of law for the United States and Canada. Also contains links to sources of commentary and practice aids.
>
> CataLaw, www.catalaw.com/. A catalog of catalogs of worldwide law on the Internet. It aids legal research by arranging all indexes of law and government into a uniform, universal, and unique metaindex.
>
> FindLaw, www.findlaw.com. Geared to the lay public.
>
> Global Legal Information Network, www.glin.gov/. From the Law Library of Congress, a database of laws, regulations, judicial decisions, and other complementary legal sources contributed by governmental agencies and international organizations. Includes official full texts of published documents in their original language.
>
> Legal Information Institute, www.law.cornell.edu/. From Cornell Law School, a very useful compilation of a wide variety of legal materials (primarily U.S.), such as state statutes on health, www.law.cornell.edu/topics/state_statutes. html#health.
>
> WashLaw, www.washlaw.edu/. Links to U.S. and international legal research on the Web.

The following texts provide good explanations and examples of how to research the law and how to conduct different types of legal analysis and reasoning:

Charles R. Calleros, *Legal Method and Writing*, 5th ed. (Aspen, 2006).
Christine Coughlin, Joan Malmud, and Sandy Patrick, *A Lawyer Writes: A Practical Guide to Legal Analysis* (Carolina Academic Press, 2008).
Susan Herskowitz, *Legal Research Made Easy*, 4th ed. (Sphinx Publishing, 2005).
Roy M. Mersky and Donald J. Dunn, *Legal Research Illustrated*, 8th ed. (Foundation Press, 2002).
Helene S. Shapo, Marilyn Walter, and Elizabeth Fajans, *Writing and Analysis in the Law*, 5th ed. (Foundation Press, 2008).
Amy E. Sloan, *Basic Legal Research: Tools and Strategies*, 3rd ed. (Aspen, 2006).

Lawmakers, judges, practitioners, scholars, and students of the law regularly contribute to legal knowledge through the production of legal and policy articles, comments, treatises, and instructional texts. It may be difficult for a nonlawyer to critically analyze legal arguments on their surface, but these materials, which include student-operated law reviews, subject-matter treatises, casebooks, and policy reviews, present broad overviews of legal subjects, allowing readers to learn a great deal on specific subjects without having to perform original legal research.

For law generally, these include legal encyclopedias (*Corpus Juris Secundum, American Jurisprudence*); annotations of law (e.g., *American Law Reports*); and condensed legal case reviews (e.g., *United States Law Week*). The authoritative legal dictionary is known as *Black's* (Garner 2004). For health law broadly the following are leading treatises and textbooks (known as casebooks):

Barry Furrow et al., *Health Law*, 2d ed. (West, 2001).
Furrow, Johnson, Jost, and Schwartz, *Health Law*, 6th ed. (West, 2008).
Lawrence Gostin, Judith Areen, Patricia King, Steven Goldberg, and Peter Jacobson, *Law, Science and Medicine*, 3rd ed. (Foundation Press, 2005).
Mark A. Hall, Mary Anne Bobinski, and David Orentlicher, *Health Care Law and Ethics*, 7th ed. (Aspen, 2007).
Mark A. Hall, Ira Mark Ellman, and Daniel S. Strouse, *Health Care Law and Ethics in a Nutshell*, 2d ed. (West, 1999).
Clark Havighurst, James Blumstein, and Troyen Brennan, *Health Care Law and Policy*, 2d ed. (Foundation Press, 1998).
Rand Rosenblatt, Sylvia Law, and Sarah Rosenbaum, *Law and the American Health Care System* (Foundation Press, 1997).

Focusing on law and medical ethics are the following:

G. J. Annas, *Standard of Care: The Law of American Bioethics* (Oxford University Press, 1993).
J. Childress and R. Gaare, *BioLaw: A Legal and Ethical Reporter on Medicine, Health Care, and Bioengineering* (University Publications of America, 1983).
Janet L. Dolgin and Lois L. Shepherd, *Bioethics and the Law*, 2d ed. (Aspen, 2009).
R. Dworkin, *Limits: The Role of Law in Bioethical Decision Making* (Indiana University Press, 1996).

Marsha Garrison and Carl Schneider, *The Law of Bioethics: Individual Autonomy and Social Regulation*, 2d. ed. (West, 2009).

Arthur LaFrance, *Bioethics: Health Care, Human Rights and the Law*, 2nd ed. (Mathew Bender, 2006).

J. Menikoff, *Law and Bioethics: An Introduction* (Georgetown University Press, 2001).

David Orentlicher, Mary Anne Bobinski, and Mark A. Hall, *Bioethics and Public Health Law*, 2nd ed. (Aspen, 2008).

D. Rothman, *Strangers at the Bedside: A History of How Law and Bioethics Transformed Medical Decision Making* (Basic Books, 1992).

W. M. Sage. 2001. The lawyerization of medicine. *Journal of Health Politics, Policy, and Law* 26: 1179.

C. Scott. 2000. Why law pervades medicine: An essay on ethics in health care. *Notre Dame Journal of Law, Ethics, and Public Policy* 14:245.

M. H. Shapiro. 1999. Is bioethics broke? On the idea of ethics and law "catching up" with technology. *Indiana Law Review* 33:17.

Michael H. Shapiro, Roy G. Spece, and Rebecca Dresser, *Bioethics and Law*, 2nd ed. (West, 2002).

For those who want a better grasp of the role of legal methods in medical ethics, the *Journal of Law, Medicine and Ethics* is an excellent place to start, as are the writings of legal and scholars in bioethics journals such as the *Hastings Center Report*, the *Kennedy Institute of Ethics Journal*, and the *Cambridge Quarterly of Healthcare Ethics*, to name just a few. Many additional articles and educational treatments of the law and its relation to medical ethics are published in medical journals (e.g., *JAMA*, *New England Journal of Medicine*); health policy journals (e.g., *Health Affairs*, *Journal of Health Politics, Policy and Law*, *Milbank Quarterly*); public health journals (e.g., *American Journal of Public Health*, *Morbidity and Mortality Weekly Reports*); and ethics/philosophy journals (e.g., *Philosophy and Public Affairs*, *Journal of Medicine and Philosophy*).

Beyond medical ethics, the connections between law and health care and public health practice and policy are so substantial that many specialty journals take this as their primary focus:

American Journal of Law and Medicine (Boston University)
Annals of Health Law (Loyola-Chicago)
DePaul Journal of Health Care Law
Food, Drug and Cosmetic Law Journal
Health Law and Policy Abstracts and *Public Health Law Abstracts* (SSRN on-line journals)
Health Matrix (Case Western University)
Houston Journal of Health Law and Policy
Indiana Health Law Review (Indiana University–Indianapolis)
Journal of Contemporary Health Law and Policy (Catholic University)
Journal of Health and Biomedical Law (Suffolk)
Journal of Health and Hospital Law (St. Louis University, AHLA)
Journal of Health Care Law and Policy (University of Maryland)
Journal of Law and Health (Cleveland-Marshall)
Journal of Legal Medicine (Southern Illinois University)

Journal of Medicine and Law
Medical Trial Technique Quarterly
Quinnipiac Health Law Journal
St. Louis University Law Journal
Seton Hall Law Review
Whittier Law Review
Yale Journal of Health Policy, Law and Ethics

✎ Notes

1. *Barber v. Superior Court*. 1983. Court of Appeal of California, 147 Cal. App. 3d 1006; 195 Cal. Rptr. 484.
2. One of the most interesting developments in the Schiavo saga, from a scholarly perspective, was the "Schiavo Timeline"—an exhaustive web-based resource compiled by a law professor and a bioethics scholar, K. L. Cerminara and K. W. Goodman, with links to a vast array of resources, including all the legal documents. Key events in the case of Theresa Marie Schiavo. Available at www.miami.edu/ethics/schiavo/terri_schiavo_timeline.html.
3. Some readers will recognize many aspects of Andrews's critique, elaborated to near-parody, in Michael Crichton's book *Next*, which takes genetic research as its subject matter.
4. For a discussion of how well legal scholars have applied standard social science methods, see, for example, Epstein and King (2002); Cross et al. (2002); Heise (2002); Revesz (2002); and Sisk and Heise (2005).
5. A leading and especially contentious example is whether gun control laws affect crime rates (Ayres and Donohue 2003).

✎ References

Andrews, L. 2006. Who owns your body? A patient's perspective on Washington University v. Catalona. *Journal of Law, Medicine and Ethics* 34 (2): 398.

Annas, G. J. 2001. The limits of state law to protect genetic information. *New England Journal of Medicine* 345:385–88.

Ayres, I., and J. Donohue III. 2003. Shooting down the more guns, less crime hypothesis. *Stanford Law Review* 55:1193.

Cross, F., M. Heise, and G. C. Sisk. 2002. Above the rules: A response to Epstein and King. *University of Chicago Law Review* 69:135.

Crump, D. 2001. How to reason about the law: Interdisciplinary approaches to the foundations of public policy. LexisNexis.

Epstein, L., and G. King. 2002. The rules of inference. *University of Chicago Law Review* 69:1.

Faden, R., Tom L. Beauchamp, and Nancy M. P. King. 1986. Consent and the courts: The emergence of the legal doctrine. In *A history and theory of informed consent*. New York: Oxford University Press.

Frey, B. S. 1997. *Not just for the money: An economic theory of personal motivation*. Cheltenham, UK: Edward Elgar Publishing.

Garner, B. A. 2004. *Black's law dictionary*. Saint Paul, MN: West.

Gilmore, G. 1977. *The ages of American law*. New Haven, CT: Yale University Press.

Goldsmith, J., and A. Vermeule. 2002. Empirical methodology and legal scholarship. *University of Chicago Law Review* 69:153–59.

Hall, M. A. 2006. The history and future of health care law: An essentialist view. *Wake Forest Law Review* 41:347, 357–62.

Hall, M. A., and S. S. Rich. 2000. Genetic privacy laws and patients' fear of discrimination by health insurers: The view from genetic counselors. *Journal of Law, Medicine and Ethics* 28:245–57.

Hall, M. A., T. R. Smith, M. Naughton, and A. Ebbers. 1996. Judicial protection of managed care consumers: An empirical study of insurance coverage disputes. *Seton Hall Law Review* 26:1055–68.

Heise, M. 2002. The past, present, and future of empirical legal scholarship: Judicial decision making and the new empiricism. *University of Illinois Law Review* 4:819.

Holmes, O. W., Jr. 1897. The path of the law. *Harvard Law Review* 10:457.

Hudson, K. L., M. K. Holohan, and F. S. Collins. 2008. Keeping pace with the times: The Genetic Information Nondiscrimination Act of 2008. *New England Journal of Medicine* 358:2661–63.

Kahn, J. P., and S. M. Wolf, eds. 2007. Symposium: Genetic testing and disability insurance. *Journal of Law, Medicine and Ethics* 35:5–89.

King, N. M. P. 1996. *Making sense of advance directives.* Washington, DC: Georgetown University Press.

Krippendorff, K. 2004. *Content analysis: An introduction to its methodology.* Thousand Oaks, CA: Sage Publications.

Leiter, B. 1997. Rethinking legal realism: Toward a naturalized jurisprudence. *Texas Law Review* 76:267.

Mazzoni, C. M. 1998. A legal framework for bioethics. Boston: Kluwer Law International.

Mendelson W. 1963. The neo-behavioral approach to the judicial process: A critique. *American Political Science Review* 57:593–603.

Morriss, A. P. 1995. Developing a framework for empirical research on the common law: General principles and case studies of the decline of employment at will. *Case Western Reserve Law Review* 45:999.

Poland, S. C. 1997. Landmark legal cases in bioethics. *Kennedy Institute of Ethics Journal* 7:191–209.

Revesz, R. L. 2002. A defense of empirical legal scholarship. *University of Chicago Law Review* 69:169.

Rothenburg, K. H. 1995. Genetic information and health insurance: State legislative approaches. *Journal of Law, Medicine and Ethics* 23:312–19.

Rothstein, M. A. 1998. Genetic privacy and confidentiality: Why they are so hard to protect. *Journal of Law, Medicine and Ethics* 26:198–204.

———. 2008a. Was GINA worth the wait? *Journal of Law, Medicine and Ethics* 36:174–48.

———. 2008b. GINA, the ADA, and genetic discrimination in employment. *Journal of Law, Medicine and Ethics* 36:837–40.

———. 2008c. Putting the Genetic Information Nondiscrimination Act in context. *Genetics in Medicine* 10:655–56.

Rothstein, M. A., and B. M. Knoppers, eds. 2005. The regulation of biobanks. *Journal of Law, Medicine and Ethics* 33:7–101.

Schneider, C. E. 1994. Bioethics in the language of the law. *Hastings Center Report* 24 (4).

Sisk, G., and M. Heise. 2005. Judges and ideology: Public and academic debates about statistical measures. *Northwestern University Law Review* 99:743, 791–93.

Stone, A. A. 1985. Law's influence on medicine and medical ethics. *New England Journal of Medicine* 312:310.

Tsosie, R., and J. L. McGregor, eds. 2007. Genome justice: Genetics and group rights. *Journal of Law, Medicine and Ethics* 35:356–462.

Tremper, C., S. Thomas, and A. C. Wagenaar. 2010. Measuring low for evaluation research. *Evaluation Review* 34:242–66.

Wolf, S. M., J. Paradise, C. A. Nelson, J. P. Kahn, and F. Lawrenz, eds. 2008. Incidental findings in human subjects research: From imaging to genomics. *Journal of Law, Medicine and Ethics* 36:216–383.

CHAPTER 9

History

SUSAN E. LEDERER

The purpose of historical inquiry is not simply to present facts but to provide an interpretation of the past. Historical methods aim generally to locate patterns and establish meaning through the rigorous study of documents and artifacts left by people of other times and other places. Historical methods can do much to enrich the understanding of how, why, and under what circumstances issues in medical ethics come to the fore and achieve national or international prominence, as well as how some issues fade away from view only to be rediscovered by subsequent observers and commentators.

In the last three decades bioethics, although explicitly interdisciplinary, has not developed an extensive collaboration with the social sciences and the humanities. In part this division reflects the tensions between normative and prescriptive methods used to approach bioethical issues and the more descriptive methods, which includes historical analysis. Historical methods also faltered in the face in the claims, especially in the 1970s and 1980s, about the absolute novelty of the ethical issues confronting society and the need for urgent innovative solutions. Yet, as historians and historical methods have documented, many of the pressing ethical issues in medicine and the life sciences have arisen in the past, reflecting competing cultural values, social roles, and political milieus. As historian Martin Pernick has compellingly demonstrated, the modern right-to-die debates over severely disabled newborns should not be considered the "unprecedented products of new lifesaving technologies." Indeed, by unearthing a silent film *The Black Stork* (1916), based on Chicago physician Harry Haiselden's controversial practice of allowing so-called defective infants to die, Pernick established how the mass media (newspapers, film, magazines) played a significant role in the early twentieth-century American debates over euthanasia, eugenics, and medical and parental decision making (1996).

Description of Historical Methods

A variety of approaches can be used for historical analyses. After the major approaches and techniques for doing so are reviewed, contemporary challenges to doing this work are discussed.

APPROACHING THE PAST

This section outlines some major historical approaches to medical ethics and bioethics. Each approach entails the identification of evidence, analysis, and the presentation of argument or interpretation, and each has contributed to a richer appreciation of issues in medical ethics and their historical roots and antecedents. These approaches differ primarily with respect to the sources used for historical reconstruction and to the analytic focus of the work. They necessarily represent overlapping domains of actors, events, and ideas; although they are discussed separately, they do not represent rigid categories.

Intellectual history

Intellectual history generally refers to the history of ideas and the development, discussion, and dissemination of these concepts. This approach is closely related to the history of philosophy. In their superb analysis of informed consent, for example, Faden, Beauchamp, and King (1986) explored how ideas about disclosure of a patient's diagnosis and prognosis were considered at the bedside, in the laboratory and in the courts over time. In so doing they were concerned with the history of ideas about responsibility in medicine embodied in oaths, codes, and treatises on medical ethics. They extended their analysis to encompass decisions about obtaining cooperation and permission from patients by examining medical case reports from the nineteenth and twentieth centuries in which physicians recorded how a particular patient had "agreed or consented" to a surgical intervention such as amputation. They noted the ambiguous character of such reports in understanding just what occurred in the doctor-patient interaction. When a physician advised the amputation of an infected leg and the patient agreed, the authors noted, "we cannot discern whether this reported 'consent' was based on accurate and adequate information. The patient may have been given pitiful information about the painfulness of the amputation, or perhaps the bleakness of the case was contrived to make acceptance of the operation inevitable" (Faden, Beauchamp, and King 1986, 54–55). Challenging the representation of past practices, in this case, problematizing the language of the terms "consent" and "agreement" is an important element of historical methodologies. It is especially important when the representation of such interactions are so one-sided. We have considerable evidence from physicians, for example, about the medical encounter. What we lack in most cases is the competing narrative or record from patients or research subjects.

Faden, Beauchamp, and King's account of the origins of informed consent illustrates how using the same evidence can yield radically different conclusions. Moreover, they demonstrate how these differing interpretations may be reconciled. Faden, Beauchamp, and King describe how after his search of a broad range of nineteenth-century documents historian Pernick concluded that truth-telling and permission seeking had long played a role in American medical practice. They contrast Pernick's case for meaningful consent practices with the bleaker picture drawn by psychiatrist Katz in his influential book *The Silent World of Doctor and Patient* (1984). Unlike Pernick, Katz characterized the long history of doctor-patient interaction as one of profound medical inattention to the desires and wishes of patients and the abject failure of the physicians to engage in mutual decision making with their patients and their families. As is the case with other methods in medical ethics, reaching different decisions or conclusions need not be seen as the outcome of inappropriate or wrongly applied methods. Historical methods necessarily involve the selection of evidence and its interpretation.

Social and cultural history

While intellectual history privileges the historical reconstruction of the idea of such concepts as autonomy, justice, rights, and informed consent, social history focuses on what is commonly understood as history from below. This has produced a history from the perspective of the infantry soldier rather than the general, the peasant rather than the royal, and in the case of medical history, this has meant turning the analytic focus from the "great doctors" to the patients who experienced medical care and their ideas and understanding of those encounters. This manner of historical method is also limited by the kinds of records and sources available.

Cultural history often encompasses both historical and anthropological approaches to the past. Like social history, it often considers the events, actors, and experiences of non-elite groups in society, and it is concerned with such concepts as power, perception, ideology, class, gender, and race. Many cultural studies expand the range of sources to include mass media—film, television, radio, newspapers, magazines, and increasingly, the Internet. In the case of medical ethics, this approach can dramatically extend our understanding of the visibility and pervasiveness of such medical practices as truth-telling in cases of cancer.

It has been generally conceded that before the 1970s most American physicians did not disclose a cancer diagnosis to their patients (Daugherty and Hlubocky 2008). Reports in the medical literature emphasize patterns of withholding the truth. In 1953, when W. T. Fitts and I. S. Ravdin analyzed questionnaires from 444 doctors in the Philadelphia area, they reported that 69 percent of their respondents indicated that they never or usually did not inform the patient of a diagnosis of cancer, 28 percent indicated that they usually informed the patient, and just 3 percent indicated that they always informed the patient (Fitts and Ravdin 1953). The two most frequently given reasons for failing to disclose the diagnosis were the "unfavorable emotional reaction" and the request from the patient's family that the doctor not reveal the diagnosis. In 1961, when Chicago psychiatrist Donald Oken conducted a survey of more than 200 physicians about disclosing a cancer diagnosis, he reported that nearly 90 percent routinely withheld such information from their patients (Oken 1961). But physicians were not the only ones with a stake in disclosing a cancer diagnosis; by broadening the historical inquiry to include popular literature, a different understanding of this medical consensus develops.

In the 1950s and 1960s several popular magazines polled both physicians and readers about the practice of telling the patient the nature of their disease. In the pages of the *Rotarian* (1950), *U.S. News and World Report* (1956), *Ladies Home Journal* (1961), *Time* (1961), and *Good Housekeeping* (1962), doctors and patients discussed ideas and practices about truth-telling and the patient with cancer, suggesting that the extent of the medical secrecy surrounding the diagnosis of cancer might be less monolithic than once supposed (Lederer 1999).

The methods of cultural history may also be especially useful in recovering aspects of the past for which there remains little documentary evidence. For example, although university libraries and medical school archives have retained the papers and manuscripts of researchers, there are few, if any, comparable records left by those individuals who participated in research (except for researchers who experimented on their own bodies). One can glean little from the published research reports that involve human subjects, but in some cases, expanding the search to the nonmedical literature can be revealing. For example, in the 1930s University of Pennsylvania physician W. Osler Abbott focused on the function and secretion of the small intestine in human digestion. He and his colleague T. Grier Miller developed a method for rapidly intubating the small intestine that entailed the patient swallowing a flexible tube twelve feet long to which a rubber ball was attached and used to inflate the tube. They practiced on themselves, they sought willing patients in the hospital wards, and during the height of the Great Depression they solicited out-of-work men in the city. Abbott described some features of this process not in a regular medical journal but instead to his fellow members of the Charaka Club, an organization of physicians who were interested in the arts and humanities. His description offers a rare glimpse into the problems of using what he described as the professional guinea pig. When he sought jobless men to come to the laboratory to swallow his intestinal tubes, Abbott offered this description of his "hunting ground":

> Picture a jobless man stalking me as I approached, the mumbled words, the pathetic glance that accompanied the touch—"willing to do any sort of work if only I could give him a job." Then the bright gleam of surprise. Two dollars for a short day's work, "Oh yes, anything would be all right—What, at a hospital? What sort of work,—Oh," and suddenly into his face would come an expression that would have warmed the heart of Boris Karloff and Bela Lugosi. One could see the color ebb away. Was I wanting to *experiment* on them in a *laboratory*? Had I sprouted bats' wings and sucked blood from my child, my prospective subjects could not have scuttled away more precipitously. (Abbott 1941; Lederer 2002)

Thus, from the investigator's perspective, the words "experiment" and "laboratory" conjure up the cinematic monsters of popular film. From the investigator's perspective we have information about the vast cultural gap that separates the investigator and his eventual guinea pigs. Abbott and Miller turned to an African American janitor who provided young African American men for the tube swallowing. Abbott jokingly describes how his black "animals" enjoyed a much larger intake of corn liquor, pork chops, and chewing tobacco than his white rats in the medical school. Even worse, the romantic antics of his "human guinea pigs" created problems with the experimental protocol of the laboratory. When a jealous "sweetheart" fired a gun at one of the young men after she saw him with another woman, the bullet lodged in his spine and made it difficult for Abbott to perform the laboratory procedure. Such events, Abbott jokingly remarked, "led me to wish at times that I could keep my animals in metabolic cages." If one confined the analysis to the published record of Abbott's scientific investigations of the secretions of the small intestine, one would certainly miss the ways in which he objectified the men and women whose bodies he relied upon for the data to advance the understanding of intestinal secretion and process.

Legal and policy history

One influential framework for understanding the history of medical ethics is a focus on law and policy. The laws of cities, states, and nations and their enforcement constrain patients, physicians, and policymakers even as they change over time. As historian Leslie Reagan demonstrated in her sophisticated analysis of the era of criminalized abortion in the United States (roughly the 1870s through the 1973 U.S. Supreme Court finding in *Roe v. Wade*), statutes outlawing abortion materially contributed to the circumstances and locations where abortion was performed and by whom. Moreover, these laws caught thousands of Americans up in criminal investigations, including physicians whose care of their female patients was compromised by the state's insistence that they obtain information from very sick women who had undergone criminal abortion. By compelling doctors to obtain what were called "dying declarations," an unusual legal means to allow the words of the dead to enter the courtroom, prosecutors sought evidence to convict both the impregnators and the abortionists. Focusing on the legal processes and court cases wherein women, men, and physicians were prosecuted for participation in abortion allows deeper insight into the lives, choices, and challenges of women and men confronted with unwanted pregnancies than relying simply on the prescriptive literature that warned couples to avoid sexual contact and illicit bodily contact (Reagan 1997).

TECHNIQUES OF HISTORICAL ANALYSIS

Historical reconstruction relies on primary sources that can be read, analyzed, interpreted, and incorporated into larger arguments about the past. For the most part, historians have access to privileged written documents; these may take the form of letters, diaries, autobiographies, books, articles, and other records. Yet the fact that something has been written down does not ensure that it is a reliable indicator of truth or reality. A critical task of the historical researcher is to scrutinize such documents, seeking to identify the biases of the document creator and being mindful of the researcher's own bias in reading these materials. Approaching documents from the past (or the present) entails questions about authorship, audience, the story line, the reason or motivation for creating the document, the intended purpose of the document, the basic assumptions (implicit and explicit) of the author, and the text's reliability.

Oral evidence

Oral evidence is another important source of information for historians. Telling stories and relating past events, ideas, and relationships has long been a means of learning about oneself as an individual and as a people. Oral history is a more structured and formal process, and most historians date the American origins of oral history to the pioneering work of the historian Allan Nevins at Columbia University. In the 1940s Nevins initiated the first systematic and disciplined efforts to preserve interviews with tape recorders, preserve the tapes, and to make these tapes available in a repository for other historians. In the 1970s tape recording the personal memories and experiences of individuals gained momentum, along with the developments in social and cultural history that privileged the narratives of those ordinary people who had more often been ignored in the traditional historiography. Along with interviews that are generally less structured and briefer, the more formal oral history provided opportunities and insights into aspects of the past for which there exists little or no documentary evidence, a means of getting at information and insights not otherwise available in the extant record. It can also be a means to integrate the experiences and the voices of those historiographically silent into historical narratives.[1]

For the historian of medicine, medical ethics, and bioethics, there are a number of significant repositories of oral history interviews. These include the large number of oral history interviews collected by the History of Medicine Division of the National Library of Medicine at the National Institutes of Health and by the U.S. Food and Drug Administration. Several American universities also maintain important collections of oral history interviews, including the Columbia University Oral History Research Office (collections include the American Society of Hematologists, whose members' recollections include the lack of concern for both human and animal subjects), the Beckman Center for the History of Chemistry at the University of Pennsylvania (which contains oral histories relating to the Human Genome Project), and the Schlesinger Library at Radcliffe College (which houses the Family Planning Oral History Collection) (Tomes 1991).

In understanding how research scientists learned about the nature and extent of their obligations to research subjects, for example, President Clinton's Advisory Committee on Human Radiation Experiments recognized that there were few or no records or documents that demonstrated the socialization of young researchers in terms of using human subjects during the four decades of the Cold War. Staff members for the Advisory Committee, with the aid of historical consultants, conducted twenty-two interviews with medical researchers whose careers began in the late 1940s and 1950s. These histories, among others, offered extensive evidence that medical researchers frequently took liberties with their sick and hospitalized patients in the decades following World War II.

Many of the researchers, for example, identified the rank opportunism that drove their use of human subjects, as well as their regret about the risks and discomforts that their unconsenting patients endured in the name of biomedical investigation. Dr. Paul Beeson, a leading internist and academic physician, described a study he had conducted as a young professor at Emory University in the late 1940s, in which he thought it might be interesting to apply the new technique of cardiac catheterization. "It would do no good for the patient," he explained, "to have a catheter placed in the heart along with a needle to obtain arterial blood. All I could say at the end," Beeson noted, "was that these poor people were lying there and we had nothing to offer them and it might have given them some comfort that a lot of people were paying attention to them for this one study. I don't remember ever asking their permission to do so" (*Human Radiation Experiments* 1996).

Oral history methods have limitations, as do other historical techniques. As Morantz, Pomerleau, and Fenichel noted in their path-breaking 1982 collection *In*

Her Own Words: Oral Histories of Women Physicians, the dialogic character of the interview can be both "a virtue and a defect." People who read oral histories must appreciate that the subject responds (generally) to the interviewer's questions, and the product is unlikely to be the same kind of account that the subject would have produced on her own or in a written autobiography. "Distortion is inherent in the process," noted Morantz and her colleagues. "Issues and incidents that the interviewee might have relegated to a footnote or passed over altogether may be pursued at length by the interviewer. Further, the give-and-take of spoken conversation lacks the tightly constructed literary quality of a written work" (Morantz, Pomerleau, and Fenichel 1982).

Archaeological and DNA evidence

Historians are often eclectic when it comes to the gathering of historical data. Some historians of medicine have turned to archaeology; others have turned to the recent advances in DNA analysis in an effort to establish the veracity of claims and counterclaims. For the historian the tools of archaeological analysis can shed light on medical and surgical practices of antiquity (Baker 2004). Understanding the practice of medicine in antiquity and the ethical norms that guided and informed such practice generally involves using evidence from surviving medical treatises, inscriptions that mention physicians and gods and goddesses of healing, biological remains (mummified remains, skeletons), and artifacts including medical and surgical instruments. As classicist Baker has pointed out, archaeologists have tended to rely on Greek and Roman medical texts to interpret the surgical functions of tools, including probes, forceps, needles, and scalpels. But examining the tools not only in their literary sense but also in their archaeological context (where they were found, in what condition they were recovered, their placement in relationship to other objects and texts) has the potential to deepen our understanding not only of their functional use but also of their symbolic importance in Greek and Roman perceptions of health and disease, the body, and the performance of healing and healing rituals.

The use of archaeological evidence, for example, serves to nuance the assumption that there existed a rigid division between secular, rational Greek and Roman medicine and "irrational" religious healing practices mediated by supernatural agents and forces. Baker considers, for example, the disposal of surgical instruments that were deliberately broken and buried, suggesting that their owners sought to eradicate the illness, bad luck, or contamination associated with them. Such a practice coexisted alongside conventions of symbolic pollution in the classical world, which outlawed both giving birth and dying in Greek healing places. Like the written medical treatises, casebooks, and inscriptions that survive from antiquity, the archaeological evidence of medical encounters—instruments, interments, and artifacts—offers the opportunity to inform understanding of the ethical practice of medicine and surgery in the past.

In the last two decades historians have turned to DNA analysis for data and evidence. In one of the most sensational efforts in the 1990s, historians sought DNA evidence in an effort to resolve the long-standing claim that President Thomas Jefferson had fathered some of the children of Sally Hemings, his enslaved companion.

Since 1802, when accusations that Thomas Jefferson had fathered a child with his slave first surfaced, historians and critics turned to both oral tradition and documentary evidence to support or deny Jefferson's paternity of Hemings's children. In 1998 researchers from the University of Leicester, Leiden University, and Oxford University compared Y-chromosomal DNA haplotypes (a combination of alleles at multiple loci that are transmitted on the same chromosome) of living male descendants of Field Jefferson (Thomas Jefferson's paternal uncle) with those of the living male descendants of Thomas Woodson, believed to be Sally Heming's firstborn son, and Eston Hemings Jefferson, her last son. These researchers concluded that molecular evidence failed to support claims that Jefferson fathered Thomas Woodson but did "provide evidence" that the president was the biological father of Eston Hemings Jefferson (Foster et al. 1998). The geneticists confirmed that an individual carrying the male Jefferson Y chromosome fathered Eston Hemings (born 1808), the last known child born to Sally Hemings. However, there were at the time approximately twenty-five adult male Jeffersons in Virginia who carried this chromosome living, and some were known to have visited Monticello, the president's home. "We cannot completely rule out other explanations of our findings based on illegitimacy in various lines of descent," the researchers conceded, even as they insisted that "the simplest and most probable explanations" for their findings was that Thomas Jefferson had fathered Eston Hemings (DuCille 2000).

DNA analysis, of course, does not resolve all the issues about the relationship between Jefferson and Hemings. Historians continue to debate the extent to which the relationship was consensual, coercive, a rape, or a liaison that provided mutual gratification (Jefferson received physical gratification; Hemings's children were released from slavery at Jefferson's death). As bioethicist Dena Davis (2004) notes, genetic research affects not just individuals but communities; the genetic evidence about the relationship between a white, male landowner and an enslaved African American woman is not just about their children, but about how we regard ourselves as Americans and how we regard Jefferson as the author of the Declaration of Independence.

CONTEMPORARY CHALLENGES

The development of bioethics and the institutionalization of protections for patients and research subjects have created new and, in some cases, onerous, challenges for the historian of medicine and medical ethics. Two significant concerns for historians are the nature and extent of institutional review board (IRB) oversight and permission and the concerns about confidentiality expressed in congressional protections for patient privacy.

IRB oversight

Since the 1990s the federal regulation and oversight of social science research, including history, has become increasingly contested. Established in the 1960s, American institutional research boards (IRBs) were originally convened to address issues that arise in medical research with human subjects. From the start, however, some prominent participants believed that the surveys, questionnaires, and interviews conducted by social scientists should be subjected to oversight. "It's not the scientist who puts a needle in the blood stream who causes the trouble," observed James Shannon, who directed the National Institutes of Health from 1955 to 1968. "It's the behavioral scientist who probes into the sex life of an insecure person who really raises hell."[2]

Until the 1990s, however, many social science researchers did not submit protocols for IRB approval or were considered exempt under IRB regulations either by the institution or by the individual researcher. In 1995 the Office for Protection from Research Risk at the National Institutes of Health effectively expanded IRB oversight to include such fields as oral history, journalism, and folklore, which were once thought to be immune from regulatory jurisdiction.

For their part most historians have vehemently resisted the requirement that they, like their colleagues in the social sciences and the biological sciences, submit their proposals and protocols to their institutional review board. In part this reluctance reflects the sense that historians have developed their own standards and safeguards for both sound methodology and ethical attention to the needs of the human participant. In 1968 the Oral History Association codified, following an exhaustive and deliberative process, a set of principles and protocols to guide work in oral history. Subsequently expanded (1979) and revised (1989–90, 1998–99), these principles, also known as the Evaluation Guidelines, outline the responsibilities of interviewers to the individual subject, to the public, and the profession. In collaboration with the Oral History Association, the American Historical Association, the leading organization of professional historians, produced a shorter document, Statement on Interviewing for Historical Documentation, for those specifically using oral history in their scholarly projects.

Historians have also resisted the equation of oral history with human subjects research conducted in the laboratory or the clinic. When she testified in 2000 before the President's National Bioethics Advisory Commission, historian Linda Shopes explained:

> I think it is important to state that for historians, oral history is not understood as research on human subjects, but rather research with other human beings: an oral history interview is an interactive process, in which the questions of the historian/interviewer elicit the responses of the narrator, which in turn influence the historian's subsequent questions. Historians view oral history as a unique kind of primary source: the quality of the interview depends as much on the methodology employed and the relationship between interviewer and narrator, as it does on the significance of the events being recalled and the sharpness of the narrator's memory.[3]

Part of the unique quality that historians see is the paramount need for critical inquiry rather than protection of the human subject. Many historians have been stunned when they have been requested from their local IRB to refrain from asking questions of a sensitive nature (for example, aspects of the subject's criminal history or their use of illegal substances) because of the "risks and discomfort" the interviewer might experience in the oral interview (Berridge 1979). For historians this raises the prospect that the current federal regulations seemingly proscribe controversial, difficult, or challenging topics in historical research. "The need to treat individual narrators with honesty and respect is not the issue here; nor is the need to apprise them of the nature and purpose of any interview," Shopes (2000) insisted. "What is at issue is the notion of critical inquiry, inquiry that does challenge, that may be adversarial, that may even 'expose,' as interviews with Klansmen and women and with Nazi collaborators, for example, have done."[4]

Despite repeated efforts and failed strategies to accommodate the needs of oral historians and the protections of the IRB process, both sides remain frustrated. After he attended the annual Public Responsibility in Medicine and Research meeting in November 2006, E. Taylor Atkins described the efforts to clarify previous federal statements on whether or not oral history is subject to review by IRBs. As a historian who has served on his university's IRB, conducted oral history research, and even made modest attempts to ease the strains between IRBs and historians and other social scientists, Atkins is unusual in that he identified both the benefits and losses in ensuring that oral history protocols be submitted for IRB approval. "As unimpeachable as the OHA's own Professional Guidelines may be," Atkins observed, "I think it is arrogant to assume that oral historians have nothing to learn from other disciplines with regard to the ethical treatment of human subjects. If nothing else, they can become more sensitized to the possibilities for psychological or social harm that may result from oral history interviewing." Atkins cites as an example the requirement by his local IRB that investigators from the psychology department who are pursuing research into childhood abuse or some other trauma be "either qualified to directly provide appropriate counseling or intervention" or able to provide a list of appropriate social services. "How many oral historians have the expertise or qualifications to handle a situation in which an informant with PTSD [post-traumatic stress disorder] experiences distress during an interview? How many would have a list of counseling services at hand in case it was necessary?" argues Atkins. At this time, however, such issues and responsibilities remain unresolved, and historians are encouraged to consult their institutional IRB before proceeding with oral histories and interviews.

Privacy

Congressional passage of the Health Insurance Portability and Accountability Act (HIPAA) in 1996 has brought additional challenges for those who wish to pursue historical methodologies relating to health care, doctors, nurses, patients, and hospitals. For historians the problem became acute when HIPAA went into effect in 2003 because medical archives and the records they contain were no longer easily accessible to researchers. As historian Susan Lawrence has noted, the Privacy Rule, one of the specific provisions of HIPAA, is the first major American regulation that protects the privacy of deceased individuals in perpetuity (Lawrence 2007). Historians interested in health care, medical ethics, and bioethics are interested in records in which there is individually identifiable health information. Moreover, the Department of Health and Human Services implemented a system in which responsibility for the supervision and oversight of the HIPAA Privacy Rule was delegated to the institutional review board. Already overburdened and underresourced for its workload, some IRBs established privacy boards that were charged with protecting the privacy rights of individuals. As in the case of IRB approval for oral history projects, access to private materials becomes more difficult when the data are socially sensitive. Asking historical questions about procedures like removal of the tonsils or the use of over-the-counter drugs is very different than posing similar questions about sexually transmitted disease, mental illness, and narcotic abuse. Because IRBs and privacy boards are independent institutions, there can be enormous variability in the kinds of records and information available to historians.

☙ Critiques of Historical Analysis

History, like other disciplines, has been ravaged on the rocks of relativism and by the claims that there exist no absolute truths (past, present, or future). Truth, the argument goes, is always relative to some particular frame of reference, culture, or language. Such an argument strikes at the core of the historical disciplines that had privileged the concept of historical objectivity. The objective historian, in this formulation, is a disinterested or neutral observer who is able to bring an even-handed and judicious analysis to events and actors in the past and to provide an interpretation that accords with the realities of the past.[5] The relativist critique fundamentally challenges the objectivist position; it reiterates, in the words of L. P. Hartley, that "the past is a foreign country," that we are all travelers to the past, and that we bring our own cultural baggage with us (Lowenthal 1985).

In the history of medicine much of the relativist turn has been conducted in the discussion of illness as a social construct. Extreme proponents of the relativist position challenge not only the reality of disease and the apparent objective reality of disease entities, but they also question the legitimacy of the cultural authority vested in physicians, who had traditionally developed and maintained such diagnostic categories. This epistemological and political challenge that dominated much of the social and cultural history of disease in the 1970s and 1980s lost much of its cachet with an increasing appreciation of the biological factors in disease and its effects. As historians Rosenberg and Golden (1992) have noted, the HIV epidemic contributed significantly to this change: Given a fatality rate of close to 100 percent (referring to the early days of the epidemic), the disease "helped create a new consensus in regards to disease, one that finds a place for both biological and social factors and emphasizes their interaction. Students of the relations between medicine and society live in a necessarily post-relativist decade" (Rosenberg and Golden 1992). Rosenberg is perhaps overly optimistic about the fortunes of post-relativism. The critique of historical approaches has been far reaching and has served to delegitimize much academic history.

☙ Notes on Resources and Training

There is a growing literature on the history of medical ethics and bioethics. One useful starting point is the *Cambridge World History of Medical Ethics* (2009), which includes chapters and entries on the historical development of medical ethics around the world from antiquity to the present (Baker and McCullough 2009). The volume offers both a comprehensive bibliography and an appendix with biographies of major actors in the history of medical ethics.

The National Library of Medicine (part of the National Institutes of Health) houses historical collections, which include selected digitized material relating to the history of medicine. Taken from the manuscripts and books collections, the prints and photographs collection, historical films and videos, and the Digital Manuscripts Program, these digitized materials cover a spectrum of centuries and cultures from medieval Islam to contemporary biomedical research and are available at the website (www.nlm.nih.gov/hmd/). The NLM History of Medicine website has links to other important online resources, including manuscripts and oral histories.

A large number of programs offer advanced training in history of medicine and history of science. History departments around the country and abroad also offer both master's programs and doctorates in history that include research and writing in medical history and the history of biomedical ethics. The American Association for the History of Medicine (AAHM) is a scholarly association devoted to the study of the history of health, healing, and disease. The association's membership includes not only historians but also doctors, nurses, and other health professionals, librarians, curators and archivists, and graduate students in history and the health sciences. Each spring the AAHM hosts an annual meeting that sponsors workshops, seminars, lectures, and luncheons and that includes more than one hundred presentations of recent research and scholarship on the history of healing, health and disease (www. histmed.org/). The *Bulletin of the History of Medicine* is the official publication of the American Association for the History of Medicine and the Johns Hopkins Institute of the History of Medicine. Published quarterly, each issue spans the cultural, social, and scientific aspects of the history of medicine around the world.

◌ Notes

1. For two useful guides to oral history, see Donald A. Ritchie, *Doing Oral History: A Practical Guide* (New York: Oxford University Press, 2003); and Sandra Lewenson and Eleanor Krohn Hermann, eds., *Capturing Nursing History: Guide to Historical Methods in Research* (New York: Springer Publishing, 2008).
2. Quoted in Zachary M. Schrag, "How Talking Became Human Subjects Research: The Federal Regulation of the Social Sciences, 1965–1991," *Journal of Policy History* 21 (2009): 3–37.
3. Linda Shopes, Pennsylvania Historical and Museum Commission, "Remarks before President's National Bioethics Advisory Commission," April 6, 2000. A full transcription of the National Bioethics Advisory Commission is available online at www.bioethics.gov/.
4. Ibid.
5. An excellent starting point for this expansive discussion is Peter Novick, *That Noble Dream: The "Objectivity" Question and the American Historical Profession* (Cambridge: Cambridge University Press, 1988) and the enormous commentary this book fostered.

◌ References

Abbott, W. Osler. "The Problem of the Professional Guinea Pig," *Proceeedings of the Charaka Club*, 10, 1941, 249–260, at pp. 251–52.
Atkins, E. Taylor. 2006. Forum on IRBs: Oral History and IRBs: An Update from the 2006 HRPP Conference, American Historical Association website. www.historians.org/perspectives/issues/2007/0703/0703vie2.cfm, accessed 2/9/09.

Baker, Patricia. 2004. Roman medical instruments: Archaeological interpretations of their possible "non-functional uses." *Journal of the Social History of Medicine* 17:3–21.

Baker, Robert B., and Laurence B. McCullough, eds. 2009. *Cambridge world history of medical ethics*. Cambridge: Cambridge University Press.

Berridge, Virginia. 1979. Opium and oral history. *Oral History* 7:48–58.

Daugherty, Christopher K., and Fay J. Hlubocky. 2008. What are terminally ill cancer patients told about their expected deaths? A study of cancer physicians' self-reports of prognosis disclosure. *Journal of Clinical Oncology* 26:5988–93.

Davis, Dena S. 2004. Genetic research and communal narratives. *Hastings Center Report* 34:40–49.

DuCille, Ann. 2000. Where in the world is William Wells Brown? Thomas Jefferson, Sally Hemings, and the DNA of African-American literary history. *American Literary History* 12:443–62.

Faden, Ruth, Tom L. Beauchamp, and Nancy M. P. King. 1986. *A history and theory of informed consent*. New York: Oxford University Press, 54–55.

Fitts, W. T., and I. S. Ravdin. 1953. What Philadelphia physicians tell patients with cancer. *Journal of the American Medical Association* 153:901–4.

Foster, E. A., M. A. Jobbing, P. G. Taylor, P. Donnelly, H. P. de Knij, R. Micreset, T. Ferjal, and C. Tyler-Smith. 1998. Jefferson fathered slave's last child. *Nature* 396:27–28.

Human Radiation Experiments: Final Report of the Advisory Committee on Human Radiation Experiments. 1996. New York: Oxford University Press, 83.

Katz, Jay. 1984. *The silent world of doctor and patient*. New York: Free Press.

Lawrence, Susan C. 2007. Access anxiety: HIPAA and historical research. *Journal of the History of Medicine* 62:422–59.

Lederer, Susan E. 1999. Medical ethics and the media: Oaths, codes and popular culture. In *The American Medical Ethics Revolution*, ed. Robert Baker, Arthur Caplan, Linda Emanuel, and Stephen Latham. Baltimore: Johns Hopkins University Press, 91–103.

———. 2002. "Porto Ricochet": Joking about germs, cancer, and race extermination in the 1930s." *American Literary History* 14:720–46.

Lowenthal, David. 1988. *The past is a foreign country*. Cambridge: Cambridge University Press.

Morantz, Regina, Cynthia Stodola Pomerleau, and Carol Hansen Fenichel, eds. 1982. *In her own words: Oral histories of women physicians*. New Haven, CT: Yale University Press, xii.

Oken, Donald. 1961. What to tell cancer patients. *Journal of the American Medical Association*, 175:1120–28.

Pernick, Martin S. 1996. *The black stork: Eugenics and the death of "defective" babies in American medicine and motion pictures since 1915*. New York: Oxford University Press.

Reagan, Leslie J. 1997. *When abortion was a crime: Women, medicine, and law in the United States, 1867–1973*. Berkeley: University of California Press.

Rosenberg, Charles E. 1986. Disease and social order in America: Perceptions and expectations. *The Milbank Quarterly* 64 (Supplement 1): 34–55.

Rosenberg, Charles E., and Janet Golden, eds. 1992. *Framing disease: Studies in cultural history*. New Brunswick, NJ: Rutgers University Press.

Tomes, Nancy. 1991. Oral history in the history of medicine. *Journal of American History* 78: 607–17.

CHAPTER 10

Literature

TOD CHAMBERS

As medical ethics has become a profoundly multidisciplinary field, perhaps one of the most unexpected disciplines to have been added to the field's methodological alchemy has been literary theory. The introduction of literary theory into medical ethics becomes intelligible when one understands that literature scholars, like philosophers and theologians, were brought into medical schools and hospitals at the end of the twentieth century to help humanize clinical practice. Many of these literature scholars, as well as their colleagues in the other disciplines, who were grouped together into what became known as the medical humanities, thought of themselves as part of a distinct social movement aimed at reforming contemporary medicine (Carson, Burns, and Cole 2003). The discipline of literature and medicine could have developed as an interest in the hermeneutics of a practice, as happened for literature and science, and located itself within traditional liberal arts colleges (see, for example, Montgomery Hunter 1991; Montgomery 2005; Charon 2006), yet its development within medical education meant that literature scholars needed to relate their teaching and scholarship toward the practical end of producing better physicians and nurses. These scholars brought into the clinical setting both the objects of their discipline (literary texts) and the methods used in analyzing these objects (literary criticism) in order to foreground what Anthony Moore refers to as the "missing medical text," that is, patient stories (1978).

This attempt toward reform through literature was but one of a series of curriculum reforms within American medical schools. These periodic medical education reforms, according to Renée Fox (1999), have all been attempts to influence the nonbiological features of contemporary clinical practice, each claiming to have the magic bullet to cure medicine of its overemphasis on treating bodies and not patients. Psychiatry was featured in the 1950s and 1960s, community medicine in the mid 1960s, and medical ethics during the 1970s. Fox points out that there is a "historic logic" to these reforms in that each of these disciplines entered medical schools during a time marked by the intellectual flowering of each discipline and the broader society's interest in the perspective each brought to medicine. Although not explicitly mentioned in Fox's analysis, literary studies was brought into medical education during the 1970s, which was a time of expanding academic capital for literary theory (Eagleton 1983). This belief in literature's efficacy was ironic, for it occurred just as academic literary studies was rejecting the moral value of literature and striving instead to become more scientific and objective (see also Trautmann 1992, 7; Davis and Womack 2001).

The first literature scholar to be hired as a full-time faculty member of an American medical school was Joanne Trautmann Banks at Pennsylvania State University in Hershey in 1972, four years after that university hired the first full-time medical ethicist, the philosopher K. Danner Clouser. These two firsts are noteworthy—they represent how literature and medical ethics became odd pedagogical bedfellows within medical schools. Like the literature scholars, medical ethicists were brought into the medical setting for assistance with issues of morality. Literature was thought to improve the moral sensibilities of health care professionals, and medical ethics was viewed as providing ways for resolving moral dilemmas. But even at the start of their tenure in medical education, literature scholars often found themselves teaching formal medical ethics courses, and medical ethicists were using literature in the teaching of medical ethics. At first literature scholars drew upon the traditional approaches in medical ethics, but they found over time that their discipline not only provided additional data for philosophical analysis but also provided an alternative approach to ethics. Some believed that literature studies supplemented the perceived failings of traditional ethical methods; others thought literature studies were superior to those traditional approaches. This move from helpful assistant to clinical expert was not greeted with automatic acceptance by their philosopher–colleagues. In a special issue of *The Journal of Medicine and Philosophy* on literature and medical ethics, one of its editors, Clouser, wrote a critique of these new approaches by stating that when the literature scholars provided ways "to enrich the details of issues and cases," that there was nothing else for philosophers to say but "thank you." If these literature scholars, however, wished to "challenge the methods, concepts, or theories of morality itself," then they would be going outside of their area of expertise. In other words, philosophy can critique the usefulness of literature but literature cannot critique philosophy, for only philosophy can do that for itself (1996, 324). The literature scholar and coeditor of the special issue, Anne Hawkins, wrote a vigorous rejoinder that could be summarized as suggesting, "There were more things in medicine and ethics, Clouser, than are dreamt of in your philosophy" (1996).

While literature scholars agreed with Clouser that their field could provide medical ethics with useful literary texts, they claimed that their field could also assist and criticize the methods of medical ethics through what I will refer to as the literature analogy. The literature analogy entails the metaphorical extension of reading and writing to the encounter with medical ethics problems and treats such problems as analogous to literary texts. When literature scholars analyze moral problems in this manner they are essentially arguing that these problems have characteristics that are best thought of as being textual—an approach that has been taken in other fields as well (Rabinow and Sullivan 1987). While all the approaches discussed in this chapter use either literary texts or the literature analogy, each of the approaches draws upon different texts or different aspects of the analogy. Rather than having a single characteristic that all these techniques share, the term "literary analogy" can be thought of as a Wittgensteinian family resemblance term. That is to say, no single approach contains all the qualities of literature as a method in medical ethics, but all of them share features with other literature approaches. It should also be noted that a number of these approaches have been at times referred to as narrative ethics, but as we shall see there are some literature methods for medical ethics that do not use or rely upon narrative, so it would be inaccurate to refer to literature approaches by this nomenclature.

Description of Literature Methods

The most conventional way that literature has been brought into medical ethics analysis is the use of literary texts, often by notable authors, as richly told examples of moral dilemmas in medicine. It has also been argued that reading literature, regardless of its subject matter, can assist us to develop empathy. Medical ethics scholars have drawn not only upon the subject of literary studies but also from the methods of analyzing literature. Narrative theory can provide tools for the analysis of moral problems as well as a method for critiquing bioethics practice. Finally, medical ethicists have discussed ethical analysis not only as a type of reading but also as a type of writing.

LITERATURE AS "THICK CASES"

Even prior to the explicit advent of such approaches as narrative ethics, literary works were used in the teaching and analysis of moral problems. A number of short stories have become a part of the medical ethics canon and are treated in ways that are substantially different from how they are treated within literary criticism. These stories have been seen as supplements to the traditional ethics case genre. The ethics case has traditionally drawn upon the model of the medical case, and because of this it often carries elements of the medical case that are not necessarily useful in the discussion of moral problems (Chambers 1999). The genre of the medical case has arisen to aid in the diagnosis of medical problems and as a way for members of the medical team to communicate (Banks and Hawkins 1992). Whether consciously or not, medical ethicists have often adopted this genre to explore moral issues, but in doing so, they have also adopted the narrative features of the case: for example, passive voice, clinical focus, and flat tone. To provide richer cases, that is, cases that can more powerfully evoke the emotional terrain of these problems, ethicists have often drawn upon the literary narratives of such physician–writers as William Carlos Williams, Richard Selzer, Perri Klass, Rafael Campo, John Lantos, and Abraham Verghese.

An example is the following ethics case.

> The patient is a seven-year-old girl who presents following three days of fever. The patient denies a sore throat but refuses to be examined. In order to determine the diagnosis, the father restrained the daughter as the physician forced open her mouth for the examination. On inspection, the throat appeared to be infected.

Essentially, this is a retelling of William Carlos Williams's short story "The Use of Force." The style used to tell the story is akin to that of the medical case, but, in doing so, this style leaves out the narrator's complex feelings toward the situation. Here is a portion of the story as created by Williams:

> The damned little brat must be protected against her own idiocy, one says to one's self at such times. Others must be protected against her. It is social necessity. And all these things are true. But a blind fury, a feeling of adult shame, bred of a longing for muscular release are the operatives. One goes on to the end.
>
> In a final unreasoning assault I overpowered the child's neck and jaws. I forced the heavy silver spoon back of her teeth and down her throat till she gagged. And there it was—both tonsils covered with membrane. She had fought valiantly to keep me from knowing her secret. She had been hiding that sore throat for three days at least and lying to her parents in order to escape just such an outcome as this. (1984, 59–60)

In Williams's version, we see the events through the point of view of what narrative theorists refer to as a dramatized narrator, that is, a narrator who is identified to some degree and who becomes for the reader, whether explicitly part of the story or not, a character. In the clinical retelling of this story, the narrator is undramatized, hidden, and effaced from the action of the tale. In Williams's original, the narrator is the physician, and by having the story related through the perspective of one of its characters, the reader can judge not merely the rightness of the action but also the rightness of how the action was carried out. One can provide a convincing philosophical argument that children may not have any right to refuse treatment and that with the consent of parents one may force a child to undergo a procedure, but Williams's story grants one insight into the moral complexity of actually carrying out that philosophically permissible act.

One of the features of literature that medical ethicists have rarely attended to is that the prose narratives used as cases are not merely artistic representations of events but also a form of argumentation (Walsh 1995). Because fiction does not require that one be anchored to actual events—and in fact can be defined by its ability to go beyond the actual (Cohn 2000)—the author should be understood to not merely be presenting actual events but rather representing a particular way of seeing the world. As Charon (2001) relates: "Stories about physicians and patients can be invented. When William Carlos Williams wrote 'The Use of Force,' he was not writing a chart note after making a housecall, even though the 'real' Dr. Williams might have visited a young girl with diphtheria in his Rutherford, New Jersey, general practice.... Instead, these writers created fictional worlds that corresponded roughly, perhaps, to authorial experiences but transcended them to express aesthetic vision and artistic coherence" (83).

One manner in which an author of fiction is able to persuade readers to view the world from a particular slant is through the construction of a particular narrator. There is always some space between the narrator of events and the actual author (Booth 1983). And in some instances the author may not share the values or worldview of the narrator. The degree to which the events portrayed are actual or fictional (or some combination of both) matters because readers expect that the values and worldview of the narrator in nonfiction are essentially the same as those of the actual author. Yet in many works of fiction used as medical ethics cases it has been left largely ambiguous whether the narrator and the author are the same individuals. For example, Richard Selzer's "Brute" has been used as a case for the discussion of using force against a patient. At first this may seem to be the same territory as seen in Williams's "The Use of Force," but the narrator of Selzer's story has been seen by some scholars as a clearly racist individual (King and Stanford 1992). If the narrator and the author in the tale are the same, then the moral import of the story changes quite dramatically, even if, and perhaps especially if, Selzer does not intend the narrator to be viewed as racist.

READING LITERATURE AS PRAXIS

Aristotle thought that while the young could become accomplished in particular forms of knowledge such as geometry and mathematics, practical knowledge required an extensive knowledge of particulars, which could come only with experience. One could argue that the best one could do for the young would be to provide lists of moral rules to follow until they acquired the necessary experience. Similarly, any form of medical ethics that argues for the superiority of Aristolean character over Kantian rules has no way to provide the necessary extensive experiences with patients to develop the moral sensibility of the virtuous physician. Literature scholars argue, however, that literature can provide these experiences. With so much attention to the importance of simulations and virtual forms of education, literature can be said to be doing analogous work. Montgomery (1991) submits that "literature gives readers and audiences a chance to see life as other people experience it. Students can learn something of what it is like to be ill or dying or of another race or class or gender, and they can also glimpse what it is to be a physician" (66). Pellegrino holds that well-crafted literature permits the reader vicarous experiences, and in doing so, "the student physician can experience something of what it is to be ill, in pain, in anguish, or dying" (1980, xvi).

Like Pellegrino, Charon argues that the reading of literature can provide a method for the development of empathy. She is, however, more specific regarding the kinds of skills that are transferred from reading to caring. She contends that the reading of serious fiction develops narrative skills by which medical students can learn to see the world through the eyes of the other, and she believes that the same skills that are brought to interpret a piece of literature—"close attention to language, diction, metaphor, and reader response"—are the very skills that a health care professional needs to develop in order to understand and care for patients. In this her narrative medicine brings together the literature analogy and the notion of using literary texts as teaching aids: reading actual literature gives one the skill to "read" patients.

Charon gives an example of caring for an elderly woman, H. B., who has become oddly concerned with catching TB from her neighbor. In the midst of this encounter, the patient tells an unusual tale of her neighbor's recent marriage to a HIV-positive prisoner who is half her age. To understand her patient, Charon creates a form of intertextuality reading between her patient and Félicité, a character in a Flaubert short story. Intertextuality, or the weaving together of two texts, permits Charon to transfer what she learned in understanding Flaubert's narrative to provide a hermeneutic key to understanding her own patient: "As I realized the similarity in emotional landscape between the two stories, I could think more clearly about the potential meaning of the neighbor's marriage" (1993, 156). The special internal knowledge furnished by fiction provides an interpretative map to understand the nonfictional stories of others, which cannot by their very nature permit an internal understanding.

Literature provides not merely a way to understand the ill and thus act in an ethically appropriate manner but also rich examples of how health care professionals respond to morally problematic situations. This is not simply the use of literature as ethics case examples but a means by which one can view moral issues in relation to the everyday life of a health care professional. In his classic essay on justifying the teaching of literature to medical students, Coles argues that because of their focus on the everyday and the ordinary, the work of novelists—as opposed to the very useful but sometimes rarefied analytic work of philosophers—should be our primary source for "examining the trials and temptations that intervene ... in a doctor's life" (1979, 445). For Coles the literary works that can assist physicians "in exploring a kind of medical ethics that has to do with the quality of a lived life" include George Eliot's *Middlemarch*, F. Scott Fitzgerald's *Tender Is the Night*, Sinclair Lewis's *Arrowsmith*, and Walker Percy's *Love in the Ruins*. In *Middlemarch* Eliot's Dr. Lydgate must confront the temptations of wealth in relation to his ideals. The choices made by Dick Diver concerning his relationship with a patient in *Tender Is the Night* are ones that continually reverberate throughout his life. Coles's decision to examine this everyday ethics through the novel is significant, for the novel as a genre, as opposed to the case study, can provide a rich explication of moral dilemmas within the context of the everyday world of the health care professional (Chambers 2000). The novel's ability to permit readers to see particular dilemmas within the prosaics of a character's everyday life is the reason it was celebrated by such literary critics as Mikhail Bakhtin. He argued that the novel permits the reader to situate "the moments to be considered in the network of all concerned persons, together with their histories and perceptions, and describing all these events with their multivalent social milieu" (Morson and Emerson 1990, 27).

The novel is free from the needs of realism. As E. M. Forster observed, "The historian deals with actions, and with the character of men only so far as he can deduce them from their actions. He is quite as much concerned with character as the novelist, but he can only know of its existence when it shows on the surface" (1985, 45). When historians go beyond the surface, they potentially leave themselves open to a range of criticisms. Fiction writers can construct a narrative in a way that portrays events through the perspectives of people other than themselves.

In *Transparent Minds*, Cohn argues that it is the move to go under the surface that defines fiction as fiction, so that "the special life-likeness of narrative fiction—as compared to dramatic and cinematic fictions—depends on what writers and readers know least in life: how another mind thinks, another body feels" (1983, 5–6). When nonfiction writers such as Truman Capote, Thomas Wolfe, and Norman Mailer take what they have learned about real people and then narrate not merely the physical world but the psychological experience of that physical world, they essentially have fictionalized the real world. This is perhaps why the exact fictional status of the stories of such physician–writers as Williams and Selzer is difficult to determine. Fiction grants us access to the internal world of others and thus to a method for knowing another that is simply not possible in other forms of representation.

Reading literature provides a model not only for understanding the internal world of patients and physicians but, as Hawkins argues, it can also foreground the way intuition and tacit knowledge are as important to our moral decision making as the warrants of casuistry and the syllogisms of logic. She states that "literature validates a concept of ethics that draws upon intuition, emotion, and imagination—faculties that, I would argue, are essential components in sound ethical decision making." For Hawkins, literature can "strengthen and train the non-rational faculties of mind" (1994, 285). It is not that Hawkins is advocating that we abandon rationality or deductive thinking but rather that ethics must take into account all of the features that we think of as part of the entire human self. Hawkins observes that one finds throughout literature moments of sudden insight, or epiphanies. Such epiphanic knowledge can be found in lyric poetry, haikus, drama, and prose fiction. Hawkins gives the moment of sudden transcendent peace at the end of Tolstoy's "The Death of Ivan Ilych" as an example of an epiphanic moment in literature (1997, 160). The knowledge acquired ephiphanically does not come through a systematic rationalistic series of steps, ideas that are the natural evolution of prior proven propositions, but instead occurs in a flash, breaking into our world without preparation.

READING ETHICS CASES

In her often-cited essay "Narrative Contributions to Medical Ethics," Charon (1994) argues that medical ethicists should develop "narrative sensitivity," and this sensitivity consists of becoming cognizant to the way moral problems are constructed and interpreted. She identifies in medical ethics deliberation four narrative stages: recognition, formulation, interpretation, and validation. Charon observes that the first stage, recognition, entails sensitivity to what may be hidden from our view. Without recognition, we can lose the person in treating the body and lose the ethics in grappling with the medical case. In the formulation stage, the ethics case narrative is constructed. "The literal writer . . . determines the perspective from which the case will be seen, chooses the traditions within which to locate the case, judges the elements that are contributory and noncontributory, and established the cognitive and affective maps with which readers will follow the narrative trail" (1994, 267). In the third stage, the ethicist becomes a critical interpreter of the case that has just been constructed. During the interpretation stage, the ethicist becomes particularly attentive to the potential multitude of interpretations of the narrative. The final step is that of validation. Charon argues that we have an ethical obligation to test out our interpretations. She notes that while there exist clear criteria for validating medical and literary interpretations, we do not yet have such criteria for moral decisions. One potential method that she recommends for validation is casuistry, the making of explicit comparisons and contrasts between particular ethics cases and established paradigms (see chapter 7).

Narrative theory also provides a method for critical self-reflection regarding the representation of medical ethics cases. One of the primary ways in which medical ethicists test out their ideas is through case narratives, and understanding the data requires attending to narratological elements of a case. That is, it means that we must recognize that cases are stories and thus are influenced by the rhetorical nature of stories, such as plot, perspective, character, and voice (Chambers 1999). For example, ethics cases tend to have what is termed in narrative theory "undramatized narrators." In narratives in which the narrator is made explicit, that is, explicitly employs or suggests the presence of a speaker, the reader is made "conscious of an experiencing mind whose views of the experience will come between us and the event. When there is no such 'I' . . . the inexperienced reader may make the mistake of thinking that the story comes to him unmediated" (Booth 1983, 152). Medical ethics cases are generally told through an undramatized narrator and this choice tends to deflect a reader from questioning the veracity of the account. When moral theories focus on motivation or perception, as virtue ethics, this form of narrator itself makes an argument against the viability of using this type of perspective in the analysis of a moral problem (Chambers 1999). All narrators taint stories and shape them toward particular ends, and medical ethics cases are no exception.

WRITING THE PATIENT'S STORY

Howard Brody has described the work of the physician in narrative terms as the "joint construction of narrative." Physicians must first learn to "read" the patient's story and then assist in a rewriting of that story.

> The physician who takes stories seriously will . . . adopt as a working hypothesis that the patient is asking a question like the following: "Something is happening to me that seems abnormal, and either I cannot think of a story that will explain it, or the only story I can think of is very frightening. Can you help me to tell a better story, one that will cause me less distress, about this experience?" If this formulation seems overly wordy, a shorter form of the patient's possible plea to the physician might be, "My story is broken; can you help me fix it?" (Brody 1994, 85)

For Brody, this narrative construction is the best method for maintaining the moral relationship of physician and patient. His notion of a broken story that needs repair relies upon a conception of the human self as narratively constructed. This narrative-based understanding of the human self is indebted to the work of such philosophers as Alasdair MacIntyre and Charles Taylor. In *After Virtue*, MacIntyre urges a return to an Aristotelian ethic based on virtue; he argues that for virtue to be "intelligible" or have any genuine traction in our lives, the self must itself be part of some unity. It is through narrative that a human life possesses this unity.

When it comes to medical ethics, however, this notion of the narrative self is used in response to another's, rather than one's own, life project (Chambers 2008, 130). The work that Brody and others promote is the repair of another's self, whose narrative self has been profoundly damaged by illness. Narrative ethicists have criticized traditional medical ethics for viewing moral issues in terms of a notion of the self as simply composed of unrelated isolated incidents, or what has been referred to as the punctual self. Unlike the philosophers discussed above, narrative ethicists are not interested in developing their own virtue through narrative. Instead, they employ this notion of the narrative self so that they can assist in the care and decisions of sick people, people for whom sickness has profoundly disrupted their life story. Miles and Montgomery were among the first to argue for the importance of the life story in resolving medical ethics problems. They viewed narrative ethics as a corrective to a predilection within medical ethics to ignore the most vital aspects of a person's life—those features that occur outside the medical encounter. From a physician's perspective, a person's story begins with the patient's entrance into the world of the clinic. The notion of past history is reserved solely for the past medical problems and not those features of a person's history that make him who he is.

This method of narrative ethics seeks to replace the focus on the genre of the medical case with that of the life story.

> It [narrative ethics] recognizes the importance of circumstance and historical setting in medical cases. It understands that narrative coherence must be constructed from a person's history of moral choices and relationships with others. This, rather than theoretical consistency, will determine how family, patients, and health care workers evaluate meaning and duties in clinical situations. It shifts the weight of the standard for evaluating ethics problems from "well-reasoned solutions" to "well-lived lives." (Miles and Montgomery Hunter 1990, 63)

Brody argues that this notion, which he calls a "life-span narrative," can be useful for medical ethics. He draws on this concept in analyzing those moral problems that occur at both the beginning and the end of the life story, infancy and old age (Brody 2003). Both infants and the elderly find themselves in states of dependence upon others but from opposed narrative perspectives. Infants have little control of their lives, for their lives are being written by others. The elderly can be in positions in which they are losing the control of their narratives, for their increasing dependence on others can make them the subjects of the scripts of others. Brody refers to the differing degrees of dependence in narrative construction as coauthorship. He notes that in old age we may find ourselves following the scripts that a younger self has written for this present older self. Brody argues that once we begin to think in terms of narrative consistency, these two parts of the life story trajectory become more readily contextualized. Such concepts as best interest and respect for autonomy are unable to show how we experience life as a narrative motion toward an expected end. Lacking this understanding is a bit like knowing how the pieces of chess move but not having a sense of what is at stake in playing.

Arthur Frank also argues that the patient's story should be at the center of medical ethics. He cautions, however, against the expectation that method of narrative ethics produces categorical and unambiguous directions for resolving moral problems. "Instead, what is offered is permission to *allow the story to lead in certain directions*" (Frank 1995, 160). For Frank, narrative has a logic of its own that, once acknowledged as an acceptable methodology, can be used by the health care professionals to assist in making decisions for patients when they are unable to present events for themselves. While such a narrative technique can be helpful for health care professionals, Frank cautions that "ill people do not tell their stories so that medical workers can make decisions" (1995, 161), for Frank believes that such an expectation once again views medical ethics from the perspective of the health care professional rather than from the perspective of the patient. For patients, their illness narratives have a much greater moral claim. Frank argues that patient stories should be understood within a larger frame of communal commitment to understanding and recognizing the suffering of others, as well as the healing power of telling and listening to stories of suffering.

Frank's particular take on narrative ethics has been profoundly shaped by the fact that he views morality and medicine from the perspective of the patient rather than from that of the health care professional. Within one year, Frank had two life-threatening illnesses, and his book, *At the Will of the Body* (1991), was both a memoir and a series of reflections on his illness experience. In *The Wounded Storyteller* Frank develops a more formal and systematic exploration of how narrative, illness, and ethics become intertwined for what he refers to as the "remission society." This new society is the result of the state of contemporary medicine, for at this time many of our illnesses are not cured by medicine (or "cured" by death) but have become chronic entities. Frank asserts that patients must move from being the passive recipients of medical care to becoming active storytellers who use their illness narratives to reshape their sense of self and to transform their listeners by the telling of their stories. "As wounded, people may be cared for, but as storytellers, they care for others" (Frank 1995, xii).

Unlike those who see patients as people who possess stories, Frank views patients as active agents who have a moral duty to tell their illness stories, and the rest of us have a moral duty to listen to their stories. Narrative ethicists have tended to view persons as being distinct and separate from others, but Frank views patient stories as embedded in a communal obligation to tell and to listen. As noted above, Frank is critical of an instrumental view of patient stories for medical ethics; they do not exist to help resolve the problems of health care professionals. For Frank, illness divests us of our voices and in becoming storytellers we are able to repossess our voices in this new self-story. Frank places the medical ethicists in the position of being listeners to illness narratives and thus radically decenters (or perhaps recenters) medical ethics.

For many of the theorists mentioned in this chapter, literature and narrative are assumed to be positive forces within human life, and thus their presence or absence signifies either a rich or poor moral world. Hilde Lindemann takes a far more agnostic stance toward narrative. From her perspective, narratives are simply additional tools of the human animal and can be as easily used for oppression as for liberation. Unlike those theorists who believe that literature can provide a method that fully replaces moral philosophy, Lindemann holds that literature and philosophy need each other. She argues that a grasp of the nature of narrative is essential to understand the nature of the human self, and the methods of philosophy provide the critical tools to evaluate the moral status of those narratives. Each is necessary but not sufficient for the construction of a robust sense of self.

Lindemann's concept of the narrative self differs in three ways from those already discussed in this chapter. First, she does not believe that the self needs to be defined by a single life narrative, and her model accepts the possibility of a multitude of simultaneous narrative identities. The reason for this more pluralistic view is related to a second key difference. She observes that our identity is not merely constructed of stories we tell ourselves but also of stories that others tell us and tell each other about us; identity is thus a "complex interaction of narratives from a first-, second-, and third-person perspective" (Lindemann Nelson 2001, 152). Third, Lindemann is not content that narrative cohesiveness or coherence is the primary way in which we should evaluate the worth of a narrative self. Instead, she asserts that narratives need to be evaluated by their ability to provide strong explanatory force, a correlation to action, and heft. One of the reasons she does not believe that coherence provides the necessary justification for any evaluation is because she is aware that our selves are the result of not solely individual mythopoesis but also the influence of others. Because we are not the sole author of ourselves, we are the potential victim of oppressive narratives of others. When a self adopts a master narrative that essentially construes the person as inferior or essentially damaged, then we have a duty to construct a new narrative, or in Lindemann's terms, a "counterstory."

❧ Critiques of Literature Methods

Here I examine critiques of the four ways in which literature has been used in medical ethics, which were described earlier. But since so many of these methods derive their perspective from the literature analogy, it seems necessary to review potential criticisms of the use of the analogy itself. In his essay "Blurred Genres: The Refiguration of Social Thought," Clifford Geertz (1983) observes that there have been three analogies from the humanities that have been drawn upon to help explicate social life: drama, game, and text. The text analogy, which Geertz himself advocated, is the conceptual cousin of the literature analogy. In the social sciences, our social lives are "read" in the same manner in which we read texts. While the text analogy in the social sciences has received general acceptance, it has also been criticized for its potential myopia. Michael Jackson warns against "fetishizing texts," for he states that while conceiving of social interactions as being like texts may make sense for academics, for those who do not define their world through their relation to texts, such a claim simply "sounds absurd," especially to those who understand their lives as serial face-to-face interactions (1989, 184). Imagine another form of humanities scholar being invited into the medical world, scholars who emphasize the other two of Geertz's analogies. What would it mean to think of medicine and medical ethics as drama or performance ? How much more would be revealed if we consider medicine as a game? Many advocates of narrative ethics seem to perceive their analogy not so much as an analogy but rather as a natural component of ethics and, by doing so, rarely acknowledge the limits and danger of this analogy.

ETHICS CASES VS. LITERARY CASES

In an examination of the use of literature as ethics cases, James Terry and Peter Williams caution against any naïve adoption of literary texts in the analysis of medical ethics. Their concern lies primarily in that the two disciplines do not share common goals. The goals of medical ethics include the identification and analysis of a moral problem toward the final end of providing recommendations for a course of action. "Extraneous elements of the case that should not influence the argument or decisions are usually isolated, ignored, or removed. Ambiguity is resolved or controlled as much as possible by collecting all relevant facts, defining important terms, making premises explicit, and proceeding in the analysis carefully, step by step" (Terry and Williams 1988, 3–4). The goals of literature, they report, are to "produce entertainment and aesthetic pleasure," "promote sensitivity and empathy," and "display ambiguity." Terry and Williams provide three examples in which they compare a literary story to an ethics case. For example, they examine Williams's "The Use of Force" in relation to a similar issue illustrated by a standard ethics case, and they conclude that the Williams story complicates the issue of medical paternalism in a manner that is missing from the case presentation. Here the Williams story exemplifies the drive of the literary to produce ambiguity, and in doing so, it thwarts the medical ethicist from providing an appropriate analysis. There is an essential flaw in this critique in that Terry and Williams believe there is a simple and clear dividing line between literary and the nonliterary texts. In their discussion of the medical case they observe, "There are even some unusual literary touches in the way the case is written" (9). Their analysis depends upon there being a "natural" or "unaesthetic" language that can be used for medical ethics in contrast to the aesthetic, ambiguity-driven language of the artist.

THE UNIVERSAL AND THE PARTICULAR

One of the sharpest critiques of using literature as a praxis in moral decision making entails a questioning of the need for this link between literature and medical ethics. Tom Tomlinson asks, "isn't it by talking to the actual patient, seeing his real suffering, feeling sympathy for her genuine plight, that we cross the bridge between the patient on the one side and the doctor, nurse, or ethicist on the other? A vicarious literary experience or second-hand story would be a poor substitute" (1997, 125). One of the features of literature that Tomlinson seems to be unaware of is that literature reveals the internal world of patients that can at times remain hidden or unarticulated. Tomlinson also points out that there is a "have your cake and eat it, too" quality to the argument of those who are in favor of using literature in this way. On the one hand, those who advocate using literature contend that what one learns from literature are the particularities and impossibility of constructing universal rules for analyzing individuals. On the other hand, they suggest that what one learns from literature informs how one should respond to the particular patient at hand. Literature's advocates appear to argue that literature is useful to show what cannot be reduced and, at the same, that it is useful because one can apply these particularistic values across stories. An advocate for this approach could respond that what is applied across stories is not the particular meaning but a specific method of understanding the particularities of a patient's narrative.

THE SPECTER OF RELATIVISM

The notion that an awareness of narrative can contribute to medical ethics has generally not received strong negative criticism. As John Arras observes, the approach to narrative ethics as proposed by Charon reinforces the status of moral principles and provides a way to make these principles "work better" (1997, 70). The use of narrative theory to criticize the field of medical ethics has understandably received more negative attention. One of the most common concerns about seeing all medical ethics cases as tainted by the theoretical perspective of the teller is that it potentially leads to moral relativism (Kuczewski 2001). If we cannot separate the rhetoric of the case narrative from that of the philosophical position proposed to resolve the dilemma, then the entire enterprise of medical ethics, that is, an applied form of ethics, can be considered itself under suspicion. From this perspective, to adopt a narrative approach to medical ethics is also to accept a view that all of medical ethics is simply an activity with no grounding in objective truth; everyone's story is simply an attempt to rhetorically support a particular theory rather than test out a theory. Yet this criticism can be answered by observing that attending to the rhetorical features of medical ethics is actually to attend to the human qualities of this very human enterprise; it is simply an honest acknowledgment of the contingent nature of knowing in medical ethics (Chambers 2001).

THE VALIDITY OF THE LIFE STORY

Criticisms of the life story approach can be divided into those who attack the empirical truth of the claim of a storied self and those who are critical of the claims that such an approach does not require external normative principles. In "Against Narrativity," Galen Strawson charges that the notion of the self as structured as a narrative is empirically false. It is not, Strawson claims, that there are not individuals who experience their lives as a narrative but the universalizing of such a notion seems to him false because there are individuals—and he counts himself as one of them—who experience their lives in an "episodic" manner. He writes, "one does not figure oneself, considered as a self, as something that was there in the (further) past and will be there in the (further) future" (2004, 430). It should be noted that Strawson is critical not only of the claim that we construe our selves through narrative but also that we should do so. Another empirically based criticism against the notion of the life story comes from the observation that this genre seems extraordinarily difficult to find in the wild (Chambers 2008). If, as it is claimed, the human animal naturally understands itself in relation to a life story, it seems quite odd that there are few instances, if any, in our life in which we actually tell our "life story," even to ourselves. We certainly tell stories about ourselves but the kind of life-story project promoted by narrative ethicists seems to exist only in the minds of narrative ethicists.

But if we were to put aside the empirical claim and agree that even if it did not happen, it should happen, then, it has been argued, narrative ethicists must still rely upon "top-down" principles in order to determine which stories are better than others. Thus, narrative ethicists would need to rely upon the sort of principlism (see chapter 3) from which they seek to distance themselves. Tomlinson observes that when narrative ethicists identify how to act in relation to a life narrative, they appeal to the notion of unity or coherence, but they seem unable to state what makes a life coherent without appealing to "extranarrative ideals" (1997, 130–32). Arras questions the self-validating nature of Frank's postmodern narrative ethics, for by privileging the patient's story simply because it is the patient's, one cannot objectively determine the validity of any particular telling. By doing so, one "risks sacrificing ethics at the altar of personal self-development" (Arras 1997, 81). Lindemann's notion of the counterstory seems to provide a response to these criticisms in that she does not privilege the patient's story (for the patient's story can be corrupted by an oppressive master narrative), and she advocates for extranarrative philosophical evaluations for determining the relative value of different stories.

❧ Notes on Resources and Training

There are two notable collections that provide a good overview of how literature can be used in medical ethics. Hilde Lindemann's edited collection *Stories and Their Limits: Narrative Approaches to Bioethics* (Lindemann Nelson 1997) remains a seminal collection of the various perspectives on the use of literature and narrative in medical ethics. The book includes essays by many of the scholars discussed in this chapter. The second collection, *Stories Matter: The Role of Narrative in Medical Ethics*, edited by Rita Charon and Martha Montello, includes a section titled "Narrative Components of Bioethics," which tries to provide examples of literary techniques that can assist in resolving moral problems, including particular attention to voice, context, time, character, plot, and reader. Although essays on literature and medical ethics can be found in most bioethics journals, some journals are notable for the particular attention they have paid to this topic. *Literature and Medicine*, the flagship journal of the discipline of its title has, since its inception, included articles about medical ethics, in particular, and the issues of the relations of literature to morality, in general. The journal *Theoretical Medicine and Bioethics* has been a key forum for the examination of hermeneutics in medical ethics. The *Hastings Center Report*, the *Journal of Clinical Ethics*, and the *Journal of Medical Humanities* have maintained an ongoing interest in literary approaches to medical ethics as well as narrative bioethics.

If one were interested in graduate work that focuses on literature as a method in medical ethics, the best environment would be medical humanities programs. Although at this time there are a number of master's degree programs in medical ethics, few of these programs provide the necessary training in literature in order to enable one to receive adequate training in the literature method. However, there are programs that equally emphasize medical ethics and medical humanities, and these programs often include literature as a distinct approach to moral problems in medicine. Examples of these types of graduate programs include those at the Institute for Medical Humanities at the University of Texas Medical Branch, Galveston; the Medical Humanities and Bioethics Program at Northwestern University; and the Narrative Medicine Program at Columbia University's College of Physicians and Surgeons.

There are several notable intensive courses, including a National Endowment for the Humanities course on Medicine, Literature, and Culture at Pennsylvania State University in Hershey, and a course on Case Narrative and the Construction of Objectivity at Northwestern University's Feinberg School of Medicine. Courses and workshops of this nature are also offered at the American Society for Bioethics and Humanities meetings. Anne Hudson Jones proposes that narrative competence can occur in less-formal training as well (2002, 163). She recommends that medical ethicists could attain some degree of competence by attending university literature department seminars. She also notes that reading groups led by literature experts could provide an excellent forum for developing these skills.

References

Arras, J. D. 1997. Nice story, but so what?: Narrative and justification in ethics. In *Stories and their limits: Narrative approaches to bioethics*, ed. H. Lindemann Nelson. New York: Routledge.

Banks, J. T., and A. H. Hawkins, eds. 1992. *The art of the case history, literature and medicine*. Baltimore: Johns Hopkins University Press.

Booth, W. C. 1983. *The rhetoric of fiction*. 2nd ed. Chicago: University of Chicago Press.

Brody, H. 1994. My story is broken; can you help me fix it? Medical ethics and the joint construction of narrative. *Literature & Medicine* 13 (1): 79–92.

———. 2003. *Stories of sickness*. 2nd ed. Oxford and New York: Oxford University Press.

Carson, R., C. Burns, and T. Cole, eds. 2003. *Practicing the medical humanities: Engaging physicians and patients*. Hagerstown, MD: University Publishing Group.

Chambers, T. 1999. *The fiction of bioethics (reflective bioethics)*. New York: Routledge.

———. 2000. Why ethicists should stop writing cases. *Journal of Clinical Ethics* 11, no. 3 (Fall): 206–12.

———. 2001. Of course I am a relativist and so should you be. *American Journal of Bioethics* 1 (4): W14.

———. 2008. Toward a naturalized narrative ethics. In *Naturalized and narrative bioethics*, ed. H. Lindemann and M. Walker. Cambridge: Cambridge University Press.

Charon, R. 1993. The narrative road to empathy. In *Empathy and the practice of medicine: Beyond pills and the scalpel*. New Haven, CT: Yale University Press.

———. 1994. Narrative contributions to medical ethics. In *A matter of principles?* ed. E. R. DuBose, R. Hamel, and L. J. O'Connell. Valley Forge, PA: Trinity Press International.

———. 2001. Narrative medicine: Form, function, and ethics. *Journal of Internal Medicine* 134 (1): 83–87.

———. 2006. *Narrative medicine: Honoring the stories of illness*. Oxford and New York: Oxford University Press.

Clouser, K. 1996. Philosophy, literature, and ethics: Let the engagement begin. *Journal of Medicine and Philosophy* 21 (3): 287–302.

Cohn, D. 1983. *Transparent minds: Narrative modes for presenting consciousness in fiction*. 1st Princeton paperback printing, with corrections. Princeton, NJ: Princeton University Press.

———. 2000. *The distinction of fiction*. Johns Hopkins Paperbacks ed. Baltimore: Johns Hopkins University Press.

Coles, R. 1979. Occasional notes. Medical ethics and living a life. *New England Journal of Medicine* 301 (8): 444–46.

Davis, T. F., and K. Womack, eds. 2001. *Mapping the ethical turn: A reader in ethics, culture, and literary theory*. Charlottesville: University Press of Virginia.

Eagleton, T. 1983. *Literary theory: An introduction*. Minneapolis: University of Minnesota Press.

Forster, E. M. 1985. *Aspects of the novel*. San Diego: Harcourt Brace Jovanovich.

Fox, R. C. 1999. Is medical education asking too much of bioethics? *Dædalus* 128 (4): 1–25.

Frank, A. W. 1995. *The wounded storyteller: Body, illness, and ethics*. Chicago: University of Chicago Press.

Geertz, C. 1983. *Local knowledge: Further essays in interpretive anthropology*. New York: Basic Books.

Hawkins, A. H. 1994. Literature, medical ethics, and "epiphanic knowledge." *Journal of Clinical Ethics* 5 (4): 283–90.

———. 1996. Literature, philosophy, and medical ethics: Let the dialogue go on. *Journal of Medicine and Philosophy* 21 (3): 341–54.

———. 1997. Medical ethics and the epiphanic dimension of narrative. In *Stories and their limits: Narrative approaches to bioethics*, ed. H. Lindemann Nelson. New York: Routledge.

Jackson, M. 1989. *Paths toward a clearing: Radical empiricism and ethnographic inquiry, African systems of thought*. Bloomington: Indiana University Press.

Jones, A. H. 2002. The color of the wallpaper: Training for narrative ethics. In *Stories matter: The role of narrative in medical ethics*, ed. R. Charon and M. Montello. New York: Routledge.

King, N., and A. Stanford. 1992. Patient stories, doctor stories, and true stories: A cautionary reading. *Literature and Medicine* 11 (2): 185.

Kuczewski, M. G. 2001. In search of an honest case. *The American Journal of Bioethics: AJOB* 1 (1): 44–45.

Lindemann Nelson, H., ed. 1997. *Stories and their limits: Narrative approaches to bioethics, reflective bioethics*. New York: Routledge.

———. 2001. *Damaged identities, narrative repair*. Ithaca: Cornell University Press.

Miles, S. H., and K. Montgomery Hunter. 1990. Commentary. *Second Opinion* 15:60–63.

Montgomery, K. 1991. How to be a doctor: The place of poetry in medical education. *Second Opinion* 16:65–77.

———. 2005. *How doctors think: Clinical judgment and the practice of medicine*. New York: Oxford University Press.

Montgomery Hunter, K. 1991. *Doctors' stories: The narrative structure of medical knowledge*. Princeton, NJ: Princeton University Press.

Moore, A. R. 1978. *The missing medical text: Humane patient care*. Carlton [Australia] Forest Grove, OR: Melbourne University Press; distributed by International Scholarly Book Service.

Morson, G. S., and C. Emerson. 1990. *Mikhail Bakhtin: Creation of a prosaics*. Stanford, CA: Stanford University Press.

Pellegrino, E. D. 1980. Introduction: To look feelingly—The affinities of medicine and literature. In *Medicine and literature*, ed. E. R. Peschel. New York: N. Watson Academic Publications.

Rabinow, P., and W. M. Sullivan, eds. 1987. *Interpretive social science: A second look*. Berkeley: University of California Press.

Strawson, G. 2004. Against narrativity. *Ratio* XVII:428–52.

Terry, J. S., and P. C. Williams. 1988. Literature and bioethics: The tension in goals and styles. *Literature and Medicine* 7:1–21.

Tomlinson, T. 1997. Perplexed about narrative ethics. In *Stories and their limits: Narrative approaches to bioethics*, ed. H. Lindemann Nelson. New York: Routledge.

Trautmann, J. 1992. Can we resurrect Apollo? *Literature & Medicine* 1 (1): 1–18.

Walsh, R. 1995. *Novel arguments: Reading innovative American fiction, Cambridge studies in American literature and culture; 91*. Cambridge, UK; New York: Cambridge University Press.

Williams, W. C., and R. Coles. 1984. *The doctor stories*. New York: New Directions.

CHAPTER 11

Sociology

RAYMOND DE VRIES

It might have been otherwise . . .

—*Jane Kenyon*

In her poem *Otherwise* Jane Kenyon (1996) describes the events that mark a pleasing but ordinary day in her life, reminding herself and her readers that for any number of reasons it "might have been otherwise." This sensibility—that the things that we assume to be a normal or natural part of life easily could be otherwise—is a defining feature of the sociological perspective. When sociologists look at some part of the social world—be it a classroom, a criminal court, a soccer match, or an ethics committee meeting—they recognize that the activity in question might have been otherwise: given a different set of social and cultural conditions, the way we educate children (or conduct legal proceedings or behave at sporting events or deliberate on ethical questions) would, in fact, be otherwise.

This unique sociological sensibility has much to offer to medical ethics. Sophisticated techniques for collecting and analyzing data about human behavior developed by sociologists are sometimes seen as the primary—if not the only—contribution of the discipline to the study and practice of medical ethics. But these techniques are not the defining feature of sociology. Quantitative and qualitative research methods (discussed elsewhere in this book) are not the sole possession of sociology; indeed, they are approaches to research used by practitioners in a number of social sciences and health services disciplines. Research methods are the tools of sociology but they tell us very little about the way sociologists approach the study of the social world. This chapter explores how the distinctive sociological way of seeing the world—the sociological imagination (Mills 1959)—can be brought to bear on matters of ethics in medicine.

Description of Sociologic Methods

The relationship between sociology and ethics is peculiar. Classical social theorists, those who created the discipline of sociology, had an explicit concern with morality, with the moral glue that held members of society together. More recently pioneers in medical sociology often examined issues in health care with direct ethical import. But, in spite of this disciplinary history, sociologists have, until recently, avoided the study of the emergence, operation, and import of medical ethics and its offspring, bioethics.

SOCIOLOGY AND MORALITY: THE MORAL BASIS OF SOCIETY

Sociology was born out of a desire to understand the moral foundations of society. Although some see shadows of sociological thinking in the work of Plato, most historians locate the origin of sociology in the nineteenth century, crediting August Comte, a French thinker, with establishing the discipline in its modern form.[1] Comte and other nineteenth- and twentieth-century pioneers of sociology lived through a period of rapid and profound social change. Industrialization, urbanization, secularization, the rise of capitalism, and the advent of mass democracy caused unprecedented physical, social, and psychological dislocation. This dislocation made visible previously taken-for-granted aspects of social life, raising the questions that became foundational for the new discipline: What is the nature of the moral fibers that hold members of society together? How do changing economic and social situations alter the obligations of humans to each other and to themselves? What are the social and human consequences of the shift from traditional to rational forms of authority?

In their efforts to understand how members of modern societies sorted out how to best live together in new social circumstances that altered ideas of right and wrong, early social scientists studied and wrote about religion, law, politics, the economy, and science. In his *Division of Labor in Modern Society*, for example, Durkheim presented his vision of the social forces that bind individuals together in a society. Responding to Tönnies's gloomy depiction (1957) of the changes wrought by modern life—where small and friendly *gemeinschaft* societies were giving way to the larger and impersonal *gessellschaft*—Durkheim offered a positive view of urbanization and industrialization as a transition from mechanical to organic solidarity.

According to Durkheim, older societies were united in a mechanical, automatic way: He found evidence of this in their legal systems, which responded to the violation of norms by lashing out with repressive sanctions. The offender was punished to exact retribution. In modern societies, Durkheim argued, people are connected organically—each dependent on the other in a complex division of labor. This type of society is characterized by a system of restitutive law: When a norm is violated the *conscience collectif* responds by addressing the imbalance created. The goal is to restore the status quo ante, not to punish the offender.

For his part, Max Weber was interested in the slide toward rationality that came with modernity. In examining the causes and consequences of modern rationality, Weber focused on values. Much of his work is an effort to understand why and how values persisted and changed and how they influenced forms of rationality in modernizing societies. In his classic *Protestant Ethic and the Sprit of Capitalism*, Weber (1992) shows how Protestant doctrines about the afterlife shaped values and thereby promoted individual behaviors that allowed the flourishing of Western capitalism. Weber also explores the proper place of values in the work of politics and science in his well-known essays, "Politics as a Vocation" and "Science as a Vocation" (in Gerth and Mills 1946).

MORAL ISSUES IN MEDICAL SOCIOLOGY

The interest in values and morality found in classical sociology also is evident in the work of the pioneers in the subfield of medical sociology. In the early to mid-1950s, a number of sociologists in the United States turned their attention to the study of patterns of diseases, social conceptions of health and illness, the functioning of medical systems, and the health care professions (Bloom 2002). While medical sociologists of the 1950s, '60s, and '70s did not explicitly study medical ethics, much of their work touched on moral issues in medical care. Consider, for example, the work of Talcott Parsons. Parsons, a social theorist whose work helped to define the new field of medical sociology, described medicine as an important system of social control. For Parsons (1951, 428–79) illness was a type of deviance, a threat to the stability of society. Those guilty of deviating from legal norms were sent to legal institutions (courts, prisons, parole offices) intended to rehabilitate them and integrate them back into society; the sick—violators of the norms of health—were treated and rehabilitated by the institutions of the medical system (doctors' offices and hospitals).

Other pioneers in medical sociology showed a similar concern with the moral questions that permeate illness and its treatment, although they, like Parsons, rarely mention an explicit interest in ethics. Included in this work are studies of medical education that describe the "fate of idealism" and explore how students "negotiate" the demands of coursework and examinations (Merton, Reader, and Kendall 1957; Becker et al. 1961); ethnographies of work in the hospital that reveal how death is thought about, managed, discussed, and revealed to next-of-kin and others (Sudnow 1967); research on the medical profession that shows an unfavorable balance between the self-interest of professionals and the interest of patients (Freidson 1970); studies of stigma and so-called total institutions that expose the underside of the treatment given those who are not seen as normal (Goffman 1961a, 1963); and analyses of the medicalization of deviance that describe how the control of certain behaviors moved from legal to medical institutions (Conrad and Schneider 1980). Each of these now-classic studies in medical sociology focuses on issues important to medical ethics. Although not labeled as such, truth-telling, conflict of interest, patient autonomy, and organizational ethics are among the ethically relevant topics explored by these sociologists.

Implicit interest in the morality of medicine became more explicit in the 1970s, when sociologists made a turn toward a more conscious study of ethical issues in health care, looking at medical experiments, organ transplantation, and medical errors. In the first half of the decade Barber and his colleagues (1973) and Gray (1975) were involved in sociological studies of human subjects in medical research. Their work was important to the conduct of science and relevant to the social sciences, but it failed to inspire other sociological studies of research ethics or medical ethics.

Bosk's (1979, 2003) *Forgive and Remember*—a study of the response to errors in surgery and surgical residency—is widely regarded as one of the first studies to look directly at medical ethics. Contrary to what most laypeople would expect, Bosk discovered that the technical mistakes of surgical residents (e.g., leaving a surgical instrument in the body of a patient) were taken less seriously, and the offender was less severely punished (if punished at all) than were normative errors—violations of the rules governing the relationships between students and their teachers. His book was ahead of its time, coming as it did before the most recent incarnation of medical ethics—bioethics—had a foothold in the clinic. Bosk is aware of this. He acknowledges that when he started his work he had "never heard of bioethicists"; and when, toward the end of his research, he did learn of this new enterprise, he was highly skeptical of its success. Bosk shows us how moral quandaries were resolved before the formal and organized presence of ethics in hospitals. Had he done his study ten years later—when bioethicists and ethics committees had begun to populate the world of medicine—we would have been able to see how the moral problems of surgeons were (or were not) influenced by "the new moral authority at the bedside" (Rothman 1991).

The research of Fox—studies of medical experiments and organ transplantation—straddled the lab and the clinic. Her two monographs, *Experiment Perilous* (1959) and *The Courage to Fail* (1974, with Judith Swazey) preceded Bosk's book, but they are less studies of ethical problem solving than they are examinations of uncertainty and stress in medical practice. In her books Fox exhibits a tone that is, to say the least, respectful of medicine. Trained under Parsons, her view of physicians emphasizes their role in rehabilitating the sick, their sense of responsibility toward patients, and their unwillingness to exploit patient vulnerability. In an otherwise glowing review of *The Courage to Fail*, Fred Davis (1975, 420) faults Fox for "viewing the terrain of illness from the seemingly heroic stance of the research physician doing battle at the furthermost frontiers of clinical practice." As her work continued, however, Fox's attitude changed. By the time of her publication of *Spare Parts* (1992, with Swazey), Fox had—like her fellow sociologists and society around her—become skeptical about the motives of physicians and the place of ethics in medicine. She and Swazey close their book by announcing their "withdrawal from the field" of organ transplantation, an act taken to separate themselves from "the human suffering and the social, cultural and spiritual harm . . . [transplant medicine] . . . has brought in its wake" (210).

By the 1990s sociological and historical research with an explicit focus on the moral problems of medicine—and their description and resolution by the new interdisciplinary field of bioethics—had begun. Medical historian David Rothman offered his history (1991) of how law and ethics transformed medical decision making, and sociologists entered medical settings with the stated intent of seeing how ethical problems were handled. Zussman examined decision making in intensive care units (1992); Bosk watched genetic counselors at work (1992); and Guillemin and Holmstrom (1986), Anspach (1993), and Mesman (2002) looked at moral deliberations in neonatal intensive care units. This decade also is marked by the first anthologies that have a specific focus on social science perspectives on medical ethics. In 1990 Weisz edited a collection that examined clinical encounters of the ethical kind, ethics in the public arena, the institutions and ideology of medical ethics, and medical ethics and social science. In 1998 De Vries and Subedi collected a series of articles on the social sources of bioethics, the social organization of bioethics, doing bioethics, and the place of sociology in bioethics.

Chambliss's classic study of nursing and ethics (1996) offers a slight variation on the sociological examination of moral issues in medical care. Unlike his colleagues, Chambliss did not start out with the intent of exploring medical ethics; instead his ethnography of nursing led him to notice the moral dimensions of hospital life and the many ways ethics gets used in organizations. His refusal to allow others to define what was and was not an ethical problem gave him a perspective on medical ethics that was missing in other studies. Because he looked for ethical problems outside of their normal venues, he was able to demonstrate convincingly that ethical problems are not discrete, one-at-a-time events that occur between patients, families, and doctors; rather, they are predictable outcomes of social organization. For example, in his graphic account of the emergency treatment given to a woman who was bleeding internally as a result of an ectopic pregnancy—he paints a vivid picture of pools of blood, a fetus that unexpectedly pops out of the woman's belly, and staff members crying and sick—Chambliss never once mentions informed consent or moral questions about the disposition of the fetus or other issues so obviously ethical. Instead he reflects on the moral order of the hospital and the emergency room and comments on what he calls the "morality of cynicism."

In the first decade of the new century, sociological studies of the new profession of bioethics began to appear. In 2002 Evans's examination of the role of bioethicists in the public debate over human genetic engineering (HGE)—*Playing God*—was published. Drawing on ideas developed by Weber (1947, 1968), Evans accuses bioethicists of conspiring with scientists to shrink the debate from a theological one focused on the ends of human life (in Weber's terms a "substantive rationality") to a more secular and "thin" debate centered on proper techniques and means (or "formal rationality" as described by Weber). In his study of the debates about, and regulatory documents governing, the use of HGE, Evans noticed how the debate about this biotechnology changed. Whereas ethicists used to focus on the questions related to the influence of HGE on what it means to be human, bioethicists asked how HGE can be accomplished without violating the principles of autonomy, beneficence, and justice. Evans sees this "thinning" of the debate as an effort by bioethics to claim jurisdiction over an area once controlled by theologians.

In 2008 Fox and Swazey published their autobiographical analysis of the rise of bioethics, *Observing Bioethics*. Drawing on their involvement with the profession of bioethics and their study of matters ethical, the authors detail the social factors associated with the creation of bioethics, show how the field subtly incorporated American values, examine the export of bioethics from the United States to other countries (both developed and developing), and evaluate the politics of bioethics made evident by the "culture wars" in ethics associated with President Bush's Council on Bioethics. Each theme of their book underscores the sociological truth that morality is socially generated, socially organized, and socially deployed.

The turn to sociological research that self-consciously explores issues in medical ethics has sometimes obscured the fact that contemporary research in medical sociology, like the pioneering work done in the 1950s, '60s, and '70s, continues to explore ethically relevant aspects of medicine and health. Because there now exists a sub-field within medical sociology—the sociology of medical ethics (or bioethics)—more general works get defined out of the ethics category. Consider Klinenberg's study of deaths among the elderly in the 1995 Chicago heat wave, for example (2002). Klinenberg presents a "social autopsy" of these deaths that goes beyond the obvious (that is, those who died lacked access to air conditioning). Instead he explores the social conditions—fear of crime, lack of community centers, insufficient attention by city government and public utilities to the needs of older, poor citizens—that led to the isolation of the elderly in their overheated apartments. He concludes: "Medical science can tell us little about the social conditions that affect the course of our lives and the context of our deaths. Excessive use of the medical microscope obscures or makes invisible the social pathologies that generate illness and disease" (234).

Similarly, my study of the influence of culture on regulations that govern maternity care, although not explicitly focused on the ethics of medicine, nevertheless describes the social sources and moral consequences of professional competition (De Vries 2004a). I conclude that we must pay attention to our shared cultural beliefs if we are to make American health more just: "Any effort to change health care systems—be it to make them more efficient, more just, more compassionate, less costly, or less prone to error—must consider the way culture is implicated in the current organization of care" (212).

As with earlier research on medical education, the breaking of bad news and the (re)definition of illness, studies of this type are rife with conclusions about the morality of medicine, but—lacking specific identification as works in ethics—they are not likely to make it to reading lists of those interested in medical ethics.

More recently sociologists are doing studies that treat medical ethics and bioethics as just another part of the medical-social-cultural complex. In her study of the changing nature of medical research, Fisher (2009) looks at the clinical trial industry, challenging the simplistic story that sees profit-minded pharmaceutical companies as the sole cause of the harms perpetuated by drug studies. While not absolving the drug trial industry, her research details the social, cultural, and political conditions that conspire to create the current (and, according to her, flawed) system for testing and marketing of new drugs. In the course of her research, Fisher looks at classical problems in research ethics, including subject recruitment and informed consent, but her analysis of these problems is embedded within her larger concern with the neoliberal ideas—with their emphasis on free markets and faith in the ability of the private sector to solve public problems—that shape the delivery of health care.

Singh explores parental decisions to resort to the use of drugs to control their sons' behaviors (2005, 2007). She details the way parents use the moral language of authenticity and personal freedom to justify their approval of drug therapy for their children. Singh's research is not focused on bioethics per se, but it serves as critique of the field. She concludes (2005, 46, emphasis added):

> Parents' decisionmaking processes around Ritalin doses involve a daunting array of social, psychological, ethical and cultural resources. But such complexity more adequately represents the *moral framework* within which parents will make current and future decisions about neuro-enhancing drugs for their children. . . .

Can applications of moral theory to the problems of neuro-enhancement be relevant without an appreciation of the meaning and significance of behavior, context and moral concepts for those making treatment decisions? The failure of bioethical analyses to properly grasp and grapple with the moral dilemmas of Ritalin treatment for parents of children with ADHD suggests not.

These examples of sociological interest in ethics and morality demonstrate the sociological imagination at work. We now can ask: What are the common features of these studies in classical theory and medical sociology? What does it mean to think like a sociologist, to bring the sociological imagination to bear on the questions of medical ethics?

DEVELOPING AND USING THE SOCIOLOGICAL IMAGINATION

The term "sociology" is a hybrid of Latin (*socius*) and Greek (*-logie*), a peculiar etymology that suits the discipline well. Sociology was conceived by its founders as something new and different, a discipline that stood apart from and above other fields of study, a discipline that could integrate and synthesize knowledge generated by other human sciences. We who practice sociology are proud of this slightly irreverent, Johnny-come-lately aspect of our field. Berger notes (1963, 43–47) that "unrespectability" is part and parcel of sociological analysis; that is, good sociology is characterized by a cynical view of existing organizations, institutions, and sociocultural practices.

But sociology is not simply an untrained, undifferentiated cynicism. It is a distinctive approach to understanding human behavior, a fact that is sometimes difficult to see because, like most other academic disciplines, sociology is divided into myriad schools, orientations, and topic areas, each of which can be crossed with others to create ever finer distinctions between those who do sociology. Thus, there is a group of sociologists who study organizational behavior using ethnographic methods to focus on gender issues. This group will have little or no interaction with those who study organizations using survey methods, especially if the researchers use surveys to focus on the origins and effectiveness of management strategies. Underneath this academic diversity, however, lies a common orientation, a shared basis of sociological insight. This common orientation is best described in two brief and clearly written introductions to the field: Mills's *The Sociological Imagination* and Berger's *Invitation to Sociology*. Both texts were written in the midtwentieth century before the field was as finely fractured as it is now; both are still widely used in college classrooms.

Writing in the late 1950s, Mills was disappointed with the state of sociology. He identified two baleful trends in the discipline: grand theory—an effort to describe universal patterns of human behavior (often written in dense, nearly indecipherable prose) and abstracted empiricism—the development of ever more sophisticated techniques of measuring behavior with no concern for meaning of those behaviors, for how those behaviors might be related to larger social and historical conditions, or for how the data thus collected may be (and can be) used. For Mills the movement in these two directions was a movement away from the genius of the sociological approach. Done well, Mills asserts, sociology examines the links between biography and history; those possessed of a sociological imagination understand the difference between personal troubles and public issues. For example, Mills asks: Is unemployment a personal trouble or a public issue? He explains that it could be either:

> When in a city of 100,000 only one man is unemployed, that is his personal trouble, and for its relief we properly look to the character of the man. But when in a nation of 50 million employees, 15 million men are unemployed, that is an issue and we may not hope to find its solution within the range of opportunities open to any one individual. The very structure of opportunity has collapsed. Both the correct statement of the problem and the range of possible solutions require us to consider the political and economic institutions of society, and not the merely personal situation and character of a scatter of individuals. (1959, 9)

According to Mills, those who would realize the promise of sociology must ask three kinds of questions about their object of study (6–7):

1. What is the structure of this particular society as a whole? (What are its essential components and how are they related to one another?)
2. Where does this society stand in human history? (What are the mechanics by which it is changing? How does any particular feature we are examining [e.g., medical ethics] affect, and how is it affected by, the historical period in which it moves?)
3. What varieties of men and women now prevail in this society and period? (And what varieties are coming to prevail? In what ways are they selected and formed, liberated and repressed, made sensitive and blunted?)

For Berger the essence of sociology is found in three fundamental features of the sociological consciousness: an inclination to debunking; relativity; and (as mentioned above) unrespectability. Berger advises would-be sociologists to develop what Nietzsche called the "art of mistrust," the ability to see through common understandings and definitions of social situations. Among the many ways it can be deployed, this debunking attitude allows a sociologist to identify the ways in which a group's ideology serves its vested interests. Berger explains: "We can speak of 'ideology' when we analyze the belief of many American physicians that standards of health will decline if the fee-for-service method of payment is abolished, or the conviction of many undertakers that inexpensive funerals show lack of affection for the departed" (1963, 41).

Good sociologists, according to Berger, use relativity as an analytic tool; they understand, for example, that "identities [and] ideas are relative to specific social locations: 'Catholicism may have a theory of Communism, but Communism returns the compliment, and will produce a theory of Catholicism. To the Catholic thinker the Communist lives in a dark world of materialist delusion about the real meaning of life. To the Communist, his Catholic adversary is helplessly caught in the 'false consciousness' of a bourgeoisie mentality" (1963, 51).

As Berger points out, a method of analysis that combines debunking and relativizing cannot help but have an air of unrespectablity. It is no surprise that sociologists—who "refuse to be impressed, moved or befuddled by official ideologies," and whose studies of communities "look at the social reality of the community not only from the perspective of city hall, but also from that of the city jail"—are seen as "outsiders" by those they study (44, 46). It is this unrespectable, outsider point of view that allows those who do sociology to generate the insights that help us move beyond official and taken-for-granted (and usually beneficent) explanations of the way organizations and institutions are organized and influence our lives.

Those with a sociological imagination have a moral commitment to challenge "hierarchies of credibility" (Becker 1967) to weigh equally the accounts of a social situation given by the disenfranchised (e.g., a poor and uninsured hospital patient) and the enfranchised (e.g., a member of a hospital ethics committees). There is, of course, what I call a "morality of method" in all the disciplines that contribute to the work of medical ethics (De Vries 2009). Philosophy, for example—especially in its Anglo-American version—is morally committed to clarity and logic. When asked to examine conflicts of interest in medical research, the philosophical imagination seeks precision in the meanings and categories of the terms employed ("conflict" and "interest") and considers the application of moral theory to problems created by these conflicts. Given the same situation, the sociological imagination begins by exploring the social history of the concept of "conflict of interest," its uses (and abuses), the way the term gets operationalized, and who gains and who loses as a result of the policies governing these conflicts. Both approaches are vital to the work of medical ethics, and in fact, the work of each benefits from the challenges of the other. Sociologists are forced to be more rigorous in their development of typologies, and philosophers are forced to make their definitions fit with empirical reality.

Notice how the sociological studies of morality described above exemplify the sociological imagination. First, all these studies consider morality in the context of the larger society, linking what might otherwise be considered private troubles to larger public issues. Fisher shows how the market-based medical system in the United States creates the private troubles of research subjects (2009); and Klinenberg explains how social policies and cultural trends that isolated older, poor city residents accounted for the death of elderly Chicagoans in the heat wave (2002). Second, all these sociologists challenge taken-for-granted explanations of social arrangements. Weber demonstrates that religious beliefs did far more than provide answers to questions about spiritual matters—they also created the conditions for the development of economic systems; Bosk discovers that the teachers of surgical residents were more interested in their moral character than their technical competence; Evans argues that bioethicists abetted ethically problematic research by shifting the terms of the debate from "thick" questions about human nature to "thin" questions about the creation of guidelines and regulations.

THE USES OF SOCIOLOGY IN MEDICAL ETHICS

Sociology is most useful to medical ethics when it is done in a way that balances the use of both its methodological tools and its socially and historically grounded concepts: using only the tools of sociology results in the abstract empiricism feared by Mills; using only the conceptual apparatus of the discipline generates grand theory detached from empirical reality.

In an earlier essay I described the different uses of sociology for medical ethics by distinguishing sociology *in* medical ethics from sociology *of* medical ethics (De Vries 2004b). Sociologists in medical ethics are collaborators. They lend their sociological skills to medical ethics, using their discipline to help medical ethicists solve the quandaries they face. This variety of sociology measures the things medical ethicists need to have measured: Are research subjects really informed after they sign an informed consent? What do research subjects understand (and want to understand) about researchers' conflicts of interest? What does (some section of) the public think about genetic testing? On the other hand, sociologists of medical ethics see the emergence of medical ethics as an opportunity to answer sociological questions, to enhance our understanding of organizations, roles, values, rituals, and the place of medicine and the biosciences in society. Where sociologists in medical ethics lend their skills to the work of medical ethics, sociologists of medical ethics operate from independent positions. They are outsiders, debunkers. They remain far enough above the fray to see how the currents of history shape social movements, disciplines, organizations, nations, and the biographies of individuals.[2]

Abstract empiricism in medical ethics

Sociologists who work in medical ethics—that is, social scientists who apply their tools to questions posed by medical ethicists—are at risk of falling into the problem of abstract empiricism. Consider, for example, the difference between the work of Henderson and her colleagues (2006) and that of Fisher (2009). Both use the tools of social science to look at the experience of research subjects: the Henderson group operates from what I have termed the "in" perspective, while Fisher's work uses the "of" approach.

The Henderson team is interested in the problem of therapeutic misconception (TM)—the problem that occurs when research subjects misconstrue their involvement in a clinical trial as therapy. To explore the causes of TM, they interviewed sixty-eight adults who were subjects in early-phase gene transfer research. They used their interview data to create a composite measure of the presence and extent of TM on the part of a research subject and then correlated TM scores with characteristics of the subjects and the study. They discovered that three variables predicted a subject's TM score: level of education, disease type, and communication by study personnel about the likelihood of benefit. Notice how Henderson et al. "keep their heads down"; that is, they limit their research and analysis to features of the subjects and the clinical trial. Although they acknowledge that "disease is a complex, multifaceted variable that encompasses not only individual- and study-level factors, but also the socially and culturally determined meanings associated with particular diseases" (251), they make no effort to understand how the interests of research subjects or the organization of clinical trials are related to cultural ideas about health care (and the value of medical therapies as a response to disease) or the organization of the health system in the United States.

For her part Fisher gives away her "of" perspective in the title of her book: *Medical Research for Hire: The Political Economy of Pharmaceutical Clinical Trials* (2009). Her research locates the experiences of research subjects—their desires, their needs, and their understandings of clinical research—in the context of a market-based health care system. She shows how the behavior of all those involved in clinical trials—pharmaceutical companies that must protect their data from the prying eyes of competitors, physicians who supplement their income by running drug trials in their private practices, study coordinators who must find a way to balance their desire to care for their patient/subjects with the demands of gathering "good" data, and research subjects who often see clinical trials as a way to get health care—is shaped by the historically situated organization of health care in twenty-first-century America. She takes seriously Mills's admonition that good sociology must consider: Where does this society stands in human history, and How does the drug trial industry affect (and how is it affected by) the historical period in which it moves?

The "in" approach of Henderson et al. can be used to improve the practice of gaining consent from research subjects, but the revision of consent forms and modification of the practices of researchers offers only a partial step toward the goals of medical ethics related to ensuring that health care and the life sciences are done in a way that respects persons and promotes justice. The broader net cast by Fisher—her research reveals how the lives and decisions of research subjects as well as the guidelines meant to protect them are products of this historical moment—provides the fundamental information necessary to promote more ethical medicine.

There is an irony here. Sociologists who begin with questions of their own—questions not given to them by medical ethicists or shaped by the field of medical ethics—are more likely to discover social facts that are important to medical ethicists. Admittedly, the findings generated by sociologists "of" medical ethics are more difficult to translate into social policy: it is far easier to develop a set of regulations for institutional review boards than it is to alter the historical conditions responsible for the organization and delivery of health care. But lacking information offered by the use of the sociological imagination, medical ethicists will likely fail to understand the mechanics of the system (including the ways they are implicated in the system) they wish to change.

Grand theory in medical ethics

If abstract empiricism—the collection and analysis of data with no consideration of historical context—creates a problem for medical ethics, so too does the development of ideas and theories with no attention to their fit with empirical reality. Most often critiqued in this regard—by sociologists and others—is the "principlist" approach that is widely used to solve the ethical quandaries of medicine.

While there are a number of sophisticated theoretical approaches for solving the moral problems of medicine—including casuistry, narrative ethics, feminist ethics, and care ethics—many deliberations that occur in hospital ethics committees, in committees that advise professional bodies, and in research ethics committees invoke the four principles of autonomy, beneficence, nonmaleficence, and justice (Beauchamp and Childress 2001). This is no surprise. Principlism provides a means of recognizing and resolving ethical dilemmas. Such routinization of ethical deliberation makes organizational sense. Medical ethicists must find a way to collect information, strip away confounding factors, and zero in on the essential issue in question. Clearing away the clutter provides clarity for medical ethics but also obscures the social origins of the facts that are brought to bear in ethical deliberation.

When asked to consider ethical problems associated with gene therapy, for example, medical ethicists ask about risks and benefits of the procedure, scrutinize the informed consent process, question the effects of altered genes on the population, and consider who will and will not have access to new treatments. They do not tend to ask about the more foundational issues:

- How did this medical practice and the science that supports it come to be (that is, what are the social and cultural forces that produced genetic therapies as opposed to other approaches to disease)?
- What influences the desires and demands for these therapies by patients and their families?
- How does this approach to disease reflect the desires and anxieties of caregivers?
- How does the social location of medical ethics—in the worlds of medicine, science, and in the larger culture—influence ethical judgment?

In distilling the facts of the case of gene therapy—about risk and benefit, personal autonomy, and justice—consultant bioethicists ignore the way these facts are produced by cultural ideas, social structures, organizational constraints, group norms, and social relationships. Of course, to add this layer of analysis and concern to ethical deliberation is organizationally impractical. But these issues arguably should be part of the conversation. Parallel, sociological analyses of the social conditions that create ethical quandaries can be used by medical ethicists to expand their vision of the causes and the solutions to moral problems.

From the sociologist's perspective, principlism also suffers from the problem of cultural fit. Advocates of principlism claim that abstract principles can float above, and yet account for, the peculiarities of culture. They argue that regardless of our cultural differences we can all agree that nonmaleficence is a good thing, even if you and I define harm differently. In the United States autonomy is conceived in a radically individualist manner, but in other cultures we can adjust the idea to incorporate more familial and communal ideas of autonomy. In the atomistic United States a free and independent individual should (must?) determine her care, while in more communal societies autonomous decisions occur in consultation with, or by decision of, recognized authorities.

Pushed too far in this direction the principles become meaningless. Can we really speak of autonomy if a treatment decision for an adult woman is made by others? Philosophical deliberation on the principles that guide ethical decisions is, of course, important. But sociologists are more interested in how a particular set of principles came to predominate and what happens when those carefully derived principles move into the world: How do they get used? Who uses them? What (cultural, institutional, organizational, corporate, or individual) purposes do they serve? Seen from the point of view of sociology, the principles are empty vessels into which cultural meanings are poured. Sociologists are more interested in how the vessel was created and what is put into it than they are in the vessel itself.

MISUSING SOCIOLOGY: HOW TO AVOID
SOCIOLOGICAL REDUCTIONISM

Sociologists who work in the field of medical ethics are fond of using the image of the mirror to describe their work. According to Turner (2009) sociologists who study medical ethics use the "mirror of social science" to provide "more 'realistic', empirically 'honest', 'grubby' accounts of social life" (84). But Turner is skeptical about the application of this mirror to medical ethics: "The trope of the mirror has its limitations. . . . The problem . . . is not that social scientists provide a mirror upon whose surface we can see bioethics with all its flaws. Rather, the chief limitation with sociological and anthropological analysis of bioethics to date is that too often social scientists offer a 'Fun House' mirror in which bioethics is, if not quite unrecognizable, at least bent out of shape" (84).

Turner has a point. Like other academics we sociologists tend to be reductionistic, to see the world through the lens of the discipline to which we have devoted our lives. This tendency is shared among the disciplines of medical ethics. In fact, the inclination toward disciplinary reductionism is aggravated in medical ethics, where members of each discipline vie for the last word on what is morally right and wrong (Chambers 2000). Thus philosophers who do medical ethics tell us social scientists: "You can't get an *ought* from an *is*," and we social scientists respond, "You can't get an *ought* from an *ought*!" (that is, logical arguments are culturally contingent). Practitioners of X-Phi (experimental philosophy) tell old-fashioned moral philosophers, "Philosophize all you want, in the end all your notions of right and wrong are predicted by your bio-, psycho-, socio-situation." We sociologists may, in fact, be more inclined than most to be defensive about our discipline, given that we have not always had the warmest welcome from medical ethicists, being variously accused of resentment, arrogance, and "baiting bioethics" (De Vries 2004b).

In spite of this disciplinary defensiveness, the interdisciplinarity of medical ethics can and should be a corrective to disciplinary reductionism. We who bring the insights of sociology to the work of medical ethics must remember that our disciplinary approach is just one among the many that contribute to this important task, and that empirical evidence can only do so much (Leget, Borry, and De Vries 2009). Moral decisions are not determined solely by empirical facts. In his comment on the morning-after pill, Callahan reminds us that the evidence that drives moral decision making requires more than empirical data:

> I am in favor of the [morning-after] pill, which I think useful for women. Yet that is my *ethical* judgment, not a scientific judgment. The scientific evidence indicates that the morning-after pill is highly, if not perfectly, effective in preventing pregnancy; it works. The ethical question then becomes: ought it to be made available over the counter? I say yes. Those opposed take a different position, but it is not in any way interference with science or a distortion of scientific evidence to take that position. It is the use of one moral view to object to another moral view, which is surely acceptable in [American] society. (2006)

Similarly, those in the United States who oppose capital punishment are quick to point out that the facts support their position. Sociological research shows that the death penalty does nothing to deter crime, reduce the murder rate, or save government money. These things are all empirically true, but one's answer to the question "Is it ethical to use the death penalty?" rests in more than facts.

Nevertheless (and wanting the last word for my discipline), the insights of sociology and its way of seeing the world with fresh, debunking, relativizing eyes remain important to the moral work of medicine. Going back to the metaphor (or, in Turner's words, the "trope") of the mirror, the reflection offered by sociological analysis may appear to be one found in a funhouse, but the image that appears distorted can be valuable to those who see themselves in a new light.

This is certainly true for the important sociological concept of role-distance. The story of its development is a classical illustration of the sociological imagination at work. Wandering through a park not far from the Berkeley campus of the University of California, sociologist Erving Goffman stopped to watch children on a merry-go-round. He noticed that unlike the younger riders, older boys on the merry-go-round acted with more abandon—holding on with one hand (or going hands-free), not taking the role of merry-go-round rider seriously. Younger children were fully engaged with the role, clinging to their steeds, smiling and enjoying the sights and sounds of the machinery. This observation led Goffman to develop the idea of role-distance. He pointed out that on the merry-go-round (and elsewhere in society) some actors take their roles seriously, while others display their superiority by acting in a way that shows they will not be limited by the expectation of the role they find themselves in (1961b). Goffman went on to explain that, like the older children on the merry-go-round, surgeons in the operating room often acted in ways—listening to (and singing along with) loud music, joking and bantering with the surgical staff—that put distance between their real selves and the role of surgeon. When confronted with this mirror of their behavior, surgeons recognized something about the way they played their role that they had not seen before, which allowed them to understand something new and important about their relationship to patients and colleagues.

So too with medical ethics: Sociologists can help medical ethicists answer the empirical questions posed by their work, but more importantly, sociologists *of* medical ethics can help the field reflect on the meaning and value of their work. The sociological imagination allows medical ethicists to see that—like all social activities—medical ethics "might have been (and can be) otherwise." Armed with this insight, medical ethicists can assess the ways their efforts do and do not help ensure that health care and the life sciences are done in a way that respects individuals and promotes justice.

ᴄ᳐ Notes on Resources and Training

How can one develop and cultivate a sociological point of view on medical ethics? To begin, one must understand how a sociological view of the world differs from the perspectives offered by other disciplines in the social sciences. I have briefly sketched these differences in my description of the sociological imagination, but this is no substitute for reading original texts. Particularly useful to newcomers to this way of thought are two introductory texts: Berger's *Invitation to Sociology* and Mills's *The Sociological Imagination*. Writing before the fracturing of sociology into myriad schools of thought, these authors describe in elegant prose the essence of the sociological method.

Once introduced to the sociological way of thought, the next step is to find articles and texts that apply that way of thought to issues in medical ethics. Over the past twenty years at least five anthologies that explore social science (not just sociological) approaches to issues in medical ethics have been published (Weisz 1990; De Vries and Subedi 1998; Hoffmaster 2001; De Vries et al. 2007; Rothman, Armstrong, and Tiger 2007). Other places to look for examples of the application of the sociological imagination to medical ethics include journals of medical sociology/health sociology and bioethics, including the *Sociology of Health and Illness*, *Social Science and Medicine*, *Perspectives in Biology and Society*, the *Hastings Center Report*, and *Cambridge Quarterly of Health Care Ethics*.

Many programs that offer a master's degree in bioethics include training in empirical ethics, but this does not necessarily mean that students will learn how to do sociological analysis. Perhaps the best route for those seriously interested in thinking sociologically about medical ethics is graduate training in medical sociology. The American Sociological Association lists graduate programs by areas of emphasis (see www.asanet.org/cs/root/leftnav/careers_and_jobs/graduate_training_in_sociology). My recommendation is to find a school that has a scholar (or, better yet, a few scholars at one school) whose work you admire and find inspirational and apply to study there.

Notes

1. The French essayist Emmanuel Joseph Sieyès first used the term "sociology" (*sociologie*) in an unpublished work in 1780 (Guilhaumou 2006), but Comte is credited with coining the term in its modern sense in his *Cours de philosophie positive* (1838). Several centuries before either of these French thinkers, Ibn Khaldūn (1332–1406), a Muslim scholar from North Africa, wrote several books of history rich in sociological insight (Enan 2007).
2. This paragraph is adapted from De Vries, 2004b, 283.

References

Anspach, R. 1993. *Deciding who lives: Fateful choices in the intensive care nursery*. Berkeley: University of California Press.

Barber, B., J. Lally, J. L. Makarushka, and D. Sullivan. 1973. *Research on human subjects: Problems of social control in medical experimentation*. New York: Russell Sage Foundation.

Beauchamp, T. L., and J. F. Childress. 2001. *Principles of biomedical ethics*. 5th ed. New York: Oxford.

Becker, H. 1967. "Whose side are we on?" *Social problems* 14:239–47.

Becker, H., B. Geer, E. C. Hughes, and A. Strauss. 1961. *Boys in white: Student culture in medical school*. Chicago: University of Chicago Press.

Berger, P. 1963. *Invitation to sociology*. Garden City, NY: Anchor.

Bloom, A. 2002. *The word as scalpel: A history of medical sociology*. New York: Oxford.

Bosk, C. 1979. *Forgive and remember: Managing medical failure*. Chicago: University of Chicago Press.

———. 1992. *All God's mistakes: Genetic counseling in a pediatric hospital*. Chicago: University of Chicago Press.

———. 2003. *Forgive and remember: Managing medical failure*. 2nd ed. Chicago: University of Chicago Press.

Callahan, D. 2006. Bad arguments for good causes: The morning-after pill. *Bioethics Forum* September 22 (www.bioethicsforum.org/morning-after-pill.asp).

Chambers, T. 2000. Centering bioethics. *Hastings Center Report* 30 (1): 22–29.

Chambliss, D. 1996. *Beyond caring: Hospitals, nurses, and the social organization of ethics.* Chicago: University of Chicago Press.

Comte, A. 1838. *Cours de philosophie positive.* Vol. 4. Paris: Bachelier.

Conrad, P., and J. Schneider. 1980. *Deviance and medicalization: From badness to sickness.* St. Louis: Mosby.

Davis, F. 1975. The courage to fail (book review). *The American Journal of Sociology* 81:417–20.

De Vries, R. 2004a. *A pleasing birth: Midwives and maternity care in The Netherlands.* Philadelphia: Temple University Press.

———. 2004b. "How can we help? From 'sociology in' bioethics to 'sociology of' bioethics." *Journal of Law, Medicine and Ethics* 32:279–92.

———. 2009. Why can't we all just get along? A comment on Turner's plea to social scientists and bioethicists. *Cambridge Quarterly of Health Care Ethics* 18:43–46.

De Vries, R., C. Bosk, L. Turner, and K. Orfali, eds. 2007. *The view from here: Social science and bioethics.* London: Blackwell.

De Vries, R., and J. Subedi, eds. 1998. *Bioethics and society.* Upper Saddle River, NJ: Prentice Hall.

Durkheim, E. 1984. *The division of labor in society.* New York: Free Press.

Enan, M. A. 2007. *Ibn Khaldun: His life and works.* New York: The Other Press.

Evans, J. 2000. A sociological account of the growth of principlism. *Hastings Center Report* 30 (5): 31–38.

———. 2002. *Playing God: Human genetic engineering and the rationalization of public bioethical debate.* Chicago: University of Chicago Press.

Fisher, J. 2009. *Medical research for hire: The political economy of pharmaceutical clinical trials.* New Brunswick, NJ: Rutgers University Press.

Fox, R. 1959. *Experiment perilous.* Glencoe, IL: Free Press.

Fox, R., and J. Swazey. 1974. *The courage to fail.* Chicago: University of Chicago Press.

———. 1992. *Spare parts: Organ replacement in American society.* New York: Oxford.

———. 2008. *Observing bioethics.* New York: Oxford.

Freidson, E. 1970. *The profession of medicine: A study of the sociology of applied knowledge.* New York: Dodd, Mead.

Gerth, H., and C. W. Mills. 1946. *From Max Weber: Essays in sociology.* New York: Oxford.

Goffman, E. 1961a. *Asylums: Essays on the social situation of mental patients and other inmates.* Chicago: Aldine.

———. 1961b. *Encounters.* Indianapolis: Bobbs-Merrill Co., 85–152.

———. 1963. *Stigma: Notes on the management of spoiled identity.* Englewood Cliffs, NJ: Prentice Hall.

Gray, B. 1975. *Human subjects in medical experimentation: A sociological study of the conduct and regulation of clinical research.* New York: Wiley.

Guilhaumou, J. 2006. Sieyès et le non-dit de la sociologie: du mot à la chose. *Revue d'histoire des sciences humaines* 15:117–34.

Guillemin, J., and L. Holmstrom. 1986. *Mixed blessings: Intensive care for newborns.* New York: Oxford.

Henderson, G., M. Easter, C. Zimmer, N. M. P. King, A. Davis, B. Rothschild, L. R. Churchill, B. Wilfond, and D. Nelson. 2006. Therapeutic misconception in early-phase gene transfer trials. *Social Science and Medicine* 62:239–53.

Hoffmaster, B., ed. 2001. *Bioethics in a social context.* Philadelphia: Temple University Press.

Kenyon, J. 1996. *Otherwise: New and selected poems.* St. Paul, MN: Graywolf Press.

Klinenburg, E. 2002. *Heat wave: A social autopsy of disaster in Chicago.* Chicago: University of Chicago Press.

Leget, C., P. Borry, and R. De Vries. 2009. "Nobody tosses a dwarf!" The relation between the empirical and normative re-examined. *Bioethics* 23:236–45.

Merton, R., G. G. Reader, and P. L. Kendall. 1957. *The student-physician: Introductory studies in the sociology of medical education.* Cambridge, MA: Harvard University Press.

Mesman, J. 2002. *Evaren pioniers: Omgaan met twijfel in de intensive care voor pasgeborenen* [*Experienced pioneers: An ethnography of the intensive care unit for newborns*]. Amsterdam: Aksant.

Mills, C. W. 1959. *The sociological imagination.* New York: Oxford.

Parsons, T. 1951. *The social system.* Glencoe, IL: Free Press.

Rothman, B. K., E. M. Armstrong, and R. Tiger. 2007. *Bioethical issues, sociological perspectives.* Amsterdam: Elsevier.

Rothman, D. 1991. *Strangers at the bedside: How law and bioethics transformed medical decision making.* New York: Basic Books.

Singh, I. 2005. Will the "real boy" please behave: Dosing dilemmas for parents of boys with ADHD. *American Journal of Bioethics* 5 (3): 34–47.

———. 2007. Clinical implications of ethical concepts: Moral self-understandings in children taking methylphenidate for ADHD. *Clinical Child Psychology and Psychiatry* 12:167–82.

Sudnow, D. 1967. *Passing on: The social organization of dying.* Englewood Cliffs, NJ: Prentice Hall.

Tönnies, F. 1957. *Community and society (Gemeinschaft und Gesellschaft).* East Lansing, MI: Michigan State University Press.

Turner, L. 2009. Anthropological and sociological critiques of bioethics. *Bioethical Inquiry* 6:83–98.

Weber, M. 1947. *The theory of social and economic organization,* trans. A. M. Henderson and T. Parsons. New York: Free Press.

———. 1968. *Economy and society,* ed. G. Roth and C. Wittich. New York: Bedminster Press.

———. 1992 (1930). *The Protestant ethic and the spirit of capitalism.* New York: Routledge.

Weisz, G., ed. 1990. *Social science perspectives on medical ethics.* Dordrecht, The Netherlands: Kluwer.

Zussman, R. 1992. *Intensive care: Medical ethics and the medical profession.* Chicago: University of Chicago Press.

CHAPTER 12

Qualitative Methods

HOLLY A. TAYLOR, SARA CHANDROS HULL,
AND NANCY E. KASS

Qualitative research methods are particularly well suited for understanding values, personal perspectives, experiences, and contextual circumstances, all of which are concerns of medical ethics. The term "qualitative research" is used broadly to refer to text-based, nonstatistical methods. Generally, qualitative methods involve asking open-ended questions of a relatively small number of informants to gather data to address particular research questions. Although qualitative data can be gathered to test hypotheses, more typically the research questions addressed by qualitative methods are discovery oriented, descriptive, and exploratory. Qualitative methods expand understanding of what types of experiences, beliefs, or attitudes exist.

This chapter provides an overview of common approaches to qualitative research and frequently used qualitative data-collection techniques, and describes when it is appropriate to use each technique. Drawing upon our own qualitative research experiences as well as published studies of qualitative research in medical ethics, we discuss specific examples of qualitative research in medical ethics. We also present a critique of qualitative research, including its advantages and limitations, to help researchers maximize the quality of their own work and readers critique research conducted by others. Finally, we review the skills and training needed by qualitative researchers and suggest additional resources for those interested in using qualitative methods for empirical research in medical ethics.

Description of Qualitative Methods

A researcher must make a series of decisions before embarking on an empirical study in medical ethics. These decisions can be broken down into at least five steps. First, the researcher must identify a research question. Second, depending on the nature of the research question, the researcher must decide whether qualitative or quantitative methods (or some combination of these methods) are warranted. Third, if a qualitative approach is selected, the researcher must decide whether to follow a traditional qualitative research approach, such as phenomenology, ethnography, grounded theory, or qualitative description to guide the overall study design, or whether a hybrid of approaches is more appropriate. Fourth, the researcher must select which specific data collection techniques are best for addressing the study's specific aims. Fifth, the researcher must decide upon an analytic plan to make sense of the data collected. The following sections review these steps in more detail.

SELECTING A RESEARCH QUESTION

The choice of a research question may be stimulated by personal or professional experience, a review of the literature, or a specific assignment or charge. A researcher may want to explore why particular experiences, beliefs, or attitudes exist, or to estimate the proportion of individuals with those particular experiences, beliefs, or attitudes. For example, a researcher may want to know how many physicians support the legalization of physician-assisted suicide, or a researcher, instead, may want to know why physicians do or do not support such a policy. Research can be initiated when a previous understanding of a phenomenon is lacking or gaps appear in results from previous work.

EMPIRICAL APPROACH

Once the research question has been identified, the next decision for a researcher to make is how best to answer the research question. The phenomenon under study, the goal of the study, and the experience, interests, and expertise of the researcher direct the selection of the most appropriate approach for a particular project. First, a broad decision regarding the use of qualitative and/or quantitative approaches must be made. If a qualitative approach is appropriate, the next decision involves the type of qualitative approach to take. These two decisions frame the overall design of the study and guide the collection, analysis, and interpretation of the data collected.

Qualitative or quantitative or both?

Qualitative and quantitative methods are quite different from each other, both in terms of the types of questions they can answer and in the specific steps taken to answer them. Quantitative methods are most appropriate when some previous understanding of a phenomenon exists; they are used to estimate the proportion of individuals with particular experiences, beliefs, or attitudes and to explore statistical associations between these experiences, beliefs, and attitudes (i.e., outcomes) and various sociodemographic characteristics or other hypothesized predictors of such outcomes. Accurate estimates generally require conducting research with large numbers of respondents. In quantitative research, respondents are sampled to be a subset of a larger population of interest. Results, then, are intended to be generalized to the larger population from which the research sample was drawn. As a simple example, one might do a quantitative study on advance directives by interviewing all patients newly admitted to a certain hospital to find out what proportion have heard of advance directives and what proportion have completed one. Quantitative approaches are described in greater detail in chapter 14 of this volume.

Qualitative methods help to explain why certain experiences, beliefs, or attitudes exist (Creswell 1998, 17–18) and allow the researcher to provide an in-depth description and exploration of a phenomenon about which nothing or little is already known. For example, one could follow up on the quantitative approach described above by approaching a subsample of those who chose to complete an advance directive and those who have not and conduct in-depth interviews with them to discover why they have or have not completed an advance directive. The goal of interviewing the subsample would not be to generalize to the larger quantitative sample but to develop a deeper understanding of why patients choose to have an advance directive or not. The results of these interviews could lead to a follow-up survey to test whether and how the factors are considered in patient decisions with the intent of generating generalizable results. Table 12.1 compares the relative purposes and goals of qualitative versus quantitative methods.

Although it is common to defend the merits of a quantitative approach over a qualitative approach and vice versa (Carr 1994; Kvale 1996), the distinct features and strengths of these approaches should be viewed as complementary rather than competing. Mixed-methods research that employs both qualitative and quantitative techniques is increasingly common in health-related research (O'Cathain, Murphy, and Nicholl 2007). Combining approaches in a single mixed-methods project can serve

TABLE 12.1   Comparison of Qualitative and Quantitative Methods

Category	Qualitative Research	Quantitative Research
General Research Focus	Description, documentation, and analysis of patterns, values, worldview, meanings, beliefs, and attitudes. Totality of experiences in natural or particular contexts.	Measurement of controlled or manipulated variables by experimental and other methods. Causal and measurable relationships.
Scope	Generally broad, holistic, and comprehensive; worldview.	Particularist, narrow, and limited focus. Controlled. Excludes more than includes.
Research Goal	Development of understandings and meanings of what one sees, hears, experiences, and discovers through a variety of sensual observation-participation modes. Obtain a full and accurate "truth" from people.	Testing hypotheses to obtain measurable outcomes among variables under study. Precision and objective findings.
Sources of Data	Participants, informants, role takers, and respondents.	Objects, subjects, cases, data banks, code numbers, and figures.
Domains of Analysis	Can reformulate and expand focus of study as one proceeds. No predetermined, a priori judgments. Open discovery. Flexible and dynamic. Moves with people, context, situation, or events.	Predetermined. A fixed design. Prejudgments and a priori position taken. Rigid and fixed categories. Nondynamic. Fixed and planned sequence of research design to reduce variations.

Note: Adapted from Leininger 1985 and Creswell 1994.

several purposes: to corroborate data and enhance the validity of findings (triangulation); to help clarify or elaborate upon analytic results and fill in gaps in knowledge; and to guide the development of subsequent research steps (for example, additional sampling, data collection, and analysis techniques). Mixed-methods studies often use the two methods sequentially. A researcher could conduct a focus to identify themes to be included as domains in a quantitative survey. A researcher could conduct a quantitative survey and then identify a range of respondents with whom to conduct an open-ended interview. In other cases mixed-methods studies use both approaches within the same instrument. An interview, for example, may have a series of closed-ended (quantitative questions) and then ask respondents to elaborate through open-ended responses, providing more detail on why they had a certain attitude, how they reacted to a certain experience, and the like. The mixed-methods paradigm is relatively new, and an emerging body of critical literature has begun to evaluate the advantages and challenges associated with merging approaches that stem from different epistemological traditions (Miller and Fredericks 2006; O'Cathain, Murphy, and Nicholl 2008).

DECIDING AMONG VARIOUS QUALITATIVE RESEARCH APPROACHES

That a particular research question is best addressed by qualitative methods still leaves open many choices for the researcher. Different qualitative research approaches have been developed by different academic disciplines. Philosophers, anthropologists, and sociologists, among others, have developed empirical approaches (also known as paradigms or traditions) that reflect their theoretical background and the intended goal of their inquiry. We consider here four approaches that influence the majority of qualitative research conducted today: phenomenology, ethnography, grounded theory, and qualitative description (Creswell 1998; Morse and Field 1995; Sandelowski 2000). The parent academic discipline, type of research questions, methods, and other data sources corresponding to each of these approaches are displayed in table 12.2.

Phenomenology

Phenomenology has its roots in philosophy. As applied to qualitative research, phenomenology seeks the essence of lived experience. A researcher engaged in a phenomenologic study relies heavily on in-depth interviews with individuals who are familiar with the phenomenon of interest. The individuals who are identified as appropriate subjects are asked to describe fully their personal, subjective experiences regarding a particular phenomenon. The goal of the researcher taking a phenomenologic approach is to produce a narrative that allows the reader to share in the experience described by the participants in the study.

For example, a researcher may want to draw on the phenomenologic approach to better understand the experiences of pregnant women who discover they are carrying fetuses with life-threatening genetic disorders. Using this approach the researcher would talk in-depth with several women who have experienced this phenomenon in order to learn enough to describe these women's experiences accurately. A reader of the final product of the study would have an appreciation of the women's lived experience.

TABLE 12.2   Comparison of Major Qualitative Research Approaches

Tradition/ Approach	Parent Discipline	Types of Research Questions	Methods	Other Data Sources
Phenomenology	Philosophy (phenomenology)	Meaning questions— eliciting the essence of experiences	Taping conversations; written anecdotes of personal experiences	Phenomeno-logical literature, philosophical reflections; poetry; art
Ethnography	Anthropology	Descriptive questions—of values, beliefs, and practices of a cultural group	Unstructured interviews; participant observations; field notes	Documents; records; photographs; maps; genealogies; social network diagrams
Grounded Theory	Sociology (symbolic interactionism)	"Process" questions— experience over time or change; may have stages or phases	Interviews	Participant observations; recording of memos; diary
Qualitative Description	Naturalistic Inquiry	Descriptive questions—of everyday events	Interviews; focus groups	Participant observations; documents; artifacts

Note: Abstracted from Morse and Field (1995) and Sandelowski (2000).

Ethnography

Ethnography has its roots in anthropology and has as its goal the description of a particular culture. A researcher engaged in traditional ethnography becomes immersed in a culture as a participant observer. The researcher may also conduct interviews and collect documents that allow him or her to better understand and describe that culture. The product of these activities is a rich description of cultural beliefs and practices. As compared with the product of a phenomenologic approach, the reader of an ethnographic report would know about how individuals in a particular culture carry out their daily activities or how a community interacts and what usual practices are but would not know how individuals who make up the community or culture felt about participating in a particular task or their experience of a particular cultural tradition.

A classic example of an ethnographic approach to a question in medical ethics is found in Fox's *Experiment Perilous* (1959), a book that provides a rich description of the lives and activities of patients with metabolic disorders and the physicians who care for them in an academic hospital. Based on months of observation and informant interviews, Fox describes the culture of academic medicine and research.

Grounded theory

Grounded theory has its roots in sociology, specifically symbolic interactionism, and has as its goal the exploration of the social and psychological processes related to a particular phenomenon. A researcher uses a grounded-theory approach to discover and develop a theory that explains the particular process of interest. To this end the researcher conducts in-depth interviews with those who are familiar with the process of interest and asks questions about steps and/or components that are relevant to that process. Additional interviews are conducted as the researcher identifies and defines the core of the theory he or she believes may explain the process of interest. Data collection is completed when the theory is elaborated. The reader of a report of a project guided by this approach is introduced to a theory that attempts to explain a single process that is relevant to a particular individual or group but finds out little about the cultural context within which the process occurs.

For example, a researcher interested in the process by which cancer patients make decisions regarding their enrollment in an early-phase clinical trial may want to consider an approach guided by grounded theory. The researcher might conduct successive open-ended interviews with patients until a theory regarding patients' decision-making patterns begins to emerge. The product of the investigation will be a theory about the process of decision making that can be tested among other groups of patients approached to enroll in early-phase trials.

Qualitative description

According to Sandelowski (2000) qualitative description has its roots in naturalistic inquiry. The report of a qualitative descriptive project remains close to the data collected. That is, in contrast to the products of projects that adopt approaches described above, the product of a project that takes a qualitative descriptive approach is less interpretive. Researchers taking a qualitative descriptive approach have as their goal a summary of their data, whereas those who adopt the approaches described above have as their goal the representation and interpretation of the data collected in other terms.

For example, a researcher taking a qualitative descriptive approach to the research question, "Why do physician-scientists choose to approach some eligible patients to offer enrollment in a clinical research protocol and choose not to approach other eligible patients?" may conduct interviews with the health care providers and produce a report on what she was told by the physician–investigators. A researcher taking a grounded theory approach toward the same question may conduct interviews as well as observe discussions among health care teams who are considering which patients to offer enrollment. The goal of the grounded theory approach is to represent that data collected as a theory about how decisions are made by physician-scientists.

Empirical researchers in medical ethics who use qualitative methods (ourselves included) tend to identify their projects in ways that focus on the data-collection technique, such as qualitative interview studies or focus group studies, rather than on the approach taken. Some methodologists argue that a qualitative project undertaken without clear, informed commitment to one of these broad approaches (such as phenomenology, ethnography, or grounded theory) is ill advised (e.g., Morse 1991).

We take a less stringent view and believe that qualitative research is valid even in the absence of such commitment or, indeed, with a clear commitment to a hybrid of approaches, as long as researchers appreciate the limitations of the approach they choose. For example, a study that relies solely on focus group data will generate more tentative conclusions than a study that draws upon well-established ethnographic techniques and includes multiple sources of data. At the same time, an in-depth ethnographic study requires substantial resources and time, whereas a focus group study is a more efficient and feasible approach to examine a narrow set of issues within a short timeframe.

DATA COLLECTION

Qualitative research involves a variety of data-gathering techniques. The decision to collect existing data or create one's own depends largely on the types of research questions being asked (see table 12.2). In the section below we describe three general sources of data for qualitative research: existing documents, observation, and interviews. For each we provide an overview of the purpose and characteristics of the technique and examples of empirical research using each of these techniques.

Document review

Documents are an important source of data for qualitative research because they provide a stable, written record of events and decisions.[1] Public documents that may be relevant to research in medical ethics include official correspondence, legislation, minutes of meetings, written reports, proposals, progress reports, consent forms, newspaper editorials, films, videos, and advertisements. Private documents such as personal correspondence, diaries, and autobiographies are also potential sources of data for qualitative research.

By way of example, the Advisory Committee on Human Radiation Experiments (ACHRE) reviewed and analyzed documents from federally funded research proposals involving human subjects. The documents reviewed for this study included the original grant proposal and the corresponding institutional review board (IRB) documents, such as the research protocol, consent forms, and IRB correspondence. The purpose of ACHRE's review was to evaluate how well these documents described informed consent procedures, the balance of risks to potential benefits for the subject, and subject selection and recruitment. An evaluation form was used by ACHRE researchers to rank how well each of these aspects was addressed in the available documentation (ACHRE 1995). A similar approach was used to evaluate the documentation associated with a large multicenter clinical trial to examine variability in IRB review (Silverman, Hull, and Sugarman 2001).

A study that examined how the prospect of benefit is described in informed consent forms for human gene transfer studies utilized aspects of both quantitative and qualitative methods. The study reviewed materials from 321 studies and counted the number of times potential for direct benefit was mentioned in the materials and whether the nature of the direct benefit described was neutral (e.g., you may or may not benefit), referred to a surrogate endpoint (e.g., tumor shrinkage) or a clinical endpoint (e.g., remission). In addition the investigators found it common for different sections of the same consent form to provide inconsistent information regarding the potential for direct benefit (King et al. 2005).

Document review also can be used to complement other sources of qualitative or quantitative data. Yin explains that an important use of documents "is to corroborate and augment evidence from other sources" (1994, 81). For example, a study on reproductive decision making among adults with cystic fibrosis compared the language contained in educational pamphlets to the language used in interviews with affected adults and their health care providers in discussing reproduction (Hull and Kass 2000).

Observation

In observational research the researcher visits a site where an activity or behavior of interest is occurring. This might include on-site clinic observations of interactions between patients and their clinicians, or of how researchers engage in an informed consent process with potential research participants. Two techniques used in observational research include participant observation and direct observation. In participant observation (see chapter 13), the researcher becomes an insider and plays an active role in the activity or behavior being observed. For example, a participant observer might be a member of a committee or a care provider. This is not intended to be deceptive—all members of a group being observed should understand that research is occurring.

In direct observation, on the other hand, the researcher is an outsider and attempts to observe behaviors passively without contributing to them. The goal of direct observation is to "watch a subject, group of subjects, or a set of interactions and record their behavior as faithfully as possible" (Bernard 1995, 311). Although the researcher does not become involved in the activities and behaviors being observed, subjects are often aware that the researcher is recording their behavior. The researcher records field notes in both kinds of observational research—concurrent with the observation, if possible.

Direct observation can serve as a formative data-collection stage to orient the researcher to the topic under study. We have used this technique in the preliminary phases of research to learn more about the clinical settings in which the subsequent phases of the research were to be conducted. This involved spending many hours observing the various activities that occurred in the clinic in preparation for conducting interviews with clinic patients and staff (Hull and Kass 2000; Taylor and Kass 2001, 2002). Direct observation can also serve as the primary data-collection technique in a study. In an effort to refine ethics curriculum directed at pediatric residents, Moon et al. (2009) conducted formative in-depth interviews followed by the direct observation of residents presenting their patients to their preceptors to describe the common ethical issues encountered in routine medical practice.

A variation of observational research involves audio recording naturally occurring interactions between physicians and patients. This method of data collection differs from direct observation because the researcher need not be present while the behavior of interest is taking place. For example, to examine how information about early-phase oncology trials is presented to patients and how this relates to what patients understand, conversations in which a physician offered a patient the option to enroll in an early-phase clinical trial were recorded. Information conveyed by the physician to the patient as documented on the recording was then compared to patients' responses to questions on a close-ended survey and during an in-depth interview (Kass et al. 2008).

Interviews

Interviews allow researchers to ask individuals about their beliefs and experiences and what they think and feel about particular issues. The interview is a kind of conversation between a researcher and an informant (or group of informants) that seeks to elicit the informant's understanding, knowledge, and insights about a particular topic (Rubin and Rubin 1995). Personal interviews and focus groups, two types of interviews commonly used in research in medical ethics, are explored in this section.

Personal interviews. A personal, in-depth interview involves an interaction between two people: a researcher and an interviewee, or informant. Informants are often people who have a common background or experience, such as patients with a particular condition, health care providers, or research subjects. In-depth interviews vary in the degree to which they are structured because different purposes are achieved with the various degrees of structure. Unstructured interviews begin with a topic and perhaps a few specific questions that allow the interviewer to identify and explore new questions and topics throughout each interview and the research process. The trajectory of an unstructured interview is informant driven. Structured interviews, on the other hand, ask each informant the same set of open-ended questions. The trajectory of a structured interview is interviewer driven. Between these two extremes, a semistructured interview balances structured and less-structured components. The semistructured interview tends to be interactive, with the interviewer asking follow-up questions based on the specific comments of each informant.

The interview field guide includes a basic set of questions that should be covered in the course of an interview. The field guide is particularly useful when more than one interviewer is involved in a study to ensure that different interviewers cover the same general topics. The field guide for an unstructured or semistructured interview includes a basic set of questions to be asked of everyone and usually does not specify a particular order in which these questions need to be asked. It also leaves room for the interviewer to ask extensive follow-up questions. Because of the iterative nature of qualitative data collection and analysis, the interview field guide evolves over time, based upon findings from emerging data. It may be desirable to conduct follow-up interviews with previous study participants when new or more focused questions emerge during the course of a study.

When less structured interviews are planned, it is all the more important to engage in a thorough training process with interview staff. Unlike highly structured, closed-ended surveys, where interview staff must be trained to ask questions exactly as printed, qualitative interviewers must be able to think on their feet. They must understand the broad goals of the inquiry, be able to pursue and follow up on certain lines of thought raised by respondents as relevant and yet also steer interview discussions back to core areas of interest when respondents veer off into areas less relevant to the focus of inquiry.

Faden and Kass (1996) conducted in-depth interviews to examine the perspectives about reproduction from health care providers and HIV-infected women. One part of the study sought to understand health care providers' beliefs and attitudes concerning HIV infection and childbearing and how they counsel HIV-infected women about reproduction. Another part of the study sought to understand HIV-infected women's intentions concerning childbearing and how their providers discussed reproduction and childbearing with them. In these interviews women sometimes said that they both did and did not want to have children, a finding related to their own internal conflict (Faden and Kass 1996). This finding illustrates one of the major values of using qualitative research methods; this conflict would likely not have been captured using standard quantitative surveys. For example, a quantitative survey that asked women, "Do you want to have children?" would require a "yes" or "no" response, leaving no room for the possibility that both answers could be true.

To the extent possible, interviews should be conducted in a setting that is comfortable and familiar for the informants. It may be ideal to conduct interviews with physicians within the clinic or their offices, but the clinic may seem formal, sterile, and intimidating to patients who would be more comfortable and, perhaps, more candid, being interviewed at their homes or in a neutral location. However, it may not always be feasible to travel to informants' homes to conduct interviews for logistical, safety, and/or cost-related reasons. At a minimum an interview location should be convenient, private, free of distraction, and comfortable.

The use of telephone interviews, which may be logistically simpler than in-person interviews, has both potential benefits and drawbacks. Participants may feel more comfortable sharing sensitive information in the more anonymous format of the telephone interview. However, it is more difficult for the interviewer to establish rapport with participants without the ability to shake their hands, make eye contact, and observe their nonverbal response to topics and questions. Personal interviews, both telephone and in person, typically are recorded and transcribed for analysis.

Focus groups. Focus groups, or group interviews, allow researchers to gain insights into the behaviors of groups of people and to learn why they feel certain ways about specific issues (Kreuger 1994). Originally used for marketing research, the focus group has been defined as "a research technique that collects data through group interaction on a topic determined by the researcher" (Morgan 1997, 6). Focus groups are advantageous for several reasons. They are efficient, in that they allow researchers to obtain input from a large number of people in a short amount of time and to produce concentrated amounts of data. Related, focus groups tend to be less expensive to conduct than survey research (Bernard 1995, 226). In addition, in contrast to one-on-one interviews, the group setting may encourage participants to discuss issues that they might not think of on their own (Morgan 1997).

A research project may use focus groups as the primary method of data collection. For example, focus groups were conducted with study coordinators to examine how they shape the ethical conduct of the research in which they are involved. The investigators purposefully sample study coordinators from the academic, federal, and private setting to compare responses across the groups (Davis et al. 2002). Another study employed focus groups to examine what potential research subjects would like to know about the financial interests of research investigators and whether the disclosure of such interest would affect their willingness to enroll in research (Weinfurt et al. 2006).

Alternatively, focus groups can be used to support or supplement other methods of data collection. They often are used to collect preliminary data that is then used to develop interview guides or questionnaires or opportunities for the direct observation of the phenomenon of interest. In addition focus group data can provide insight into the language used by the study populations regarding the issues of interest. Bernhardt et al. (1997) conducted a series of focus groups as the first stage of a project to develop a model informed consent process for BRCA1 genetic testing. Eight focus groups, of nine to ten women each, were convened to discuss beliefs about the causes of breast cancer, their expectations of health care providers, what they would want to know if offered a genetic test, and their understanding of the benefits and risks of genetic testing.

Focus groups can be conducted with naturally occurring groups of previously acquainted persons, such as support groups, committees, or students in a class. In many cases, however, focus group participants are strangers who are recruited solely for the purpose of the research via a flier, newspaper advertisement, or other method. Ideally, focus groups include between six and twelve participants and the group moderator (Bernard 1995, 225). In addition, a notetaker/research assistant is often included as a second moderator.

Composition of focus groups is also an important consideration. It is generally thought best for participants in focus groups to be in some way homogeneous so that respondents will feel comfortable voicing their views. That is, whether or not they are familiar with each other or strangers, they usually share some attribute or experience in common. Conducting more than one homogeneous focus group facilitates analysis of differences in perspective among groups (Morgan 1997). For instance, focus group participants are often from the same background, all women or all men, or homogeneous on factors relevant to the research question, such as having the same medical condition.

The choice of moderator should be made with sensitivity to the composition of the group (gender, age, race, ethnicity, and so forth). A moderator with a similar background will generally make people feel more comfortable about revealing personal or sensitive information. A skilled focus group moderator will draw out the quieter participants and limit the more outspoken ones. The moderator's goal is to guide the topic of the conversation and to hear a range of views and experiences.

Focus groups typically are recorded and transcribed for analysis. Though expensive, the use of a stenographer can be extremely helpful in focus groups, since voices can be hard to distinguish through a recording. The stenographer attends the focus group and by using specialized equipment is able to create a verbatim transcript while attributing each comment to a specific person.

ANALYSIS

The specific analytic techniques chosen are influenced by the qualitative approach taken by the researcher, the phenomenon under study, and/or the goal of the study. However, there are three basic steps followed in virtually all qualitative analysis: immersion, data reduction, and synthesis.

One of the key ways in which qualitative and quantitative research methods differ is related to the researcher's role in data analysis. Whereas the researcher strives to remain detached and objective during the analysis of quantitative data, the researcher becomes immersed in the data during qualitative analysis. In Sandelowski's words, "researchers [who collect qualitative data] must first look at their data to see what they should look for in their data" (1995). In qualitative analysis the researcher routinely reviews the data as they are collected in order to identify what additional data are needed and when saturation has been achieved (i.e., no new information is emerging, so the data set is complete). Immersion is the necessary first step that enables the researcher to plan and complete the remaining analysis tasks.

The next step in the data analysis process usually involves data reduction. "Data reduction," a term used by Miles and Huberman (1994), refers to the process of dividing the data into more manageable units and labeling or coding the units. For example, a large interview transcript may be reduced into smaller units according to the different topics covered within the interview (e.g., views about genetic testing; views about disability; views about abortion). The mechanics of data reduction typically involve labeling topically related units of data with codes that help identify and sort the data (Coffey and Atkinson 1996). Codes are generated either from topics identified in advance (e.g., questions included in a semistructured interview guide) or from topics that emerge from the data itself. Coding of data can be done by hand (e.g., highlighting on an interview transcript the passages related to a particular topic, or "code") or in conjunction with qualitative data analysis software such as NVivo8 (2008).

Once the data have been reduced, themes and patterns can then be explored to reshape and synthesize the data into a more coherent whole. Any conclusions or hypotheses generated during this process of data synthesis are then tested within the data set. For example, a hypothesis about the relationship between two or more themes identified during data reduction is tested by reexamining the data in search of instances that contradict the proposed hypothesis. Qualitative data analysis is an iterative process: while data reduction and synthesis usually follow one another, the sequence is often repeated to create a feedback loop that continues throughout the data analysis process (Miller and Crabtree 1994).

The final product of data synthesis is determined by the qualitative approach taken or the phenomenon under investigation—or both—and the goals of the study. That is, the qualitative approach taken will influence the level of interpretation presented by the researcher. In general terms the narrative product of a project where a researcher has taken a phenomenologic or grounded theory approach will include considerably more interpretation than will the narrative product of an ethnographic or qualitative descriptive project.

Regardless of the approach taken, maintaining a record of each decision made during the data analysis process to arrive at the narrative product of the project is helpful both to the researcher and to the readers of the research (Koch 1993). An analysis road map can facilitate the replication of the study and allow readers to assess whether they agree with the researcher's synthesis and interpretation of data. In addition, when developing the final product, it is important for researchers to aim for an appropriate balance of substance (e.g., quotes) and interpretation (e.g., synthesis) to allow readers to follow the reasoning behind the analysis and determine whether they share the researcher's conclusions (Morse 1999).

SUMMARY OF STEPS IN QUALITATIVE RESEARCH

Table 12.3 introduces a potential topic for a qualitative research project—women at risk for breast cancer seeking genetic testing—and provides examples of the research question/focus, potential participants or informants, data-collection methods, and

TABLE 12.3   Comparison of Approaches in a Hypothetical Qualitative Project

Approach	Research Question/ Focus	Participants/ Informants	Data-Collection Methods	Types of Results
Phenomenology	What is the meaning of seeking genetic testing?	Women at risk of breast cancer; phenomenological literature; art; poetry; and other descriptions	In-depth conversation	In-depth reflective description of the experience of "seeking genetic testing"
Ethnography	What is the setting like when women come to seek out genetic testing?	Women at risk of breast cancer in the clinic; families; genetic counselors; clinic staff; other clinic staff who work in the setting	Interviews; participant observations; direct observations; other records such as medical charts	A description of the day-to-day events and relationships at the genetic testing clinic
Grounded Theory	What is the process like when women seek out genetic testing?	Women at risk of breast cancer; families	In-depth interviews; observations	Description of the social, psychological process in the experience of seeking genetic testing
Qualitative Description	What factors do women consider before they agree to have a genetic test?	Women at risk of breast cancer seeking a genetic test	Interviews	A description of the factors women consider before they agree to a genetic test

Note: Abstracted from Morse and Field (1995) and Sandelowski (2000).

type of results that projects guided by each of the four qualitative approaches discussed would produce.

∾ Critiquing Qualitative Research in Medical Ethics

In the following section we present a critique of qualitative research, including its scope, advantages, and limitations. Our goals are to provide researchers with tools to help maximize the quality of their own work and to assess the quality of research conducted by others. The quality or rigor of an empirical study refers to how confident one is that the findings and conclusions from that study are accurate. Methodological rigor occurs at each stage of a qualitative research project, including selection of a research question, data collection, analysis and interpretation, and writing/presentation. The concept of validity in qualitative research generally refers to the credibility of the study findings, while reliability refers to the consistency and dependability of the research process over time and across researchers and methods (Miles and Huberman 1994).

Qualitative researchers have several techniques available to them to improve the reliability and validity of their research, and critical readers of qualitative research will want to see that these techniques have been utilized. For example, peer or colleague review and member checking can improve the reliability of qualitative research findings. Peer review involves soliciting the help of colleagues or peer researchers to analyze a subset of the data and compare their findings with those of the researcher. Member checking involves sharing emerging findings with study participants to see if the researcher's description of the data is consistent with those of the participants (Creswell 1998).

The use of multiple sources of data or analytic techniques, which is known as triangulation, increases the validity of qualitative research by using complementary methods and data sources to produce converging conclusions about the phenomenon under study. When different conclusions emerge from related data sources, the researcher needs to reconsider the entire data set until all of the evidence corroborates a single set of conclusions or a reasonable explanation is discovered for the apparent divergence.

THE STRENGTHS OF QUALITATIVE METHODS

The primary strengths of qualitative research include its ability to uncover new concepts, its exploratory and explanatory roles, and its ability to provide illustrative examples of quantitative phenomena. By having informants describe phenomena in their own voices, the researcher may be less likely to impose a preconceived understanding on the results of the research. The benefits of qualitative research have been summarized in four points by Gittelsohn et al.: explorative flexibility, going in-depth, validation of information, and taking a holistic perspective (1998, 369).

Explorative flexibility refers to the researcher's ability to acknowledge assumptions and biases about the topic to be studied, enter data collection with an open willingness to learn from the study participants, and explore new questions that are likely to emerge throughout the study. Detailed information is acquired in qualitative

TABLE 12.4   Strengths and Weaknesses of Qualitative Data Techniques

Technique	*Strengths*	*Weaknesses*
Documentation	• Stable; can be retrieved repeatedly • Unobtrusive • Exact; contains exact names, references, and details of an event • Broad coverage; long span of time, many events, and many settings	• Access may be blocked • May not convey what actually occurs in practice
Observation	• Covers events in real time • Covers context of events	• Time consuming • Event may proceed differently because it is being observed

Interviews	• Targeted; focuses directly on the topic of interest
	• Provides insight into participant's perspectives
		• Potential biases related to:
		  • How researcher frames the questions, choice of vocabulary
		  • Subject's ability to recall events accurately
		  • Interviewee gives what interviewers want to hear
		  • Which informants are willing to be interviewed

Note: Adapted from Yin (1994).

research by going in-depth and conducting increasingly specific data collection, while validation of information occurs through the use of multiple data-collection methods, and sometimes returning to the same participants/informants to validate conclusions. Taking a holistic perspective using qualitative methods permits an elucidation and examination of the contextual conditions under which the topic of study occurs.

In addition to the general benefits of qualitative research, each specific data collection technique contains its own unique advantages. Documents are stable and precise, and their retrieval for research purposes is generally unobtrusive. Observation allows the researcher to examine actual events and behaviors as they occur in their natural context. Interviews allow the researcher to ask participants directly about a specific topic of interest. The strengths of the specific data-collection techniques reviewed in this chapter are summarized in table 12.4.

THE WEAKNESSES OF QUALITATIVE METHODS

Qualitative research methods are also characterized by several weaknesses or limitations. These limitations can be placed into one of two categories: the general limitations of qualitative research and the limitations of individual qualitative research techniques. An often-referenced limitation of qualitative research is its lack of generalizability. The term "generalizability," as it is commonly used, refers to use of statistical inference to determine the applicability of a study's findings beyond the research context. It is the gold standard to which the findings of quantitative research are held.

Quantitative research is designed to be generalizable; typically through selecting a random sample of subjects that represents a larger population of interest. Qualitative research is not generalizable in the same sense because it involves selecting a smaller, nonrandom, purposive sample of individuals who contribute to the generation of theories and hypotheses. Generalizability in qualitative research commonly refers to the development of a theory that helps to make sense of a phenomenon or process in one context and explains how it might differ in another context (Maxwell 1992).

Another weakness of the qualitative approach is that collection and analysis of qualitative data are influenced by the subjectivity and biases of researchers. The personal worldviews of the researchers, including biases of which they might be unaware, are reflected in how qualitative studies are conducted. But it is important to note that this is not a weakness unique to qualitative research. While it is true that quantitative research may rely on more objective methods of analysis (computer-aided statistical analysis), the selection of what research question to ask and how the researcher frames the questions to be asked can certainly be influenced by his or her personal worldview.

Each of the qualitative data-collection techniques reviewed in this chapter is characterized by specific limitations as well. For example, ACHRE's document review of federally funded research was limited in that consent documentation may not be a good surrogate for learning about the consent process (ACHRE 1995). In both observational and interviewing research, the research participants may react negatively to the researcher's presence and provide inaccurate or modified information. The limitations of these techniques are summarized in table 12.4.

❧ Concluding Comments

Numerous topics in medical ethics are appropriate to explore using qualitative methods, particularly those that seek a better understanding of values, personal perspectives, experiences, and contextual circumstances. In this chapter we have provided an overview of qualitative research methods that might serve as a starting point for those interested in using qualitative methods to conduct research in medical ethics or to those interested in becoming a more critical reader of qualitative ethics research. The decisions facing any researcher begin with selecting a research question and appropriate specific aims, which lead to decisions regarding what kind and how much data to collect. For researchers who seek to gain an understanding of the meaning of a phenomenon, of the context in which an event occurs, or why individuals act in certain ways or hold certain beliefs, qualitative research is appropriate. Qualitative researchers then must decide how best to organize and synthesize the collected data and create a product with an appropriate balance of substance and interpretation.

❧ Notes on Resources and Training

A well-trained qualitative researcher possesses theoretical sensitivity. Although this term derives from the grounded theory research tradition (Glaser 1978; Strauss and Corbin 1990), theoretical sensitivity generally applies to a researcher's ability to recognize the subtleties of meaning in qualitative data. This ability to recognize what is important in the data and give it meaning develops through personal and professional experience. An increased understanding of the phenomenon under study develops during a researcher's interaction with data collection and analysis.

Qualitative research that involves group or personal interviews requires a researcher to have excellent communication skills. Qualities such as empathy, sensitivity, and sincerity are central. The ability to build rapport, inspire trust, listen carefully, and ask questions in a sensitive manner will enable a researcher to acquire more accurate and detailed responses from interviewees. Furthermore, because qualitative researchers serve as the primary data-gathering instruments in interview research, they do not play a neutral role in data generation and analysis. Personal experiences and biases shape the kinds of questions a qualitative researcher asks. Therefore, one of the most important skills for qualitative researchers is to recognize and openly describe personal perspectives and biases that might influence the research. Achieving balance, rather than neutrality, is a goal of qualitative research (Rubin and Rubin 1995).

The role of mentoring in qualitative research should not be underestimated. Training with a mentor who is experienced in a particular kind of qualitative methodology is a critical step in becoming a good qualitative researcher. Many of the skills required to conduct qualitative research may be better conveyed through one-on-one communication rather than in written texts (Burns 1989). Although referring to methodological texts is an important component of learning how to conduct qualitative research, it is not sufficient training in itself. Sole reliance on methodological texts, without the guidance of a mentor, has been compared to learning how to drive from reading a car manual, or learning how to write from reading a computer manual (Morse 1997). Mentors may be identified among colleagues who are doing qualitative research at one's institution, at professional conferences, or from courses, workshops, and seminars.

Coursework in qualitative research offers a more formal way to review methodological texts, conduct fieldwork in a supervised setting, and develop relationships with potential research mentors and collaborators. Precise data on the extent to which courses on qualitative research methods are offered at universities and medical schools are lacking. However, schools seem to vary on the extent of courses available on qualitative research. Schools of nursing seem to offer a wider range of qualitative methods courses than do schools of medicine and public health.

For students or faculty at institutions that do not offer extensive coursework in qualitative research methods, there are several alternatives. It is advisable to look to other divisions within their institution for methodological courses. For example, departments of anthropology, sociology, and political science, as well as schools of nursing, are good places to look for qualitative coursework.

The most comprehensive qualitative research training program for health professionals of which we are aware is offered by the University of North Carolina at Chapel Hill School of Nursing. This program features a series of two preliminary courses in qualitative methods and an Annual Summer Institute in Qualitative Research (2008). The program now offers a certificate in qualitative methods to those who complete a series of three courses. The educational objectives of this particular program, displayed in table 12.5, represent a comprehensive set of goals for qualitative

TABLE 12.5 Educational Goals in Qualitative Research Coursework[a]

	Objectives
Methods	1. Describe the "qualitative attitude" toward inquiry.
	2. Compare defining attributes of selected qualitative methods.
	3. Describe method specific techniques for sampling, data collection, data analysis and interpretation and representation.
	4. Describe orientations to and techniques for optimizing validity.
	5. Describe issues surroundings techniques for ensuring the protection of research participants.
	6. Describe the features of successful qualitative research proposals.
	7. Critique qualitative research reports.
Analysis	1. Explain the varied goals of qualitative analysis.
	2. Differentiate among data preparation, data management, data analysis, and interpretation.
	3. Differentiate between case-oriented and variable oriented analysis.
	4. Describe generic technical approaches to analysis (e.g. coding, counting, quoting, visual displays).
	5. Differentiate empirical/analytic from other methodologic approaches to analysis, including qualitative content analysis, constant comparison analysis, and 'classical' ethnographic analysis.
	6. Describe issues surrounding and techniques for secondary analysis of qualitative data.
	7. Compare interpretive products, including qualitative descriptions, grounded theories, ethnographies, and phenomenologies.
	8. Describe templates or logics for writing reports of empirical/analytic studies.
Evaluation	1. Describe frameworks for qualitative evaluation, especially utilization-focused evaluation, and their utility for assessing health care practices, programs, and policies.
	2. Describe templates and techniques for combining qualitative and quantitative methods.
	3. Describe the use of qualitative methods in intervention and outcome studies.
	4. Describe issues related to triangulation in qualitative research.
	5. Describe issues relating to techniques for putting qualitative findings directly into practice.

[a]Adapted from University of North Carolina at Chapel Hill School of Nursing 1999 and 2008.

methods coursework in general. However, we want to reiterate here that coursework is not the only manner in which to receive methodological training, which can occur through mentorship, collegial support, and independent reading.

Although we have presented a broad overview of qualitative methods in medical ethics research, we were not able to go into detail on any particular aspect of these methods. Those interested in conducting qualitative research should consult methodological texts that review the overall approaches, data collection, and analysis in greater detail. The references cited throughout this chapter represent a cross section of the literature available on qualitative research, including methodological texts and journal articles. A list of general texts that we have found to be most helpful in our own research is included in appendix A.

Appendix B provides a selection of medical and/or ethics journals that have published reports using qualitative research methods. This list includes traditionally more quantitative journals (such as *JAMA*—Journal of the American Medical Association), which are increasingly likely to consider qualitative research, particularly manuscripts for research in which qualitative methods are used in a complementary way with quantitative methods.

Finally, the internet is an excellent resource for current information about qualitative research. Qualitative methods course syllabi, information about current qualitative textbooks and journals and their publishers, and online discussion groups devoted to qualitative research are all available via the internet. Because of the dynamic and ever-changing nature of the internet, information about any specific websites has not been included in this chapter.

❧ Notes

This chapter is not subject to U.S. copyright.

1. The term "document review" is used to refer specifically to the review and analysis of previously existing documents. The term "content analysis" also may be used to refer generally to the analysis of written materials. Bernard explains that "content analysis is a catch-all term covering a variety of techniques for making inferences from 'texts'" (1995, 339). According to this definition, content analysis can be used for interview transcripts that were generated as part of a research project, as well as for documents that existed outside of the research project. Because the term "content analysis" is somewhat ambiguous, we avoid using it in this chapter.

❧ References

Advisory Committee on Human Radiation Experiments (ACHRE). 1995. *The human radiation experiments*. New York: Oxford University Press.

Bernard, H. R. 1995. *Research methods in anthropology: Qualitative and quantitative approaches*. Walnut Creek, CA: AltaMira Press.

Bernhardt, B. A., G. Geller, M. Strauss, K. Helzlsover, M. Stefanek, P. M. Wilcox, and N. A. Holtzman. 1997. Toward a model informed consent process for BRCA1 testing: A qualitative assessment of women's attitudes. *Journal of Genetic Counseling* 6:207–22.

Burns, N. 1989. Standards for qualitative research. *Nursing Science Quarterly* 2:44–52.

Carr, L. T. 1994. The strengths and weaknesses of quantitative and qualitative research: What method for nursing? *Journal of Advanced Nursing* 20:716–21.

Center for Lifelong Learning, University of North Carolina at Chapel Hill School of Nursing. 2008. Summer Institutes in Qualitative Research. http://nursing.ce.unc.edu/certificates.php.

Coffey, A., and P. Atkinson. 1996. Concepts and coding. In *Making sense of qualitative data: Complementary research strategies*, 26–53. Thousand Oaks, CA: Sage Publications.

Creswell, J. W. 1994. *Research design: Qualitative and quantitative approaches*. Thousand Oaks, CA: Sage Publications.

———. 1998. *Qualitative inquiry and research design: Choosing among five traditions*. Thousand Oaks, CA: Sage Publications.

Davis A. M., S. C. Hull, C. Grady, B. S. Wilfond, and G. E. Henderson. 2002. The invisible hand in informed consent: The study coordinator's critical role in human subjects protection. *Journal of Law, Medicine, and Ethics* 30 (3): 411–19.

Faden, R. R., and N. E. Kass. 1996. *HIV, AIDS, and childbearing: Public policy, private lives*. New York: Oxford University Press.

Fox, R. C. 1959. *Experiment perilous: Physicians and patients facing the unknown*. Philadelphia: University of Pennsylvania.

Gittelsohn, J., P. J. Pelto, M. E. Bentley, K. Baltacharyya, and L. Jensen. 1998. *Ethnographic methods to investigate women's health: Rapid assessment procedures (RAP)*. Boston: International Nutrition Foundation.

Glaser, B. 1978. *Theoretical sensitivity*. Mill Valley, CA: Sociology Press.

Hull, S. C., and N. E. Kass. 2000. Adults with cystic fibrosis and (in)fertility: How has the health care system responded? *Journal of Andrology* 21 (6): 809–13.

Kass, N., H. Taylor, L. Fogarty, J. Sugarman, S. Goodman, A. Goodwin-Landher, M. Carducci, and H. Hurwitz. 2008. Purpose and benefits of early phase cancer trials: What do oncologists say? What do patients hear? *Journal of Empirical Research on Human Research Ethics* 3 (3): 57–68.

King, N. M. P., G. E. Henderson, L. R. Churchill, A. M. Davis, S. C. Hull, D. K. Nelson, P. C. Parham-Vetter, B. B. Rothschild, M. Easter, and B. Wilfond. 2005. Consent forms and therapeutic conception: The example of gene transfer research. *IRB: Ethics & Human Research* 27:1–8.

Koch, T. 1993. Establishing rigour in qualitative research: The decision trail. *Journal of Advanced Nursing* 19:976–86.

Kreuger, R. A. 1994. *Focus groups: A practical guide for applied research*. 2nd ed. Thousand Oaks, CA: Sage Publications.

Kvale, S. 1996. *Interviews: An introduction to qualitative research interviewing*. Thousand Oaks, CA: Sage Publications.

Leininger, M. M. 1985. Nature, rationale, and importance of evaluative research methods in nursing. In *Qualitative research methods in nursing*, ed. M. M. Leininger, 1–25. New York: Grune & Stratton.

Maxwell, J. A. 1992. Understanding and validity in qualitative research. *Harvard Educational Review* 62 (3): 279–300.

Miles, M. B., and A. M. Huberman. 1994. *Qualitative data analysis*. Thousand Oaks, CA: Sage Publications.

Miller, S. I., and M. Fredericks. 2006. Mixed-methods and evaluation research: Trends and issues. *Qualitative Health Research* 16 (4): 567–79.

Miller, W. L., and B. F. Crabtree. 1994. Qualitative analysis: How to begin making sense. *Family Practice Research Journal* 14 (3): 289–97.

Moon, M. H., E. Taylor, M. Hughes McDonald, and J. Carrese. 2009. Everyday ethics in the clinical practice of pediatric residents. *Archives of Pediatrics & Adolescent Medicine* 163 (9): 838–43.

Morgan, D. L. 1997. *Focus groups as qualitative research*. Thousand Oaks, CA: Sage Publications.

Morse, J. M. 1991. Qualitative nursing research: A free-for-all? In *Qualitative nursing research: A contemporary dialogue*, ed. J. M. Morse, 14–22. Newbury Park, CA: Sage Publications.

———. 1997. Learning to drive from a manual? *Qualitative Health Research* 7:181.

———. 1999. Silent debates in qualitative inquiry. *Qualitative Health Research* 9:163–65.

Morse, J. M., and P. A. Field. 1995. *Qualitative research methods for health professionals*. Thousand Oaks, CA: Sage Publications.

NVivo 8. 2008. Markham, Ontario, Canada: QSR International Pty., Ontario.

O'Cathain, A., E. Murphy, and J. P. Nicholl. 2007. Why, and how, mixed methods research is undertaken in health services research: A mixed methods study. *BMC Health Services Research* 7:85–95.

———. 2008. Multidisciplinary, interdisciplinary, or dysfunctional? Team working in mixed-methods research. *Qualitative Health Research* 18 (11): 1574–85.

Rubin, H. J., and I. S. Rubin. 1995. *Qualitative interviewing: The art of hearing data*. Thousand Oaks, CA: Sage Publications.

Sandelowski, M. 1995. Qualitative analysis: What it is and how to begin. *Research in Nursing and Health* 18 (4): 371–75.

———. 2000. Whatever happened to qualitative description? *Research in Nursing and Health* 23:334–40.

Silverman, H., S. C. Hull, and J. Sugarman. 2001. Variability among institutional review boards' decisions within the context of a multicenter trial. *Critical Care Medicine* 29 (2): 235–41.

Strauss, A., and J. Corbin. 1990. *Basics of qualitative health research: Grounded theory procedures and techniques*. Newbury Park, CA: Sage Publications.

Taylor H., and N. Kass. 2001. Factors that influence parent decision-making about enrolling their HIV-infected children in clinical research. *AIDS & Public Policy Journal* 16 (1/2): 28–42.

———. 2002. Attending to local justice: Lessons from pediatric HIV. *IRB: Ethics & Human Research* 24 (6): 9–17.

Weinfurt, K. P., J. Y. Friedman, J. S. Allsbrook, M. A. Dinan, M. A. Hall, and J. Sugarman. 2006. Views of potential research participations on financial conflicts of interest: Barriers and opportunities for effective disclosure. *Journal of General Internal Medicine* 21:901–6.

Yin, R. K. 1994. *Case study research: Design and methods*. Thousand Oaks, CA: Sage Publications.

✎ Appendix A *Recommended Texts*

GENERAL

Creswell, John W. 1998. *Qualitative Inquiry and Research Design: Choosing among Five Traditions*. Thousand Oaks, CA: Sage Publications.

Marshall, Catherine, and Gretchen Rossman. 1995. *Designing Qualitative Research*. 2nd ed. Thousand Oaks, CA: Sage Publications.

Mason, Jennifer. 2002. *Qualitative Researching*. 2nd ed. Thousand Oaks, CA: Sage Publications.

Morse, Janice M., and Peggy Anne Field. 1995. *Qualitative Research Methods for Health Professionals*. Thousand Oaks, CA: Sage Publications.

INTERVIEWS

Kreuger, R. A. 1994. *Focus Groups: A Practical Guide for Applied Research*. 2nd ed. Thousand Oaks, CA: Sage Publications.

Morgan, David L. 1997. *Focus Groups as Qualitative Research*. Thousand Oaks, CA: Sage Publications.

Rubin, Herbert J., and Irene S. Rubin. 1995. *Qualitative Interviewing: The Art of Hearing Data*. Thousand Oaks, CA: Sage Publications.

Weiss, Robert S. 1994. *Learning from Strangers: The Art and Method of Qualitative Interview Studies*. New York, NY: The Free Press.

ANALYSIS

Coffey, A., and P. Atkinson. 1996. *Making Sense of Qualitative Data: Complementary Research Strategies*. Thousand Oaks, CA: Sage Publications.

Miles, Matthew B., and A. Michael Huberman. 1994. *Qualitative Data Analysis*. Thousand Oaks, CA: Sage Publications.

Silverman, D. 2001. *Interpreting Qualitative Data: Methods for Analysing Talk, Text and Interaction*. 2nd ed. Thousand Oaks, CA: Sage Publications.

✎ Appendix B *Examples of Medical/Health and Ethics-Related Journals that Publish Qualitative Research*

Academic Medicine
Advanced Nursing Science
Bioethics
BMC Health Services Research
BMC Medical Ethics

BMJ
Cambridge Quarterly of Health Care Ethics
Genetic Medicine
Health Communication
Health Policy
IRB
Journal of the American Medical Association
Journal of Clinical Ethics
Journal of General Internal Medicine
Journal of Genetic Counseling
Journal of Medical Ethics
Journal of Medicine and Philosophy
Journal of Palliative Care
Nursing Ethics
Nursing Research
Patient Education and Counseling
Qualitative Health Research
Qualitative Inquiry
Social Science and Medicine
Western Journal of Nursing Research

CHAPTER 13

Ethnographic Methods

PATRICIA A. MARSHALL AND

BARBARA A. KOENIG

Ethnography refers to the description of cultural systems based on methods that may include a combination of intensive fieldwork, participant observation, and a range of interviewing techniques that enable investigators to identify, explore, and interpret social contexts, networks, relationships, and processes. In its broadest articulation, ethnography concentrates on ideology, beliefs, values, rituals, customs, and behaviors of individuals and communities interacting within social, economic, religious, political, and geographic environments. An important focus of ethnography is the interpretation of meanings and symbols that provide a lens for understanding how people make sense of their world. Ethnography is not, however, simply a set of tools. An ethnographic inquiry makes connections between local action and global, social, and political factors. It is tied to and based on theoretical premises about social process (Clarke 2005). It represents an interpretive approach to understanding cultural practices.

Overview

In this chapter we describe the relevance of ethnography to medical ethics. We begin with a brief review of critiques of the evolving field of bioethics that have called attention to the importance of social context and social processes for understanding and addressing moral and ethical questions in science and medicine. We then discuss a range of ethnographic methods and provide a critique of ethnography. We conclude with a list of resources and provide suggestions for further training in ethnographic methods.

SOCIAL CONTEXT, ETHNOGRAPHY, AND BIOETHICS

The emergence of the multidisciplinary field of bioethics in the 1970s was shaped primarily by scholars from philosophy, theology, medicine, and law. At that time the dominant paradigm within the field emphasized the use of the ethical principles (see, for example, Beauchamp and Childress 1979). Nevertheless, some scholars recognized the importance of the vulnerability of patients and families in relation to the authority of medical professionals and the implications of this for the application of ethical principles in medical practice (Pellegrino and Thomasma, 1981). Others demonstrated the significance of a narrative approach for understanding the moral complexities that arise in the unfolding of life's stories in sickness, health, and death (see, for example, Brody 1987; Hunter 1991). Renee Fox, a medical sociologist, was an early critic of bioethics and an advocate for the use of social science methodologies in the field (2008).

Beginning in the early 1990s anthropologists and other social scientists affirmed Fox and Swazey's critique of the foundational schema of medical ethics (1984), noting its lack of attention to the lived experience of illness, suffering, and death; its reliance on Western philosophical principles, and its limited recognition of the relevance of dominant approaches within bioethics for non-Western and resource-poor countries (Marshall 1992a, 1992b; Muller 1994; Kleinman 1995; Marshall and Koenig 1996, 2004; Kleinman, Fox, and Brandt 1999; De Vries and Conrad 1998; Turner 2003a, 2003b, 2009; De Vries et al. 2007; Gaines and Juengst 2008). Arthur Kleinman (1995) argued that an anthropological—in particular an ethnographic—approach to medical ethics has the potential to expand conventional perspectives through cultural analysis of moral conflicts found within unique local worlds. Concurrently, there was a heightened awareness of the importance of ethnographic attention to moral conflicts encountered in the social worlds in which scientific technologies are conceived and applied. A number of scholars (Jennings 1990; Hoffmaster 1992; Conrad 1994) challenged ethicists to incorporate ethnographic approaches in their philosophical analyses. Hoffmaster (1992, 1421), for example, argued that "what is needed is a different brand of moral theory, one that is more closely allied with and faithful to real-life moral phenomena. Ethnography has a vital role to play in developing a more empirically grounded theory of morality."

Some medical ethicists argued that ethics is essentially an interpretive enterprise (Carson 1990; Churchill 1990; Weisz 1990; Thomasma 1994; Hoffmaster 2001). Advocates of hermeneutical explorations of medical morality made explicit the interpretive nature of understanding ethical issues in science and medicine. Carson (1990), for example, proposed a multifaceted framework for considering moral questions in medical care. His framework incorporated elements of hermeneutics, casuistry, practical reasoning, and so-called thick description (see Geertz 1973) of cases. Such contextual models have the potential to bridge some of the fundamental tensions between the context-rich perspectives of the humanities and social sciences and the abstract reasoning associated with traditional philosophical approaches to medical ethics.

Ethnographic and other qualitative research methods provide opportunities for achieving greater sensitivity to social contexts at local, national, and global levels. As Gordon and Levin (2008, 83) write: "Ethnography contributes to bioethics by: 1) locating bioethical dilemmas in their social, political, economic and ideological contexts; 2) explicating the beliefs and behaviors of involved individuals; 3) making tacit knowledge explicit; 4) highlighting differences between ideal norms and actual behaviors; 5) identifying previously unrecognized phenomena; and 6) generating new questions for research."

Qualitative research approaches, including ethnographic methods, have been used to examine ethical issues on a wide range of topics including decisions at the end of life (Koenig 1997; Hern et al. 1998; Kaufman 2005); decision making in neonatal intensive care units (Guillemin and Holstrom 1986; Levin 1986; Anspach 1993); death in childhood (Bluebond-Langer 1980); pediatric chronic illness (Mattingly 1998); human organ and tissue replacement therapies (Sharp 1994, 2006, 2007; Lock 1995, 2002; Hogle 1999; Marshall and Daar 2000; Gordon 2001); clinical ethics consultations (Kelly et al. 1997); human genetics (Bosk 1992; Press and Browner 1998; Rabinow 1999; Rapp 1999; Konrad 2005); informed consent in clinical settings (Kaufert and O'Neil 1990; Barnes et al. 1998); the conduct of for-profit contract research organizations (Fisher 2009); and the biotechnology industry (Rabinow 1996; Rabinow and Dan-Cohen 2005). In international settings ethnographic methods have been used in studies of informed consent to research in infectious disease (Molyneux et al. 2005; Molyneux, Pashu, and Marsh 2005; Marshall et al. 2006); global health disparities (Farmer 1999); and the politics and practices of recruitment for international clinical trials conducted by the pharmaceutical industry (Petryna 2009).

Such work illustrates how ethnographic approaches to ethical questions can both elicit and help clarify the uncertain, ambiguous, and contextual features that are intrinsic to problematic moral issues that arise in clinical care and medical research. For example, Kaufman (2005) describes the profound impact of hospital procedures—including bioethics practices—on the experience of death and dying for clinicians, dying patients, and their families. In their ethnographic study of the use of life-extending cardiac interventions such as angioplasty, stents, bypass surgery, and implantable cardiac defibrillators on aging patients, Kaufman and her colleagues raise ethical questions about the meaning of advanced age and application of these technologies in critical care (Shim, Russ, and Kaufman 2006, 2009). Their findings suggest a "treatment imperative" that results in "almost inexorable momentum towards intervention that is experienced by physicians, patients, and family members alike" (Shim, Russ, and Kaufman 2009, 2). Their findings also inform bioethics scholarship, by pointing out the distance between ideal, rational choice deliberations about end-of-life decision making and actual clinical experience.

Ethnographic studies of biomedical and cultural practices in human organ replacement therapies throw into sharp relief the moral conundrums that arise when the social body—imbued with life or death, embedded in community—is transformed into a deconstructed and disarticulated body of spare parts (Fox and Swazey 1992). In her analysis of cultural influences on our understanding of the meaning of death and its timing in relation to organ transplantation in Japan and North America, Margaret Lock (2002), for example, explores the cultural and political sources of Japanese opposition to the concept of brain death compared to the acceptance of the new definition of death in North America. In the West attention is placed on the life-saving miracles of transplantation and the altruistic importance of donation, not on the source of human organs or the circumstances and practices surrounding their retrieval. Based on her ethnographic work on transplantation, Sharp (2006, 2007) coined the term "organ transfer" to call attention to the interdependency of human organ and tissue procurement, donation, and transplant practices. Sharp underscores the tension between the life-sustaining results of transplantation for organ recipients and the inevitable loss experienced by family members who donate the organs and tissues of a loved one following death.

Fundamental moral questions associated with scientific and technological advances and their clinical application are deeply contingent upon social context. In our view a robust cultural account of ethical issues in science and biomedicine must question the often unexamined assumptions underlying beliefs about the integrity of the human body and values expressed through the development of scientific and medical technologies, beliefs, and values that are negotiated within local economies and political arrangements. Detailed ethnographic accounts provide the best way to reveal complexity. Such examinations allow us to imagine alternative futures or the impact of varying social arrangements.

∾ Description of Ethnographic Methods

The breadth and scope of traditional ethnography illustrates the importance that early anthropologists placed on obtaining a holistic view of cultural worlds. In addition ethnographers emphasize the importance of an *emic* (native) perspective, which privileges the worldview of members of the culture being studied. An important goal of ethnography is to provide a comprehensive and coherent description of cultural practices, symbols, and ideas associated with a particular group or problem at a particular historical moment in time. Ethnography assumes a dynamic view of culture as action.

Ethnography is an inductive method for data collection, not a deductive approach that tests predefined hypotheses using fixed variables. It provides an analytical framework for assessing the relationship between practices observed at the local level (e.g., at an institutional, programmatic, or community level) and broader sociocultural, political, and economic phenomena. For example, an ethnographic examination of ethical problems associated with clinical practices observed at a health maintenance organization would take into account the regulatory demands of managed care at the macro level of organization of medicine in the United States. Likewise, a study of informed consent for cancer clinical trial participation may reveal that the actual decision to participate predates the ritualized informed consent discussion in the clinic (Sankar 2004).

Specific definitions of ethnography have been the subject of debate among social scientists for many years. At the heart of the controversy is an ideological divide that separates those investigators for whom ethnography represents a broad philosophical paradigm and others who view it simply as a methodology that is used when appropriate (see, for example, Atkinson 1994; Hammersley and Atkinson 1995). Early in the twentieth century, under the influence of Bronislaw Malinowski in Great Britain and Franz Boas in the United States, ethnographic fieldwork became the methodological foundation of cultural anthropology. Malinowski, renowned for his ethnographic descriptions of the Trobriand Islands in Malaysia, was clear about the ethnographer's task: "Find out the typical ways of thinking and feeling, corresponding to the institutions and culture of a given community and formulate the results in the most convincing way" (1961 [1922], 23). Documenting, analyzing, and reporting the relationship between meaning and observable action in the context of local worlds is the core of an ethnographer's job. In the development of the field of anthropology, scholars have emphasized various aspects of the enthnographic enterprise, including the focus of its inquiry and the nature of its underlying purpose (Geertz 1983; Marcus and Fischer 1986; Tyler 1996).

In 1973 Geertz published a collection of essays titled *The Interpretation of Cultures* in which he argued that ethnographers practice what he called "thick description"—descriptions of events, beliefs, and behavior, with sufficient attention to local background and meaning, so that they are comprehensible from the perspective of the people involved.

In the last three decades increasing attention has been given to the importance of critical self-reflexivity in writing ethnographies. Scholars such as Clifford and Marcus (1986) and, more recently, Denzin and Lincoln (2005), argue that it is impossible to write an objective account of someone else's cultural world because ethnographers bring to an investigation their own cultural constructions and their own worldviews and assumptions. Thus, an ethnographer's account is necessarily a secondhand account—a description of a cultural problem filtered through the interpretive lens of the ethnographer. This stands in sharp contrast to positivist biomedical approaches that speak of researcher "bias" as a problem to be corrected. Interpretive scholars accept the reality that all knowledge is "situated," informed by the inevitability of each researcher's unique cultural perspective and background. It is imperative that ethnographers maintain a reflective posture about their own beliefs and values. In the presentation of ethnographic data, researchers openly confront and describe how their background shapes interpretation.

There are many ethnographic methods that include participant observation, various types of ethnographic interviews, focus groups, archival research, life histories, diaries, and media or video analysis. In this chapter we provide brief descriptions of participant observation and ethnographic interviews.

PARTICIPANT OBSERVATION

Participant observation is the cornerstone of ethnographic research and is characterized by a period of intense social interaction and engagement between the researcher and individuals involved in the study, during which time data (e.g., field note observations, interview results, archival materials) are systematically collected. There are several examples of classic medical ethnographies in which participant observation was used to examine moral dimensions of clinical care and biomedical practice. Charles Bosk's classic text *Forgive and Remember* (1979) is based on intensive participant observation to understand the nature of medical mistakes. During his fieldwork Bosk spent considerable time with the surgeons and surgical residents, in formal and informal settings, attending rounds, and observing surgical procedures.

Ethnographies of neonatal intensive care units incorporated participant observation to demonstrate how moral tensions evolve within the cultural framework of biomedicine in caring for critically ill newborns (Guillemin and Holmstrom 1986; Anspach 1987). These investigations have shown that, despite the emphasis on an idealized partnership between parents and the health care team, physicians' opinions about therapeutic interventions often override the views of parents. Moreover, these ethnographies illustrate that evaluative judgments of an infant's diagnosis and prognosis are culturally and professionally situated. Anspach, for example, observed that nurses' judgments of a baby's future condition were based on sustained interactions with the infant, while physicians relied primarily on diagnostic information from test results to determine the infant's prognosis.

Participant observation is characterized by a continuum of roles, depending upon the context of the research, the relationships developed in the research process, and the experience and background of the ethnographer. In some studies observation, rather than participation, may be privileged. For example, in an ethnographic study of factors contributing to staff anger toward adolescent psychiatric patients hospitalized on locked wards, the investigators were primarily observers, documenting behavior and affect of staff and patients during routine activities such as group therapy sessions, meals, and free time (Scheinfeld et al. 1989). Although the ethnographers participated in informal conversations on the psychiatric units with staff and patients, they were not actively engaged as participants during group therapy or other formal activities.

In other situations ethnographers may be more active as participants because of the nature of the research and the opportunities to develop relationships with participants or because of the ethnographer's role in the community being studied. In a study of end-of-life decision making among ethnically diverse cancer patients, Koenig and the ethnographers involved in the study developed close personal relationships with a number of the participants and their families (Orona, Koenig, and Davis 1994: Barnes et al. 1998; Hern et al. 1998). Under these circumstances, it was not uncommon for the ethnographers to provide transportation to and from the hospital or to assist the families in other ways when possible.

Similarly, Marshall (1996) conducted a study on decision making surrounding which patients were considered to be appropriate candidates for heart transplantation. In weekly meetings of the Cardiac Transplant Team, it was decided who would be placed "on the list" to receive a cardiac transplant. Handwritten notes were taken during the meeting; additional comments were recorded after the meeting ended. Although Marshall was primarily an observer, because she was involved in the clinical activities of the medical center as an ethics consultant, occasionally she would volunteer or be asked for information or an opinion on a patient with whom she was familiar. In this sense Marshall was both a participant and observer at the weekly meetings of the Cardiac Transplant Team.

Although ethnographers using participant observation may begin a research project with a substantive or theoretical question, the particular focus of their inquiry evolves as they become acclimated to the field. For example, in her exploration of decisions about heart transplantation, Marshall's ongoing analysis of the ethnographic field notes revealed an interesting dynamic that occurred in situations of medical ambiguity (1992b). If a physician was invested in pursuing a cardiac transplant for a patient but results of medical tests did not clearly support a heart transplant, then a process of character construction began to unfold. This process involved a systematic attempt to promote a view of the patient as someone of good moral character, someone who was worthy of the transplant. In one case a mother of four young children was being evaluated for a heart transplant. The medical evidence to support transplantation was marginal. Her cardiologist began to call upon others at the meeting—cardiology nurses, the social worker, the pastoral care counselor—to provide "evidence" that would support the image of a good mother, a woman whose young children depended on her ability to provide for them in the future. The evidence presented was used to support a favorable decision for the patient. Marshall did not begin her fieldwork with the intention of examining the process of constructing a virtuous character in situations of medical uncertainty; instead, this process became evident through her systematic review and analysis of field observations of the meetings throughout the year. One of ethnography's strengths is generating ideas and analyses that were not conceived of in the initial project design. Ethnographers routinely move between analyzing ongoing field observations and using the results of analysis to go back to the field for further exploration of the issues that emerge.

ETHNOGRAPHIC INTERVIEWS

Different types of interviews may be used in an ethnographic study, depending upon the context and the kind of information the researcher seeks. Ethnographic interviews are designed to elicit an individual's interpretation of events, beliefs, and behavior; special attention is given to the meanings attached to cultural symbols and activities.

Informal ethnographic interviews are characterized by a lack of structure or control; these are conversations the researcher may have with individuals during the course of daily fieldwork. Informal interviewing may be used while getting settled in the field or can be used throughout the ethnographic study to build rapport or explore newly emerging topics of interest. Notes from informal interviews may be taken in the field and then fleshed out later in the day along with more substantive descriptions.

Unstructured ethnographic interviews, in contrast to informal interviews, have a topical focus but are marked by minimal control over the informants' responses. An ethnographer working in the area of HIV prevention among injection drug users, for example, used unstructured interviews to explore beliefs and practices associated with obtaining informed consent for participation in HIV prevention studies (Strenski et al. 2000). Although the general topic has been defined, there is no attempt to follow a predetermined line of questioning. Rather, the conversation follows the direction taken by the engaged and knowledgeable ethnographer based on the responses of the interviewee. Interviewers must have considerable substantive knowledge and detailed training. Notes or audio recordings may be taken during the interview, or details of the discussion may be written following the interview.

In a *semistructured interview*, a written guide is used to help the ethnographer in systematically reviewing a core set of issues. Questions are preestablished and are often followed by leads (or probes) for exploring the topic in greater detail. Semistructured interviews might be used in situations in which the researcher has only one opportunity to interview someone or needs to be sure that the same data are collected from all informants. Marshall used semistructured interviews to explore the process of informed consent for genetic epidemiological research conducted in Nigeria (Marshall 2001). A set of questions was designed to elicit information on the procedures used by tribal chiefs to let the community know that a health care study would be taking place. Respondents often would begin by providing one approach to informing the community. Additional questions elicited a range of possible strategies for alerting the community about upcoming research. This information would not have been easily accessible using a survey or questionnaire with forced choice responses.

Structured interviews are characterized by asking all research participants an identical set of questions through the use of a detailed interview schedule. A set of explicit instructions is developed for interviewers who administer the questionnaires; interview guides are piloted before use. Interviewers normally undergo a period of training in which they learn how to conduct the interview. Attention is given to the importance of adhering to the questions laid out in the instrument, collecting the data in a systematic fashion, and avoiding leading questions (i.e., the way in which the question is phrased suggests the answer).

Key informant ethnographic interviews are those interviews conducted with carefully selected individuals knowledgeable about the topic being explored. A semi-structured interview guide is often used in these interviews. In the Nigerian case study mentioned above, a list of key informants was identified that included research investigators and physicians involved in the epidemiological studies, individuals who obtained informed consent from potential participants, and participants in the research. These interviews helped to identify ethical issues relevant to the process of obtaining informed consent for genetic epidemiological research from the perspective of individuals with diverse roles in the implementation of the studies. Key informant interviews often are conducted in the early stages of an ethnographic or quantitative study to help clarify the focus of the inquiry and to provide information for the development of subsequent interview guides or surveys. As research progresses, ethnographers may return frequently to key informants.

Group interviews involve conversations with small groups of individuals from the field site selected on the basis of specific criteria (e.g., members of a support group of women with known risk factors for breast cancer; family members caring for an elderly parent with Alzheimer disease; scientists involved in international collaborative health research). Group interviews may be helpful in exploring novel issues; sensitive topics are better covered in face-to-face or telephone interviews.

VALIDITY AND RELIABILITY IN QUALITATIVE RESEARCH

Validity refers to the credibility and accuracy of the basic concepts used, the instruments developed, the data collected, and thus of the overall findings obtained in a study. Allowing informants to explain the details of their concerns or illness experience in their own terms enhances the validity of qualitative findings. Another method of determining validity is triangulation; this involves the use of multiple methods, multiple investigators, and diverse data sources to cross-check data. For example, in an ethnographic study being conducted on practices associated with advance directives in a hospital intensive care unit, results of in-depth interviews with patients might be compared with the results of key informant interviews and reviews of medical records to determine the validity of the concepts used and the data collected.

Investigators may also conduct *member checks* to determine validity. Member checks refer to the process of feeding back results of analyses to key informants to verify and affirm interpretations of the data collected. This may be accomplished by informal interviewing. Validity is a particular strength of ethnographic research because the concepts developed are based on direct interaction with research subjects.

Reliability refers to the capacity to obtain the same findings in repeat measurements. A number of approaches are used in determining reliability in research. Ethnographers cross-check the reliability of coding categories used in analyzing text data from interviews and field observations by involving several individuals working independently as judges in coding the data. *Interrater reliability* is high when thematic codes are applied in a consistent and similar pattern. A threat to reliability may occur when interview guides are revised in response to new developments in the field. This is both a potential threat and a way to ensure that the data collected capture the phenomena of interest. Information may come to light in the course of conducting interviews that necessitates changing the interview guide; changes in instruments, such as the interview field guides, result in what is called *instrumentation confound*. Thus, careful attention must be given to patterns that emerge in data collected when instruments are revised.

An additional threat to reliability occurs when there are a number of different people conducting interviews. Individual styles of interviewing vary, even when an interview guide is used. If one interviewer consistently reports certain data while another interviewer consistently reports contrasting information, it might be an indication of *interviewer bias*. These problems can be diminished when interviewers are trained to conduct the interview similarly, to see things, ask questions, and record them in more or less the same way. In ethnographic research where there are multiple interviewers, careful attention to training enhances reliability.

Trade-offs between validity and reliability must always be made. Data-collection techniques that change over time enhance validity but may sacrifice reliability, making both analysis and interpretation of data complex.

PROTECTION OF HUMAN SUBJECTS IN ETHNOGRAPHIC RESEARCH

The implementation of ethnographic research requires careful attention to the protection of human subjects. Ethnographers confront unique ethical challenges because of the unstructured nature of participant observation and because of the types of interviews conducted, which often involve the collection of sensitive personal information (Marshall et al. 1998; Marshall 1992a; Kayser-Jones and Koenig 1994; LeCompte and Schensul 1999; Singer et al. 1999; Koenig, Back, and Crawley 2003; Mosavel et al. 2005). The range of problems includes obtaining informed consent working with vulnerable populations, respecting confidentiality and privacy, and determining whether or not to intervene in a situation that occurs while in the field.

A number of questions must be addressed regarding informed consent for ethnographic research: Is written consent necessary, or will oral consent suffice? When group observations are conducted, who, if anyone, should be asked to provide consent? Deciding whether or not to seek written or oral consent is a judgment based on the nature of the research, the context of the study, and the seriousness of the risks involved for participants. It is imporant to distinguish the risks that arise from the research itself from those that arise only from confidentiality violations that result from mandated signatures on consent forms. In some cases written documentation of consent may be waived (e.g., if participants are illiterate or vulnerable because of their legal status or involvement in illicit activities, or if the research is conducted in a cultural setting in which signing a document to participate in research is viewed as inappropriate). However, IRBs that are unfamiliar with ethnography may dictate written consent for ethnographic studies, even when the circumstances require sensitivity to the vulnerability of participants or to the cultural context of the research (Marshall 2003, 2006). For example, in an ethnographic and epidemiological study of the indirect benefits of participating in a syringe exchange program, the IRB overseeing the study required signed consent forms for all injection drug users participating in the research (Strenski et al. 2000). Moreover, after conferring with legal representatives at the institution, the IRB insisted that the consent form state that, although a federal Certificate of Confidentiality (Comprehensive Drug Abuse and Control Act of 1970, Public Law No. 91–513, Section 3 [a]) had been obtained, confidentiality could not be guaranteed if there was a court order to secure research records.

In ethnographic research involving direct observation of group activities, arrangements usually are made before the initiation of the study to inform group members that the ethnographer will be present in the course of routine activities. In closed systems such as a hospital unit, an outpatient clinic, or a laboratory, a priori informed consent should be obtained from all those who are at the facility on a regular basis. Further, "in the moment" informed consent should be obtained from others, for example, patients and members of their family who cannot be approached ahead of time, as is possible with members of the hospital staff. Informed consent always should be obtained from individuals in the group who are interviewed. Whether such consent must be documented by the use of a written informed consent form depends very much on the particular situation.

In some group observations it may not be possible or necessary to obtain formal informed consent from every person present. For example, at informal gatherings of family members or staff at a nurses' station in a busy unit of a medical center, it would be intrusive to introduce the ethnographer and explain the study to every person who passed by. On the other hand, an ethnographer's presence at a family conference for an ethics consultation should be explained and permission should be obtained to observe the proceedings; if any of the family or members of the staff are uncomfortable with the observation, the ethnographer should leave. A good rule to follow is that in private interactions such as these, informed consent—not necessarily documented with a written form—should be obtained from everyone present. In semipublic places where individuals interact informally, however, it is less important to obtain consent from everyone, and it may be impossible. (Note that some public fora are specifically excluded from human subjects protection regulations; such settings, where individuals do not make the presumption of privacy, may be observed without a formal informed consent process.) Another important consideration is making certain not to affect ongoing clinical activities; the correct balance may be difficult to achieve.

At each stage of research—data collection, data analysis, and data reporting— every effort should be made to protect the privacy and confidentiality of the study participants. The data-collection strategies associated with ethnography require careful attention to the representation of individuals and communities in written transcripts derived from interviews and observations. Descriptive data collected by the ethnographer are recorded in field notes, daily logs, or diaries, using a coding system that protects the confidentiality of the research participants. Data collected in the field must also be secured out of the field setting to safeguard the identity of participants, especially if they are involved in deviant or illegal activities. In published manuscripts that include case narratives, pseudonyms are used rather than participants' names. This gesture, however, will not necessarily protect confidentiality because it may be possible to identify the individuals involved based on the details of the case and the research setting.

The question of whether the ethnographer should intervene in a problematic situation that occurs in the course of conducting ethnographic observations can be difficult. Once again, it is a judgment based on the purpose of the study, the context, and the specific event that occurs (Kayser-Jones and Koenig 1994). If ethnographers were to intervene continually in field situations that are directly related to the issue being investigated, the possibility that their research will have an impact is jeopardized since they would be unable to document the events being studied.

In some ethnographic studies, however, intervention may be the correct course of action. For example, in her two-year investigation of technology use in medical practice, Koenig (1988) conducted extensive observational fieldwork on the introduction and application of therapeutic plasma exchange (TPE), which, at that time, was an innovative treatment for autoimmune diseases. In addition to conducting interviews with key participants involved in TPE research and development, Koenig was a participant observer in TPE units and observed numerous treatments as they were carried out. An incident occurred in the course of her studies in which the TPE blood tubing broke while a patient was undergoing treatment. Koenig was the only other person in the room; she acted quickly and clamped off the machine, thereby preventing the patient from losing a large volume of blood.

Finally, ethnographers must address questions that arise in the course of obtaining approval from IRBs at local study sites (see, for example, Marshall 2003). Most IRBs do not have members with expertise in ethnographic methods. This often leads to confusion and misunderstandings concerning the research design and the protocols for implementing the study. Individuals who consider the use of ethnographic methods in medical ethics research should not make assumptions about the IRB's capacity to adequately evaluate ethnographic research. Instead, investigators might consider contacting the chair of the IRB to discuss questions that may arise in the IRB's discussion of the study. In preparing their research protocols, ethnographers need to be explicit about strategies for protecting participants from unintentional risks and harms associated with the study.

❧ Critique of Ethnographic Methods

Although ethnography is unquestionably useful in clarifying the nuanced and multifaceted realities of social life, ethnographic methods have a number of limitations. In conducting fieldwork, the investigator is unable to control contingent events. The ethnographer cannot regulate who is involved in activities or what occurs when he or she is observing or participating in ongoing social processes. Fieldwork in clinical settings, in laboratories, or in neighborhoods is defined by its openness to social process, unconstrained by an investigator's experimental model. Similarly, ethnographic interviews allow for the emergence of new avenues of exploration even when the investigator is pursuing a clear direction using an interview guide. Study variables are not predefined to the extent that they are in survey research, and this limits the amount of control the investigator has over the specific factors examined.

Another limitation associated with ethnography is that study samples tend to be smaller than when quantitative methods are used to test hypotheses and generalize the results to similar populations. Ethnographers can speak in detail about a particular group of people in a specific social setting, but their ability to generalize beyond the study sample is limited. It is important to note that generalizable results are never the main aim of ethnographic inquiry; findings may, however, be presented as generalizable in a theoretical sense, in that an ethnographic finding may be critical in informing a theoretical claim. In addition, ethnographic approaches are time consuming to implement. Ethnographers spend considerable time familiarizing themselves with the study site, conducting field observations, recording field notes, and implementing in-depth ethnographic interviews. Analyzing transcript data from field notes is significantly more labor intensive than conducting statistical analyses of survey data. Even when computer software programs are used to assist in the analysis, the ethnographer must develop coding categories for open-ended responses to questions or notes from field observations.

Finally, there is the challenge of objectivity. Some critics argue that the subjective and experiential nature of ethnography is outside the bounds of science—that ethnographic approaches lack the rigor of an experimental or clinical trial design. Ethnographers tend to be unapologetic about their methods, observing correctly that the purpose of ethnography is not to force a patient's experience into predefined categories that set limits on a social domain. Indeed, it is the very absence of these features that allows for the unique expression of a participant's perspective and for the study of social behavior in natural settings. Thus, ethnography offers a framework for collecting and interpreting data that is paradigmatically different from quantitative methods. Skilled ethnographers actively maintain a posture of reflexivity to enhance their awareness of possible biases.

ॐ Concluding Comments

Ethnographic research strategies have enormous potential for the examination of ethical issues that arise in medical practice and in the development and application of scientific technologies. Ethnography and related qualitative methods highlight the phenomenology of moral experience through detailed descriptions of beliefs and behavior in social contexts. Ethnographic research accommodates the complicated social interactions and experiences of everyday life and in this way provides a framework for a deeper and more contextualized understanding of moral challenges in medicine. Ethnographic accounts of problems in medical ethics offer the possibility of furthering our understanding of the ways in which medical morality is socially constructed and reinvented through cultural practices at particular historical moments.

❧ Notes on Resources and Training

Scholars who want to implement ethnographic research but lack experience should familiarize themselves with the relevant literature and enlist the help of others who are trained. In addition to the sources cited in this chapter, there are some basic volumes that can be helpful resources. For example, the volume edited by Russell Bernard, *Research Methods in Anthropology* (1998), provides a strong foundation, including specific information on implementing ethnographic research and analyzing qualitative ethnographic data. Similarly, Norman Denzin and Yvonna Lincoln's edited volume, *The Sage Handbook of Qualitative Research* (2005), offers a thorough treatment of all aspects of qualitative research, including ethnography. Adele Clarke's *Situational Analysis* (2005) offers a postmodern approach to grounded theory, attending to the particular historical and social geographical situations in which knowledge is embedded.

Jacoby and Siminoff's overview of empirical methods in bioethics (2008) addresses multiple qualitative approaches, including content analysis (Forman and Damschroder 2008), focus groups (Simon and Mosavel 2008), ethnographic approaches (Gordon and Levin 2008), and semistructured interviews (Sankar and Jones 2008).

Two collections of papers address the theoretical dimensions of empirical research in bioethics, with a particular focus on ethnography. A special issue of the journal *Daedalus*, "Bioethics and Beyond" (vol. 128, no. 4, fall 1999), was edited by Arthur Kleinman, Renée Fox, and Allan Brandt. The *Hastings Center Report* published a series of papers that asked, "What can the social scientist contribute to medical ethics?" (vol. 30, no. 1, January/February 2000). More recently, two additional collections of articles were published: the journal *Bioethics* (vol. 23, no. 1) contains papers that address the uses of empirical research in bioethics and the utility of empirical bioethics, and *The American Journal of Bioethics* (vol. 9, no. 6–7) contains an article by Alexander Kon, "The Role of Empirical Research in Bioethics," followed by eighteen peer commentaries.

Research that has incorporated ethnographic methods is published in a wide range of professional journals in the social sciences, education, nursing, and, less frequently, medical journals. For an example of the use of qualitative methods in a medical journal, see Carrese and Rhodes (1995). Avenues for publication of manuscripts based on qualitative and ethnographic data include: *Qualitative Inquiry* (a methods journal); *Qualitative Health Research*; *Social Science and Medicine*; *Culture, Medicine and Psychiatry*; *Medical Anthropology Quarterly*; *Sociology of Health and Illness*; *Medical Anthropology*; and *Human Organization*. Lists of journals that publish qualitative research are maintained by *The Qualitative Report* (www.nova.edu/ssss/QR/calls.html) and by the St. Louis University Qualitative Research Committee (www.slu.edu/organizations/qrc/QRjournals.html).

A number of websites provide useful information on books and other resources for ethnographic research design. For example, two general sites are www.altamira press.com and www.sagepub.com.

Individuals who are interested in training in ethnographic methods have several options. For example, the firm called Research Talk (www.researchtalk.com) offers courses and workshops for individuals with different levels of experience; the training includes introductions to software applications for ethnographic analysis (e.g., NVivo, MaxQDA, and Atlas.ti). In addition, there are ethnographic field schools (contact American Anthropological Association, www.aaanet.org) and an annual conference at the University of Alberta International Institute for Qualitative Methodology called Thinking Qualitatively that is organized by the editor of the journal *Qualitative Health Research.*

∾ References

Anspach, R. 1987. Prognostic conflict in life-death decisions: The organization as an ecology of knowledge. *Journal of Health and Social Behavior* 28:215–31.

———. 1993. *Deciding who lives: Fateful choices in the intensive-care nursery.* Berkeley: University of California Press.

Atkinson, P. M. 1994. Ethnography and participant observation. In *Handbook of qualitative research,* ed. N. Denzin and Y. Lincoln, 248–61. Thousand Oaks, CA: Sage Publications.

Barnes, D. M., A. J. Davis, T. Moran, C. J. Portillo, and B. A. Koenig. 1998. Informed consent in a multicultural cancer patient population: Implications for nursing practice. *Nursing Ethics* 5:412–23.

Beauchamp, T. L., and F. J. Childress. 1979. *Principles of biomedical ethics.* New York: Oxford University Press.

Bernard, H. R. 1998. *Research methods in anthropology: Qualitative and quantitative approaches.* 4th ed. Thousand Oaks, CA: Sage Publications.

Bluebond-Langer, M. 1980. *The private worlds of dying children.* Princeton, NJ: Princeton University Press.

Bosk, C. L. 1979. *Forgive and remember: Managing medical failure.* Chicago: University of Chicago Press.

———. 1992. *All God's mistakes: Genetic counseling in a pediatric hospital.* Chicago: University of Chicago Press.

Brody, H. 1987. *Stories of sickness.* New Haven, CT: Yale University Press.

Carrese, J. A., and L. A. Rhodes. 1995. Western bioethics on the Navajo reservation: Benefit or harm? *Journal of the American Medical Association* 274:826–29.

Carson, R. A. 1990. Interpretive bioethics: The way of discernment. *Theoretical Medicine* 11:51–60.

Churchill, L. 1990. Hermeneutics in science and medicine: A thesis understated. *Theoretical Medicine* 11:141–44.

Clarke, A. E. 2005. *Situational analysis: Grounded theory after the postmodern turn.* Thousand Oaks, CA: Sage Publications.

Clifford, J., and G. Marcus, eds. 1986. *Writing culture: The poetics and politics of ethnography.* Berkeley: University of California Press.

Conrad, P. 1994. How ethnography can help bioethics. *Bulletin of Medical Ethics* (May): 13–18.

Denzin, N., and Y. Lincoln. 2005. *The Sage handbook of qualitative research.* Thousand Oaks, CA: Sage Publications.

De Vries, R., and P. Conrad. 1998. Why bioethics needs sociology. In *Bioethics and society. Constructing the ethical enterprise,* eds. R. De Vries and J. Subedi, 233–57. Upper Saddle River, NJ: Prentice Hall.

De Vries, R., C. L. Bosk, K. Orfali, and L. B. Turner. 2007. *View from here: Bioethics and the social sciences.* Oxford: Blackwell.

Farmer, P. 1999. *Infections and inequalities: The modern plagues.* Berkeley: University of California Press.

Fisher, J. 2009. *Medical research for hire: The political economy of pharmaceutical clinical trials.* New Brunswick, NJ: Rutgers University Press.

Forman J., and L. Damschroder. 2008. Qualitative content analysis. In *Empirical Methods for Bioethics: A Primer,* ed. L. Jacoby and L. A. Siminoff, 39–62. New York: Elsevier.

Fox, R. C., and J. P. Swazey. 1984. Medical morality is not bioethics: Medical ethics in China and the United States. *Perspectives in Biology and Medicine* 27:336–60.

———. 1992. *Spare parts: Organ replacement in American society*. New York: Oxford University Press.

———. 2008. *Observing bioethics*. New York: Oxford University Press.

Gaines, A. D., and E. T. Juengst. 2008. Origin myths in bioethics: Constructing sources, motives and reason in bioethic(s). *Culture, Medicine and Psychiatry* 32:303–27.

Geertz, C. 1973. *The interpretation of cultures*. New York: Basic Books.

———. 1983. *Local knowledge: Further essays in interpretive anthropology*. New York: Basic Books.

Gordon, E. 2001. "They don't have to suffer for me": Why dialysis patients refuse offers of living donor kidneys. *Medical Anthropology Quarterly* 15 (2): 1–22.

Gordon, E., and B. W. Levin. 2008. Contextualizing ethical dilemmas: Ethnography for bioethics. In *Empirical methods for bioethics: A primer*, ed. L. Jacoby, and L. Siminoff, 83–116. New York: Elsevier.

Guillemin, J. H., and L. L. Holmstrom. 1986. *Mixed blessings: Intensive care for newborns*. New York: Oxford University Press.

Hammersley, M., and P. M. Atkinson. 1995. *Ethnography: Principles in practice*. 2nd ed. New York: Routledge.

Hern, H., B. A. Koenig, L. Moore, and P. Marshall. 1998. The difference that culture can make in end-of-life decision making. *Cambridge Quarterly of Health Care Ethics* 7:27–40.

Hoffmaster, B. 1992. Can ethnography save the life of medical ethics? *Social Science and Medicine* 35:1421–32.

———, ed. 2001. *Bioethics in social context*. Philadephia: Temple University Press.

Hogle, L. 1999. *Recovering the nation's body: Cultural memory, medicine, and the politics of redemption*. New Brunswick, NJ: Rutgers University Press.

Hunter, K. 1991. *Doctor's stories: The narrative structure of medical knowledge*. Princeton, NJ: Princeton University Press.

Jacoby, L., and L. A. Siminoff, eds. 2008. *Empirical methods for bioethics: A primer*. New York: Elsevier.

Jennings, B. 1990. Ethics and ethnography in neonatal intensive care. In *Social science perspectives on medical ethics*, ed. G. Weisz, 261–72. Philadelphia: University of Pennsylvania Press.

Kaufert, J. M., and J. D. O'Neil. 1990. Biomedical rituals and informed consent: Native Canadians and the negotiation of clinical trust. In *Social science perspectives on medical ethics*, ed. G. Weisz, 41–63. Philadelphia: University of Pennsylvania Press.

Kaufman, S. R. 2005. *And a time to die: How American hospitals shape the end of life*. New York: Scribner.

Kayser-Jones, J., and B. A. Koenig. 1994. Ethical issues in qualitative research in long-term care settings. In *Qualitative methods in aging research*, ed. J. F. Gubrium and A. Sankar, 15–32. Thousand Oaks, CA: Sage Publications.

Kelly, S., P. Marshall, L. Sanders, T. Raffin, and B. A. Koenig. 1997. Understanding the practice of ethics consultation: Results of an ethnographic multi-site study. *Journal of Clinical Ethics* 8:136–49.

Kleinman, A. 1995. Anthropology of bioethics. In *Encyclopedia of bioethics*, ed. W. Reich, 1667–74. New York: Macmillan.

Kleinman, A., R. Fox, and A. Brandt, eds. 1999. Bioethics and beyond. *Daedalus* 128(9).

Koenig, B. A. 1988. The technological imperative in medical practice: The social creation of a routine treatment. In *Biomedicine examined*, ed. M. Lock and D. Gordon, 351–74. Boston: Kluwer.

———. 1997. Cultural diversity in decision making about care at the end of life. In *Approaching death: Improving care at the end of life*, ed. M. J. Field and C. K. Cassel (Institute of Medicine), 363–82. Washington, DC: National Academy Press.

Koenig, B., A. L. Back, and L. M. Crawley. 2003. Qualitative methods in end-of-life research: Recommendations to enhance the protection of human subjects. *Journal of Pain and Symptom Management* 25:S43–S52.

Konrad, M. 2005. *Narrating the new predictive genetics: Ethics, ethnography, and science*. New York: Cambridge University Press.

LeCompte, M. D., and J. J. Schensul. 1999. *Designing and conducting ethnographic research*. Walnut Creek, CA: Altamira Press.

Levin, B. W. 1986. *Caring choices: Decision making about treatment for catastrophically ill newborns*. Unpublished PhD dissertation, Columbia University, New York, NY.

Lock, M. 1995. Contesting the natural: Moral dilemmas and technologies of dying. *Culture, Medicine and Psychiatry* 19:1–38.

———. 2002. *Twice dead: Organ transplants and the reinvention of death*. Berkeley: University of California Press.

Malinowski, B. 1961 [1922]. *Argonauts of the Western Pacific*. Reprint. New York: E. P. Dutton.

Marcus, G., and M. J. Fischer. 1986. *Anthropology as cultural critique*. Chicago: University of Chicago Press.

Marshall, P. A. 1992a. Research ethics in applied anthropology. *IRB: A Review of Human Subjects Research* 14:1–5.

———. 1992b. Anthropology and bioethics. *Medical Anthropology Quarterly* 6:49–73.

———. 1996. Boundary crossings: Gender and power in clinical ethics consultations. In *Gender and health: An international perspective*, ed. C. Sargent and C. Brettel, 205–26. Englewood Cliffs, NJ: Prentice Hall.

———. 2001. The relevance of culture for informed consent in U.S. funded international health services. In *Ethical and policy issues in international research: Clinical trials in developing countries*. Vol. 2 of *Commissioned Papers and Staff Analysis*. The President's National Bioethics Advisory Commission. Washington, DC: National Bioethics Advisory Commission, May, C1–C38.

———. 2003. Human subjects protections, institutional review boards, and cultural anthropological research. *Anthropological Quarterly* 76 (2): 281–97.

———. 2006. Informed consent in international health research. *Journal of Empirical Research on Human-Research Ethics* 1 (1): 25–42.

Marshall, P., C. Adebamowo, A. Adeyemo, et al. 2006. Voluntary participation and informed consent to international genetic research. *American Journal of Public Health* 96:1989–95.

Marshall, P., and A. Daar. 2000. Ethical issues in human organ replacement: A case study from India. In *Global health policy, local realities: The fallacy of the level playing field*, ed. L. M. Whiteford and L. Manderson, 205–30. Boulder, CO: Lynne Rienner.

Marshall, P., and B. Koenig. 1996. Bioethics in anthropology: Perspectives on culture, medicine and morality. In *Medical anthropology: Contemporary theory and method*. 2nd ed. C. Sargent and T. Johnson, 349–73. Westport, CT: Praeger.

———. 2004. Accounting for culture in a globalized bioethics. *Journal of Law, Medicine and Ethics* 32:252–56.

Marshall, P., B. A. Koenig, D. Barnes, and A. Davis. 1998. Multiculturalism, bioethics and end-of-life care: Case narratives of Latino cancer patients. In *Health care ethics: Critical issues for the 21st century*, ed. J. Monagle and D. Thomasma, 421–31. Gaithersburg, MD: Aspen Publishers.

Mattingly, C. 1998. *Healing dramas and clinical plots: The narrative structure of experience*. Cambridge: Cambridge University Press.

Molyneux, C. S., N. Peshu, and K. Marsh. 2005. Trust and informed consent: Insights from community members on the Kenyan coast. *Social Science and Medicine* 61 (7): 1463–73.

Molyneux, C. S., D. R. Wassenaar, N. Peshu, and K. Marsh. 2005. "Even if they ask you to stand by a tree all day, you will have to do it (laughter . . . !)": Community voices on the notion and practice of informed consent for biomedical research in developing countries. *Social Science and Medicine* 61:443–54.

Mosavel, M., C. Simon, D. Stade, and M. Buchbinder. 2005. Community-based participatory research (CBPR) in South Africa: Engaging multiple constituents to shape the research question. *Social Science and Medicine* 61:2577–87.

Muller, J. 1994. Anthropology, bioethics and medicine: A provocative trilogy. *Medical Anthropology Quarterly* 8:448–67.

Orona, C. J., B. A. Koenig, and A. J. Davis. 1994. Cultural aspects of nondisclosure. *Cambridge Quarterly of Health Care Ethics* 3:338–46.

Pellegrino, E. D., and D. C. Thomasma. 1981. *A philosophical basis of medical practice*. New York: Oxford University Press.

Petryna, A. 2009. *When experiments travel*. Princeton, NJ: Princeton University Press.

Press, N., and C. H. Browner. 1998. Characteristics of women who refuse an offer of prenatal diagnosis: Data from the California maternal serum alpha fetoprotein blood test experience. *American Journal of Medical Genetics* 78:433–45.

Rabinow, P. 1996. *Making PCR: A story of biotechnology*. Chicago: University of Chicago Press.

———. 1999. *French DNA: Trouble in purgatory*. Chicago: University of Chicago Press.

Rabinow, P., and T. Dan-Cohen. 2005. *A machine to make a future: Biotech chronicles*. Princeton, NJ: Princeton University Press.

Rapp, R. 1999. *Testing women, testing the fetus: The social impact of amniocentesis in America*. New York: Routledge.

Sankar, P. 2004. Communication and miscommunication in informed consent to research. *Medical Anthropology Quarterly* 18:429–46.

Sankar, P., and N. L. Jones. 2008. Semistructured interviews in bioethics research. In *Empirical Methods for Bioethics: A Primer*, eds. L. Jacoby and L. A. Siminoff, 117–38. New York: Elsevier.

Scheinfeld, D., P. Marshall, D. Beer, and K. Tyson. 1989. Knowledge utilization structures, processes and alliances in a psychiatric hospital study. In *Making our research useful: Case studies in the utilization of anthropological knowledge*, ed. J. Van-Wiligen, B. Rylko-Bauer, and A. McElroy, 201–18. Boulder, CO: Westview Press.

Sharp, L. 1994. Organ transplantation as a transformative experience: Anthropological insights into the restructuring of the self. *Medical Anthropology Quarterly* 9:357–89.

———. 2006. *Strange harvest: Organ transplants, denatured bodies, and the transformed self*. Berkeley: University of California Press.

———. 2007. *Bodies, commodities, & biotechnologies*. New York: Columbia University Press.

Shim, J. K., A. J. Russ, and S. R. Kaufman. 2006. Risk, life extension, and the pursuit of medical possibility. *Sociology of Health and Illness* 28:479–502.

———. 2009. Late-life cardiac interventions and the treatment imperative. *PLoS Med* 5(3):e7. doi:10.1371/journal.pmed.005007.

Simon, C. M., and M. Mosavel. 2008. Ethical design and conduct of focus groups in bioethics research. *Empirical methods for bioethics: A primer*, ed. L. Jacoby and L. A. Siminoff, 63–82. New York: Elsevier.

Singer, M., P. Marshall, R. Trotter, and J. Singer. 1999. Ethics, ethnography, drug use, and AIDS: Dilemmas and standards in federally funded research. In *Integrating cultural, observational, and epidemiological approaches in the prevention of drug abuse and HIV/AIDS*, ed. P. Marshall, M. Singer, and M. Clatts, 198–222. Bethesda, MD: U.S. Department of Health and Human Resources, National Institutes of Health, National Institute on Drug Abuse.

Strenski, T., P. A. Marshall, J. Gacki, and C. Sanchez. 2000. The impact of emergent syringe exchange programs on shooting galleries and injection behaviors in three ethnically diverse Chicago neighborhoods. *Medical Anthropology Quarterly* 18:415–38.

Thomasma, D. C. 1994. Clinical ethics as medical hermeneutics. *Theoretical Medicine* 15:93–112.

Turner, L. 2003a. Bioethics in a multicultural world: Medicine and morality in pluralistic settings. *Health Care Analysis* 11 (2): 99–117.

———. 2003b. Zones of consensus and zones of conflict: Questioning the "common morality" presumption in bioethics. *Kennedy Institute of Ethics Journal* 13:219–31.

———. 2009. Anthropological and sociological critiques of bioethics. *Bioethical Inquiry* 6:83–98.

Tyler, S., ed. 1996. *Cognitive anthropology*. New York: Rinehart & Winston.

Weisz, G., ed. 1990. *Social science perspectives on medical ethics*. Boston: Kluwer Academic Publishers.

CHAPTER 14

Quantitative Surveys

ROBERT A. PEARLMAN AND
HELENE E. STARKS

Quantitative study of problems in medical ethics can be quite useful. For instance, this approach to studying ethical problems has fostered increased communication and understanding between ethicists and clinicians. Ethicists have also learned about the variability in practice behaviors (e.g., how physicians sometimes provide and sometimes withhold treatment based on their own subjective perceptions of patient benefit), ethical issues that clinicians confront (e.g., requests from patients or their families for treatment perceived to be medically futile), and the difficulties that clinicians and health care organizations face when trying to implement ethics policies (e.g., the difficulties of shared decision making with regard to forgoing life-sustaining treatment). The results of multiple studies have helped ethicists reframe old questions and deliberate about new ones (Brody 1990; Pearlman, Miles, and Arnold 1993; Foglia et al. 2008). Over the last three decades, many more investigators have also started to study ethical problems in medicine in a broader sense (see chapter 2). In addition, this area of inquiry gradually became a legitimate career pathway for physicians, nurses, other clinicians, and health services researchers.

In this chapter quantitative survey methods are described and critiqued. Examples are presented to demonstrate how these methods have addressed topics of concern in medical ethics.

❧ Description of Quantitative Surveys

Developing excellent surveys requires a comprehensive research approach, including careful consideration of steps in planning and methodological options.

PLANNING A STUDY

Planning a study involves a series of steps, as summarized in table 14.1. First, it is essential to identify and to specify explicitly the goal(s) of the study (Weber and Cobaugh 2008). After these goals are specified, they should be formulated into answerable study questions (Lipowski 2008). For example, an investigator might have the goal of wanting to characterize how physicians respond to requests for assisted dying. The answerable study questions, however, might be the following: How do physicians discuss with patients (and their families) the motivation for these requests? How do physicians modify their treatment plans after hearing about patients' interest in assisted dying? Do physicians obtain other professional opinions for help in managing these requests, and if so, from whom? And how often do physicians respond affirmatively to such requests, and under what circumstances?

After the study questions are formulated, the literature should be reviewed to see whether these questions have been previously investigated (Cronin, Ryan, and Coughlan 2008). If so, one must then determine if the previous research was done well, if it involved the same population of current interest, and if the limitations of the previous study could be overcome through modifications to the study design or protocol. It is also essential to discern whether the study goals are still justified. At this time, research questions should be refined if necessary or appropriate.

After identification of the overall study objectives and resultant study questions, the research design needs to be developed. Although the design is an essential component to any research protocol, for the purposes of this chapter we concentrate on designs employing quantitative surveys, including cross sectional or longitudinal interviews.

Next, the desired target population needs to be identified, with a focus placed on those who meet eligibility criteria, where these individuals might be found, and any time considerations that must be met. The choice of the study population is influenced by the relevance of the study questions to the potential respondents, their ability to participate in the study, and the ability to recruit them. The plan for budgetary support also needs to be ascertained. If there is an available budget, this may shape the scope and format of the research. If government or foundation funding is going to be requested, then budgeting will be assessed after the development of a study proposal in which the details are specified.

The strategy for sampling also needs to be considered. With exploratory investigations, it is usually acceptable to obtain what is called convenience samples.

TABLE 14.1   Sequential Approach to Planning a Study

Step Activity
1. Select a researchable question.
2. Search and review related work, and then justify the research question again.
3. Develop hypotheses.
4. Identify instruments and data sources.
5. Develop the research protocol.
6. Identify the study population and sampling strategy.
7. Identify the study limitations.
8. Address as many procedural biases as possible.
9. Plan the statistical analyses.
10. Identify how the results will be reported.
11. Maintain notes for consideration for the discussion, interpretation, or conclusions.

Sampling patients who attend a morning clinic in which there is an available room for interviewing, interviewing all patients in a clinic, or sampling ones' professional colleagues are all examples of convenience sampling. If the purpose of the survey is to infer that the results generalize to a larger population, then more representative sampling is required. The most rigorous sampling technique that permits generalization to a larger population, since it is less likely to be biased, is *random sampling*. Random sampling means that each of the respondents chosen for the study has the same chance of being included and that no single respondent has any influence on the selection of another respondent. Random sampling can be achieved by random digit dialing, having a computer generate a list of random numbers, or using a list of random numbers (which are available in the appendices of many statistics textbooks). Other sampling strategies that promote generalizing, but are not random, include systematic sampling, stratified sampling according to a pertinent set of characteristics, and disproportionate sampling.

Systematic sampling means that the investigator chooses a selection system and applies it to the entire possible study population. For example, instead of approaching every patient in a clinic, an investigator could decide to approach the fourth and seventh patients on every clinician's roster. *Stratified sampling* is used to ensure that the study sample will have proportional representation of key respondent characteristics. For example, if educational level is thought to be a factor in opinions about completing advance directives, the investigator might stratify the sample to be sure that equal numbers of people with less than a high school education, a high school diploma, some years of college, a bachelor's degree, and postgraduate degrees are included in the study. In *disproportionate sampling* an investigator may oversample a subpopulation to ensure sufficient responses to be able to analyze this group. Some investigators question whether oversampling or disproportionate sampling truly achieves its goals.

SURVEY TECHNIQUES

Many methodological issues need to be considered when developing a survey instrument, including the mode of administration and the survey format, including whether the survey will ask stand-alone questions or prompt responses to hypothetical scenarios or vignettes.

Mode of administration

A central question in designing survey research is to choose an appropriate mode of administration. Table 14.2 presents advantages and disadvantages of different survey methods. Many factors determine whether the survey is conducted in person, over the telephone, on the internet, or by mail. Foremost is whether the study participants can hear, read, write, or own and use a computer. In addition, it is important to consider the complexity of the topic, the format of the questionnaire (e.g., vignette-based surveys are difficult to conduct over the telephone), the degree of burden of the survey itself on respondents, the desire or need for respondent anonymity or confidentiality, and the format for how the questions are answered. Last, the choice also will be influenced by budgetary and time considerations. Mail and internet-based surveys are less expensive than in-person, interviewer-administered surveys or telephone surveys but often result in a lower response rates and incomplete data.

The choice of administrative mode may be influenced by the desired sample. Telephone interviews present several challenges, including the increasing use of screening technologies (voice mail, caller ID, and call blocking) and decreasing telephone coverage of households that forgo land lines in favor of cell phones, especially among persons between the ages of eighteen through thirty. Random-digit dialing and the use of phone number lists (including both land lines and cell phones) can overcome some telephone coverage problems but require additional investments to acquire updated and reliable lists (Kempf and Remington 2007).

With mailed surveys it may be unclear who is responding within a household or whether the respondent has access to any literature that might contaminate the responses. Similarly, it may be unclear what motivates people to respond to mailed surveys, especially when there is no financial or in-kind benefit. Surveys over the Internet provide a low-cost and speedy approach to collecting data that also permits direct data entry. Internet-based surveys, however, require sensitivity about how the information might look on differently sized computer screens and with different operating systems. As a result, Internet-based surveys often require the expertise of a Web designer or the use of Web-based software (for example, SurveyMonkey, SurveyGizmo, SnapSurveys, or Zoomerang). They also require special data security considerations to protect the privacy of participants.

Often, mixed methods are employed to promote participation and/or offset weaknesses associated with a single method (Dillman 2000). For example, an introductory letter may be sent in advance to invite participation in a telephone interview. Another common rationale for using mixed methods is to reduce the costs of a longitudinal follow-up. For example, in a study that pertains to durability of attitudes over several years, an initial telephone interview might be followed with mailed or internet-based surveys. A concern with using different methods for the same questions, however, is that the different modes of administration may introduce systematic biases in the results. These include social desirability biases associated with telephone and in-person interviews or nonrandom missing data from mail or internet-based surveys inquiring about sensitive topics. Often the differences are neither anticipated nor easily explained.

Survey format

Many issues relate to how the survey itself is organized. They include considerations of ordering the topics, response formats, and the use of skip patterns. Telephone interviews typically group questions with the same introductory clauses and/or the same response categories to make it easier for respondents to answer the questions. For mail surveys, information design experts recommend leaving significant white space on the page, using a print font that is large and easy to read, and choosing paper colors that provide good contrast with the type style.

Written mail survey questionnaires often use skip patterns to guide respondents through the questionnaire. For example, if a respondent answers "yes" to a question, she goes on to the next question, but if she answers "no," she is instructed to

TABLE 14.2   Survey Methods: Advantages and Disadvantages

Survey Type	Advantages	Disadvantages
Mail	• Permits large numbers of respondents • Geographically unlimited • Absence of interviewers • Lower cost • Time convenience for respondents—can respond when they want to; start and stop as necessary • Anonymity with sensitive questions	• Limited response rate • Risk of incomplete data • Often requires multiple mailings • Reading and language barriers • Respondent identity uncertain
Internet	• Permits large numbers of respondents • Geographically unlimited • Lower cost • Direct data entry • Drop-down boxes permit immediate coding of answers • Easily incorporates skip patterns • Allows for pop-up instructions • Time convenience for respondents—can respond when they want to; start and stop as necessary	• Requires access to a computer • Requires computer literacy • Computer screens and operating systems may vary across respondents • Web design challenges • Reading, language, and physical disability barriers • Anonymity can be compromised without use of individualized access codes or passwords
Telephone	• Permits large numbers of respondents • Geographically unlimited • Respondent identified • Complete data likely • Quality assurance possible • Can obtain quick responses to time-sensitive questions	• Language and hearing barriers • Limited to people who have and answer telephones • Phone number lists often exclude cell phones • Cell phones are often assigned to individuals (not households) who may be ineligible for inclusion (e.g., minors) • Interviewer costs (training, time, and quality assurance) • Uncertainty about whether respondent is paying attention • Answering machines and caller ID foster screening, which increases nonresponse bias
Face-to-Face Interview	• Complete data very likely • Respondent identifiable • Controlled environment • Complex tasks and visual aids possible • Quality assurance possible • Good response rates	• Often limited by geographic considerations • Interviewer costs (see above) • Travel costs • Smaller number of respondents usually because of costs • Sensitive questions may be difficult to address

skip the next two questions. In self-administered mail surveys, moderate use of skip patterns is acceptable; excessive use can cause increased burden and confusion for the respondent. For example, a respondent should never have to refer to a previous page to answer a question. Neither should a respondent have to endure complicated routing between questions. An advantage of web-based surveys is that complicated skip patterns can be used that are invisible to the respondent because they are programmed into the software. This decreases the burden on respondents and increases the flexibility to tailor questionnaires to multiple subpopulations through the use of screening questions. In studies where vignettes are used to simulate clinical decision making, the questionnaire can be programmed to add details to the case based on the respondent's specific choices.

Questionnaires can be designed with or without the use of clinical cases or vignettes. When the survey does not use vignettes, the series of questions are usually grouped by topic and, when possible, placed together on the same page. There is usually a heading or introduction of some kind to signal the reader what the questions are about. When the topic changes, the next set of questions begins on a new page with a new header or introduction. When clinical vignettes are used, these are placed at the beginning of the page and then followed by a series of questions that relate to the particularities of the case.

Regardless of whether the format is a survey questionnaire or vignette, the questions usually provide closed-ended, ordered choices. This works well for eliciting information about well-defined issues or characterizing the dimensions within issues. This format, however, restricts thinking to the dimension being explored by the investigators.

Question format. The questionnaire format often is used to explore knowledge, beliefs, attitudes, and behaviors. The ideal way to study behaviors is through direct, unobtrusive observation. Questionnaires are used to obtain an approximation or self-report of behaviors since it is often logistically impractical to conduct observational studies. For example, surveys have explored physician attitudes, as well as behaviors, regarding physician-assisted dying. In a national study, Meier and colleagues (1998) mailed a survey to a national stratified probability sample of physicians. This research team discovered that approximately 18 percent of the physicians had received a request for assistance with dying and of those receiving requests, 16 percent had written at least one prescription.

The presentation of the questions is also critical to eliciting opinions. In a 2004 study Haider-Markel and Joslyn conducted a random-digit dial telephone survey with 1,200 residents of midwestern states to evaluate how changing the presentation of information (known as framing effects) influences the responses. The investigators used four different presentations of physician-assisted dying (two "pro-life" frames and two "individual rights" frames, with and without a messenger, e.g., Reverend Jerry Falwell and Dr. Jack Kevorkian) and demonstrated that both the message and the messenger are influential in shaping responses. In both cases the message was endorsed in the expected direction of the stated positions ("pro-life" being opposed to and "individual rights" being in favor of physician-assisted dying) and the messenger reinforced the message, which resulted in even stronger endorsements.

Vignette format. Clinical vignettes are used to present a standardized scenario from which respondents express their attitudes or indicate intended behaviors. They are used when the investigator wants to control for, or modify in a controlled way, many of the variables that could influence a decision or behavior. Using vignettes allows the investigator to present each respondent with the same information to test for the effect of this information on responses.

In one approach to using vignettes, the investigator specifies many of the issues within the case and then tries to characterize the other factors that might influence a behavior or decision. For example, in one study physicians were asked to respond to a standardized vignette regarding whether to withhold mechanical ventilation and allow a patient to die (Pearlman, Inui, and Carter 1982). Physicians were allowed to ask for different details about the case, such as laboratory results, spousal preferences, and the patient's functional abilities. Physicians then were asked to explain their intended behaviors. They also provided demographic information about themselves. In this study physicians who withheld the mechanical ventilator were more likely to be physicians in training or attending physicians, compared to private physicians; preferentially request social information about the patient; and believe that the hypothetical patient had a very limited life expectancy and poor quality of life.

In another approach, the investigator presents multiple vignettes with carefully modified attributes. When aspects of the case are changed, the investigator can use this variability to study the relative importance and influence of the changing characteristics on the decisions (Ludwick and Zeller 2001). For example, in one study, physician attitudes about withholding feeding tubes from nursing home patients were characterized (von Preyss-Friedman, Uhlmann, and Cain 1992). The investigators systematically modified information in the vignettes, such as the patient's age, sex, and functional status, to see how these patient attributes affected withholding of this treatment.

A third approach to case-based surveys involves asking respondents to recall a recent clinical case of their own with variables of interest to the investigator and then answer survey questions based on this specific encounter or occurrence. The advantage of using real clinical cases is that respondents are asked to report on actual behaviors as opposed to speculating as to how they might behave given a hypothetical clinical vignette. As an example, investigators conducted a study characterizing the consideration of medical futility as a rationale for writing "do not attempt resuscitation" (DNAR) orders (Curtis et al. 1995). They asked medical residents to identify who among their patients in the hospital had DNAR orders. These cases were then characterized by the residents' responses to questions about the patient's likelihood of surviving CPR (cardiopulmonary resuscitation) to hospital discharge and the current and anticipated quality of life for the patient. In another example, investigators wanted to understand how Washington state physicians responded to requests for assisted dying (Back et al. 1996). In anonymous mailed surveys, the investigators asked physicians to answer a series of questions about their most recent request. These data were analyzed in order to characterize both the patients making the requests (e.g., age, gender, disease, prognosis, symptom burden, perceived rationale for the request) and the physicians' behaviors in response to these requests (e.g., discussion, referral, refusal, psychiatric evaluation, prescriptions for symptom relief and depression, prescription for assisting the dying).

The use of vignettes in survey research gives rise to an unavoidable tension regarding their composition. Although brief, "shorthand" versions of clinical scenarios may be quick and easy to read, they are often unrealistic and do not provide enough information for a well-informed decision regarding an intended behavior. Longer, more specific vignettes permit the elicitation of more informed preferences and intended behaviors and probably have a stronger relationship between intention and true behavior (Ajzen and Fishbein 1977). For example, in studies using vignettes concerning circumstances of decisional incapacity and end-of-life decisions, a team of investigators characterized health states by providing information about cognition, mobility and ability to walk, ability to perform activities of daily living, and level of pain (Patrick et al. 1997). Similarly, they described treatments with reference to the acute or chronic condition that created the need for treatment, the nature of the treatment, its side effects, the likelihood of success, and the potential outcomes other than returning to the baseline situation.

The benefits of this approach are that study respondents have more specific details to create a mental image of hypothetical scenarios. These can reduce the likelihood of unrealistic or folk beliefs, such as the belief that patients in a coma "could catch up on their rest" or that a mechanical ventilator "was the equivalent of an iron lung." The limitation of these specific scenarios is that the preferences applied only to very specific conditions and treatments. Longer narratives may be used to convey the richer details of a case, thus making the story more complex and realistic. However, the length of these narratives may limit their use in a survey because of the time required for respondents to read and synthesize the details and the risk of cognitively overloading the reader with too much detail. Table 14.3 presents examples of levels of descriptive detail.

WRITING GOOD QUESTIONS

Writing good questions is a skill that requires practice. To write a good question, one should (a) use simple words, (b) avoid ambiguous or incomprehensible terms or concepts, (c) be brief, (d) be specific, and (e) be neutral. In addition, questions should avoid using terms that are leading, suggest a "correct" answer, or promote an answer that is socially desirable. If extra information is included that frames the question, one should try to present this information in a balanced way. For example, if the investigator is asking about treatment preferences, the question should include the likelihood of both success and failure of the treatment. This can be presented as the risk of surviving and the risk of dying. One should avoid double-barrel questions; that is, questions that ask about more than one issue at a time. Any question that contains an "and" or an "or" should be reviewed critically. Multiple-choice questions should include the full range of possible responses to avoid leaving out participants whose responses are at the bottom of the range (floor effects) or the top of the range (ceiling effects). When a questionnaire is used multiple times in a longitudinal study, questions that are insensitive to change may have limited value. Table 14.4 presents examples of poorly written questions and shows how they could be modified to make them better.

TABLE 14.3   Types of Vignettes

Clinical "Shorthand"

Imagine that you have Alzheimer disease. Would you want CPR if your heart stops?

Functional Description

Imagine that you are 82 years old and you:
- Cannot think or talk clearly, are confused, and no longer recognize family members.
- Are not in any pain.
- Are able to walk but get lost without supervision.
- Need help with getting dressed, bathing, and bowel and bladder functions.

Now imagine that your heart stops beating and you lose consciousness (black out). You could receive cardiopulmonary resuscitation (CPR), which would involve:
- Electric shocks, pumping on your chest, help with breathing, and heart medications through your veins.
- Possible side effects include broken ribs, sore chest, and memory loss.
- Possible outcomes are a 20 percent chance of returning to your baseline, a 5 percent chance of coma, or a 75 percent chance of death.

Would you want CPR in this situation if your heart were to stop beating?

Narrative

Imagine that you have severe memory loss. You sit in a chair most of the day and do not interact with others. You have full health care coverage that includes the cost of living in a nursing home, which is necessary because you cannot control your bladder or bowels and you must be spoon fed. Your family members come to visit you every two days and you enjoy their visits, although you cannot speak and do not know who they are. In addition to your memory loss, you have an irregular heartbeat. Your doctor wants your family to decide if you should receive cardiopulmonary resuscitation (CPR) if your heart suddenly stops beating. He tells the members of your family that CPR would include applying electric shocks to your chest to jump-start your heart. A breathing tube would be placed into your lungs to help you breathe, and you would receive medications through a tube placed in your veins. This would go on for 15–30 minutes until your heartbeat was restored, and you would probably go to the hospital afterward for follow-up care in the intensive care unit. You would have about a 4 percent chance of returning to your previous health condition and going back to the nursing home. What should your family advise the doctors regarding the use of CPR if your heart suddenly stops beating?

LEVELS OF MEASUREMENT

A complementary activity to writing good questions is choosing how the answers will be measured. The investigator must consider the level of specificity of the desired answers and the scaling methods. There are three principal types of measurements: nominal, ordinal, and interval. *Nominal data* categorize information without an ordered relationship. For example, the presence or absence of an advance directive, gender, and ethnic background represent nominal data. *Ordinal data* reflect an ordering of values, such as from small to large, slightly to predominantly, and none to moderate to severe. With ordinal data the size of the intervals between categories cannot be specified. In some surveys a statement is presented and a *Likert scale* is used

TABLE 14.4 The Development of Survey Questions: Draft and Revised Examples

Original Draft Question	Problem with the Question	Revised, Improved Questions
• Would you consider hastening your death by physician-assisted dying?	• The term "physician-assisted dying" is undefined.	• Have you seriously considered obtaining medications from a physician to hasten your death?
• Do you agree or disagree with the proposed policy that requires a psychiatric evaluation of patients requesting assisted dying?	• Assumes the respondent understands the basis for the proposed policy.	• Should all terminally ill patients who request physician-assisted dying see a psychiatrist to make sure that depression is not the source of the request?
• Have you considered requesting PAD or euthanasia?	• Double-barreled question: Asks two questions in one. Also uses an undefined acronym.	• Have you requested physician-assisted dying (PAD) for yourself (i.e., obtaining a prescription from your doctor with the intent of hastening your death?) (separate euthanasia question)
• Most experts recommend completion of an advance directive. To what degree do you think this is a good idea? (Responses: very much, a little, very little, not at all).	• Suggests a "correct" (or socially desirable) answer. The term "advance directive" is undefined. The response categories don't match the question.	• Do you agree or disagree with the idea that older adults should complete an advance directive (e.g., Living Will) to help guide their health care in the event they are too sick to make decisions on their own? (Responses: strongly agree, somewhat agree, neither agree nor disagree, somewhat disagree, strongly disagree.)

to facilitate responses. A Likert scale is an ordinal scale that indicates the strength of the response to a statement. Example response categories include "strongly agree," "agree," "disagree," and "strongly disagree." *Interval data* are similar to ordinal data in being ordered but also represent intervals of known size. Examples of interval data are the number of requests per year to a physician for assisted dying and the percentage of cases of perceived medical futility (from the physician's perspective) for a particular treatment.

Equal-appearing interval scales present the respondent with a series of intervals that are either labeled with ordinal descriptions for each interval or labeled only at the end points. An example of this type of question is, "On average, how bad is your pain, where 0 equals no pain and 10 equals pain as bad as it could be?" These scales are ordinal but have the appearance of being interval. Some investigators will mistakenly assume that statistics that require interval data are appropriate for these data. It is best to assume that the data are ordinal. Repeat statistical analyses can evaluate whether it makes a statistical difference when the intervals are treated as being equal. If statistical tests that assume interval data are employed, the use of such tests should be justified.

MEASUREMENT SAFEGUARDS

The methodological rigor needed to develop quantitative surveys always argues for a search for questionnaires (also referred to as instruments) that have been shown to be valid and reliable. The expression "do not re-create the wheel" is always good advice in this context. *Valid instruments* measure what is intended to be measured. Several lines of evidence establish validity. These include *face and content validity* (preliminary lines of evidence that make sense "on the face of it" without external comparative measures), *criterion validity* (showing the relationship between what is measured and other proven measurements of the same or similar phenomena), and *construct validity* (showing the relationship between two hypothetical assumptions or constructs).

Reliable data are reproducible. *Test-retest reliability* assesses the degree to which the same sample of respondents provides the same answers to a questionnaire over a short period of time (usually between two and six weeks). *Interrater reliability* is the degree to which two (or more) investigators ask the same questions or review the same data and obtain the same answers. Reliability is also determined by the *internal consistency* of the questions. This is achieved by asking about the same topic in two different but similar ways and then comparing the answers. A related concern, especially for longitudinal studies, is *responsiveness*. This is the degree to which a question is sensitive to change over time.

PILOT TESTING

Questions should be evaluated critically before incorporating them into questionnaires. When this step is left out, investigators typically invest enormous resources only to find at the end of the study that their data cannot answer their research questions. The value of pilot testing questions and questionnaires is often underappreciated, but the early effort reveals flaws in how questions are understood by respondents, the logistics of administration (e.g., how long it takes, whether skip patterns work), the feasibility of recruiting respondents, and what it takes to get completed questionnaires. The first phase of pilot testing focuses on ensuring that the respondents understand the questions and can give accurate responses that address the topic of interest. This can be done using focus groups or by having a small sample of individuals who are similar to the study population complete the questionnaire. Focus groups allow investigators to get feedback on the "big picture" issues, such as formatting, font size, paper color, sequence of the questions, and any questions that are confusing. A technique known as "cognitive debriefing" can also be used with individuals to assess the comprehension of the questions, and to understand the recall or decision strategies respondents use and how the response categories map to what respondents are trying to convey (Willis 2005). One technique of cognitive debriefing involves a "think aloud" exercise during which the investigator sits with the respondent while she is completing the questionnaire and asks her to discuss what the questions mean to her as she is answering them. The cognitive burden of individual questions or the questionnaire as a whole can be assessed during this type of debriefing. Pilot testing (or pretesting) should address the issues identified in table 14.5.

Sometimes pilot testing provides fascinating, unexpected insights. In a pilot test of vignettes depicting decisional incapacity (e.g., stoke, dementia), we identified that

TABLE 14.5   Issues Addressed in Pilot Testing of Surveys

Questions	*Questionnaire and Administration*
• Comprehension/understanding • Jargon • Appropriate reading level • Acceptability of cognitive burden • Responsiveness of the scales • Presence of floor or ceiling effects • Repeat items to assess reliability • Positive versus negative structure to assess framing effects	• Monitor the time to administer • Assess reliability: test-retest, interrater, internal consistency • Feedback on content, comprehensiveness • Assess patterns of responding due to format (e.g., sequencing, ensuring that responses are aligned to a common scale) • Check on validity (content measures what it is supposed to) • Assess response rate (by question and overall) • Observe interviewers: assume neutral roles, use exact wording, record exact responses, use nondirected probes • Ensure quality graphic design and simple, easy-to-follow formatting

patients were unwilling to imagine some psychological dimensions, such as sadness. They were willing to imagine being cognitively impaired, bedbound, and unable to care for themselves but not sad for part or most of the time. Without pilot testing we would have never imagined this selective aversion to imagining a psychological state. As a result we identified a structural limitation to the use of vignettes.

PROTECTION OF HUMAN SUBJECTS

Prior to initiating any research with human subjects, investigators must establish a protocol. IRBs critically review research protocols to ensure that the appropriate standards for conducting research are satisfied. Moreover, IRBs review the informed consent process (including a consent form if appropriate). Including a few sample questions in consent forms can give potential participants an idea of the kinds of questions they will be asked. With quantitative surveys it is prudent to include at least one example of a difficult question and one example of a sensitive question. For example, one study about advance care planning included the following questions on the consent form as examples of sensitive questions (Patrick et al. 1997): "Imagine that you develop a life-threatening illness and couldn't speak for yourself; would you want kidney dialysis for the rest of your life?" and "To what extent do you feel you are a burden on your family and friends?"

ROLLOUT CONSIDERATIONS

There are several important considerations to address to improve response rates once data collection begins. Participation is enhanced when potential respondents feel that they trust the researchers and purpose of the study, feel that they are contributing to an important endeavor, and feel that their voices and time are respected.

The following points can be included in introductory letters, consent forms, or conversations with potential respondents as ways to motivate participation and survey completion.

- Tell individuals why the study is being conducted and why it is important
- Ask individuals for their help
- Provide easy access to the survey and simple instructions
- Get key leaders to personalize encouragement to participate
- Communicate peer support for participation
- Clearly explain how anonymity or confidentiality will be managed
- Provide incentives to participate such as cash or gift cards
- For workplace surveys, arrange for individuals to complete the survey while "on the clock"
- Express thanks at the end of the survey and/or with a follow-up note, especially for longitudinal studies

Additional strategies that increase participation rates include sending individuals a prenotification about the upcoming survey; sending follow-up reminders by mail, E-mail, or telephone; and having competition between groups for greater participation.

✑ Critique of Survey Research in Medical Ethics

As in the development of any research endeavor, some critical questions to ask at the beginning of the project are, in what ways are the research questions interesting and timely, and who are the intended audiences for the results? In studies that rely on questionnaires, it is also worth ensuring that the results, regardless of the findings, should be important and noteworthy. The reason for this latter caveat is a practical one. Trainees and faculty conduct these investigations, and dissemination of the results is desirable. Thus, it is prudent to frame the research so that the results are of interest to the target audience(s).

Unfortunately, many of the empirical studies in medical ethics that employ questionnaires or vignettes exhibit poor methodological rigor. At the most fundamental level, questionnaires often are developed without consideration of hypotheses, theoretical underpinnings, or conceptual models. A common mistake is to generate one or two study questions and jump straight to a study design without stepping back and considering whether those questions capture the complexity of the problem. For example, consider the case in which an investigator wants to study the influence of uncertainty on how patients make decisions. An inexperienced investigator interested in this topic decides he will design a short questionnaire that asks patients about their general discomfort with uncertainty in decision making and whether they feel that their physicians discuss uncertainty in a balanced way. He provides a definition of uncertainty but does not provide the context of the discussions and the decisions.

Although of great interest and relevance, this study, as conceived, fails to address several important issues that would lead to a broader understanding of potential influential factors. For example, the role of uncertainty in clinical decisions may play out differently if the decision refers to a diagnostic test or a clinical decision. Other factors include whether the decision is about a lifesaving or elective intervention, the degree of uncertainty or relative likelihood of success or failure (small, moderate, large), the patient's attitudes about risk, the setting and timing of the disclosure, the clinician's comfort level with sharing uncertainty, and how the probability estimate is communicated (verbally, with visual cues, likelihood of success, likelihood of failure, and so forth).

If the investigator had limited his study to his original design, he would likely discover that his results raise more questions than provide answers. Thinking broadly before getting focused on the study or questionnaire design helps frame the issues and then forces the investigator to select explicitly which aspects of an issue are going to be explored. Thoughtful reflection is enhanced when an interdisciplinary group is incorporated into the planning stages of the research. Interdisciplinary is meant to suggest a broad array of scholars with interests that relate to the question or phenomenon. Many quality research endeavors using quantitative techniques have benefited from collaboration with anthropologists, psychologists, sociologists, philosophers, and health services researchers.

STRENGTHS OF SURVEY METHODOLOGY

Even though there are many threats to the quality of surveys, this research method has many strengths. Surveys are often simple, easy to administer, and present limited risks to the respondents. The greatest risk is usually the discomfort of being asked to consider a sensitive topic. Surveys permit analyses involving large numbers of respondents in a relatively short period of time, can be used to make comparisons between groups, and are usually cost-effective. They can serve multiple purposes, including describing the attitudes, beliefs, and behaviors of populations, patients, and health care providers. They also can be used to test hypotheses and infer generalizable associations through the use of inferential statistics.

WEAKNESSES OF SURVEY METHODOLOGY

Despite these strengths, surveys are limited in the richness of the information that can be obtained. Surveys usually only obtain a limited description of attitudes or behavior. Moreover, they are limited to the approach and resultant questions of the investigator. For a richer understanding of issues, qualitative methods need to be employed (see chapters 12 and 13).

The other weaknesses of survey methods are mostly those previously described. However, a common problem sometimes occurs with research trainees. In a paradigmatic situation, a trainee in geriatric medicine or general internal medicine embarks on conducting a survey with limited time and budget, a sketchy understanding of the conceptual basis for studying the question(s), imprecise study objectives, and inadequate resources and expertise to ensure that naïve mistakes are avoided. Rather than being an intrinsic weakness in the research method, however, this more accurately reflects a weakness in research training.

∾ Concluding Comments

Quantitative surveys have become a well-appreciated approach to studying problems in ethics. When survey methods are employed in a study, careful attention needs to be directed at the identification of the appropriate target population, the mode in which the survey is administered, and the use of clear language and simple formatting.

Interdisciplinary input in the early stages of planning can help identify the scope of the inquiry and as a consequence the questions to be addressed. Here, critical feedback from other researchers with expertise in survey methods helps ensure scientific rigor. Finally, pilot testing helps ensure that the survey results are reliable and valid.

∾ Notes on Resources and Training

To conduct survey research with scientific rigor, the investigator needs to have adequate education and training. Education needs to focus on research and survey methods, questionnaire design, cognitive and social psychology, the strengths and weaknesses of scaling techniques, psychometric properties of measurement, and the assumptions and limits of statistical tests. Training requires responsible supervision from experienced survey researchers and statisticians to ensure that reliable and valid information is obtained, that appropriate statistical analyses are done, and that the collection of data occurred voluntarily and with informed consent.

One of the more ideal situations involves a multistep process of developing a research study, only one or a few components of which would focus on questionnaire development. In many training and fellowship programs, trainees and research fellows present their early study ideas and obtain feedback and criticism. Subsequent reviews that occur prior to beginning the research focus on the choice of questionnaire design, measurements and scales, goals of pilot testing, and the results and proposed changes due to the pilot. After completion of data collection, supervision of data analyses and reporting is essential.

Another aspect of training is hands-on experience. Conducting pilot interviews and obtaining feedback is humbling and educational. Another element of hands-on experience is soliciting the impressions and hearing the experiences of the interviewers. With longitudinal studies it is imperative that interviewers be observed for drift from the original protocol. Even with closed-ended interview schedules, interviewers can get sloppy over time and skip over instructions or paraphrase questions they consider wordy or confusing. Investigators should participate in this observational review process. If the investigators are collecting primary data, their behavior should be reviewed and critiqued by someone else.

Many of the resources for conducting survey research reside within universities. In academic environments the search for assistance should not be limited to one's own clinical or departmental area. Universities usually have faculty with expertise in sociology, psychology, statistics, and questionnaire design. Depending on the topic, there also may be experts with interest in the study topic. This can include individuals with expertise in ethics and the related clinical or research entity. In addition, there are excellent textbooks that provide overviews and advice about how to conduct survey research (see, for example, Dillman 2000; Aday and Llewellyn 2006; Sue and Ritter 2007).

There are three other general approaches to identifying resources: contact academic scholars who have published in the area of interest and request their feedback on ideas and questionnaires; access resources through the internet; and communicate with graduate training programs in ethics to see if they have faculty with expertise in empirical research in ethics. A listing of graduate medical ethics programs is available through the American Society for Bioethics and Humanities (www.asbh.org). It is important to remember that interdisciplinary review often provides useful insights. Moreover, many academic faculty members provide consultations and guidance to researchers from distant sites.

∿ Note

∿ References

Aday, L. A., and J. C. Llewellyn. 2006. *Designing and conducting health surveys: A comprehensive guide.* 3rd ed. San Francisco, CA: Jossey-Bass.

Ajzen, I., and M. Fishbein. 1977. Attitude-behavior relations: A theoretical analysis and review of empiric research. *Psychological Bulletin* 84:888–918.

Back, A. L., J. I. Wallace, H. E. Starks, and R. A. Pearlman. 1996. Physician-assisted suicide and euthanasia in Washington state: Patient requests and physician responses. *Journal of the American Medical Association* 275:919–25.

Brody, B. A. 1990. Quality of scholarship in bioethics. *Journal of Medicine and Philosophy* 15:161–78.

Cronin, P., F. Ryan, and M. Coughlan. 2008. Undertaking a literature review: A step-by-step approach. *British Journal of Nursing* 17 (1): 38–43.

Curtis, J. R., D. R. Parks, M. R. Krone, and R. A. Pearlman. 1995. Use of medical futility rationale in do not attempt resuscitation orders. *Journal of the American Medical Association* 273:124–28.

Dillman, D. A. 2000. *Mail and internet surveys: The tailored design method.* 2nd ed. New York: John Wiley & Sons.

Foglia, M. B., R. A. Pearlman, J. Altemose, M. Bottrell, and E. Fox. 2008. Priority setting and the ethics of resource allocation within VA health care facilities: Results of a survey. *Journal of Organizational Ethics: Healthcare, Business, and Policy* 4 (2): 83–96.

Haider-Markel, D. P., and M. R. Joslyn. 2004. Just how important is the messenger versus the message? The case of framing physician-assisted suicide. *Death Studies* 28 (3): 243–62.

Kempf, A. M., and P. L. Remington. 2007. New challenges for telephone survey research in the twenty-first century. *Annual Review Public Health* 28:113–26.

Lipowski, E. E. 2008. Developing great research questions. *American Journal of Health-System Pharmacy* 65 (17): 1667–70.

Ludwick, R., and R. A. Zeller. 2001. The factorial survey: An experimental method to replicate real world problems. *Nursing Research* 50 (2): 129–33.

Meier, D. E., C. A. Emmons, S. Wallenstein, T. Quill, R. S. Morrison, and C. K. Cassel. 1998. A national survey of physician-assisted suicide and euthanasia in the United States. *New England Journal of Medicine* 338:1193–1201.

Patrick, D. L., R. A. Pearlman, H. E. Starks, K. C. Cain, W. G. Cole, and R. F. Uhlmann. 1997. Validation of life-sustaining treatment preferences: Implications for advance care planning. *Annals of Internal Medicine* 127:509–17.

Pearlman, R. A., T. S. Inui, and W. B. Carter. 1982. Variability in physician bioethical decision making: A case study of euthanasia. *Annals of Internal Medicine* 97:420–25.

Pearlman, R. A., S. H. Miles, and R. Arnold. 1993. Empirical research in ethics. *Theoretical Medicine* 14:197–210.

Sue, V. M., and L. A. Ritter. 2007. *Conducting online surveys.* Thousand Oaks, CA: Sage Publications.

von Preyss-Friedman, S. M., R. F. Uhlmann, and K. C. Cain. 1992. Physicians' attitudes toward tube feeding chronically ill nursing home patients. *Journal of General Internal Medicine* 7 (1): 46–51.

Weber, R. J., and D. J. Cobaugh. 2008. Developing and executing an effective research plan. *American Journal of Health-System Pharmacy* 65 (21): 2058–65.

Willis, G. B. 2005. *Cognitive interviewing: A tool for improving questionnaire design.* Thousand Oaks, CA: Sage Publications.

CHAPTER 15

Experimental Methods

MARION DANIS, LAURA HANSON,
AND JOANNE M. GARRETT

Empirical research in medical ethics is useful to determine the effectiveness of interventions deemed valuable on theoretical grounds. When researchers wonder whether ethical reasoning can influence clinical action, or whether ethical guidelines can influence clinical outcomes, they can utilize a range of research methods, from observation and description of interventions to an experimental approach in which an intervention is planned, conducted, and monitored for an expected outcome. In this chapter we will emphasize the unique aspects of experimental research that tests whether an intervention is able to affect outcomes with moral significance.

Research questions that are appropriate for experimental designs might include the following: Can an educational program improve medical students' knowledge and practice of obtaining informed consent? Does the use of pain scores, in conjunction with vital signs, result in an increased proportion of patients who receive satisfactory pain relief? Or, do programs that teach clinic staff to respect cultural diversity increase access to services for minority patients who attend primary care clinics? The investigator who seeks to answer such questions using experimental methods will design an intervention and then evaluate its effect on specified, relevant outcomes.

Although this chapter is meant to help those conducting experimental trials to do so more effectively, it is also intended for nonexperimentalists by making them aware of the important insights that such research yields for the field of medical ethics as a whole. Experimental research that demonstrated the limited effectiveness of written advance directives serves as an important example of how experimental studies can test widely held beliefs in medical ethics (Danis et al. 1991; Schneiderman et al. 1992). Anyone with an interest in medical ethics who wishes to have a well-rounded understanding of the discipline should appreciate what experimental research can contribute and know how to critically evaluate this type of research. As we planned this chapter, we incorporated the insights of Weiss about the nature of experimental research, which were particularly helpful, and many of our explanations derive from his work on randomized controlled trials (Weiss 1996).

❧ Description of Experimental Methods

The experimental method differs from other research methods in that it requires control over a phenomenon under study. The researcher assumes some control over the experience of study subjects so that experimental subjects receive an intervention and are compared with control subjects who do not receive the intervention. To the degree possible, other sources of differences between the intervention and control groups are eliminated. Experimental studies in clinical research are called clinical trials—studies that test interventions to improve health or change clinical practices. Such studies have a prospective design and require longitudinal follow-up to measure the effects of the intervention. Investigators may also study the effects of interventions designed and carried out by others, as, for example, when a new educational program or governmental policy influences clinical action. These studies, termed natural experiments, are observational rather than experimental in nature but may still offer insight into purposeful efforts to change clinical practice.

At times, results of an experiment may challenge ethicists to reexamine ethical theory. Medical ethicists often develop a systematic approach to ethical challenges encountered in the clinical setting based on theoretical principle and the reflective analysis of cases. A controlled trial of an intervention may be used to apply the approach and test its impact on desired outcomes. For example, the Study to Understand Prognoses and Preferences for Outcomes and Risks of Treatment (SUPPORT Principal Investigators 1995) was a randomized, controlled trial to test whether nurses' facilitation of communication about patients' preferences and prognosis would change the treatment experienced by seriously ill patients with short life expectancy. The design of the intervention was based on the ethical principles of autonomy and truth telling and on evidence from descriptive studies that concluded that patients preferred less aggressive life support than the current standard of care. In spite of a careful design that was consonant with current ethical thinking, the SUPPORT intervention had no significant impact on the treatment experienced by patients or their satisfaction with it. The study results challenged fundamental assumptions in clinical ethics and raised new questions about the meaning of autonomy and the translation of ethical reasoning into practice.

Conducting an experiment to test a hypothesis is a costly and laborious endeavor. Thus, it is advisable for the investigator to identify a problem worthy of this effort. Unlike descriptive studies, an experimental study is begun after substantial previous observational study and theoretical analysis in support of the intervention. Furthermore, because of their cost, experiments are generally reserved for questions of the greatest merit—interventions that, if successful, would offer significant benefit to large numbers of persons. Once convinced of the need to use experimental design, the investigator must make decisions about overall study design, design of the intervention, selection of subjects and controls, measurement of outcomes, and the plan for interpretation of the results.

STUDY DESIGN

The overall design of an intervention study may be of three types: a randomized controlled trial, a nonrandomized controlled trial, or an uncontrolled trial. In randomized trials subjects enter control or intervention groups by random assignment. Nonrandomized controlled trials include studies with historical controls who elect not to receive the intervention or other comparison groups chosen without random assignment. Uncontrolled trials study the impact of an intervention by measuring and comparing some key outcome measures for a single group of subjects before and after the intervention. Strictly speaking, the latter two study designs do not adhere to an experimental method. Subjects self-select for the intervention, potentially introducing bias if those selecting the intervention differ in important ways from those who do not select it.

Randomized controlled trials

Randomization of subjects allows investigators to study the isolated effect of an intervention. Study subjects are informed of the trial's design and purpose, and after informed consent they are assigned randomly to one of the study groups. The control group may receive no intervention, a different intervention, or usual care. Chance alone dictates group assignment, creating groups that do not differ (except by chance) in ways other than their experience of the intervention. Randomization removes known and unforeseen causes of bias that could lead to false conclusions.

Nonrandomized controlled trials and uncontrolled trials

While the randomized controlled trial is considered to be the gold standard for evaluation of the effect of an intervention, there are circumstances that limit the use of this study design. Subjects who can serve as a comparison group for measuring the effect of an intervention can be derived through other approaches. A common strategy is to use historical controls, the same or a similar group of patients who received services prior to introduction of the intervention. For example, perceived access to care could be measured before and after implementation of a new program to improve access. Researchers may also choose to use a convenience sample of control subjects from a similar population to whom the intervention is not offered, such as patients in a neighboring hospital. A third alternative is to permit subjects to elect or refuse the intervention, and use self-selected controls. Nonrandomized trials permit comparison of two study groups but strictly speaking are truly descriptive rather than experimental in design.

Nonrandomized and uncontrolled trials are useful when (a) a randomized trial would be too costly, (b) randomization is considered ethically unsound, or (c) the proposed intervention is comprehensive or complex. While randomization gives the investigator complete control over one aspect of the patient's experience or therapy, this approach is ethically permissible only when patients are willing to forgo a personal choice and when there is no clear evidence that subjects assigned to this intervention will face great risk or that control subjects will give up an effective or important intervention. Currently, for example, while clinically important information could be gained from a randomized controlled trial that compared survival and satisfaction with tube feeding versus manually assisted feeding for seriously ill patients, the trial would abrogate a patient's right to choose whether to have a feeding tube.

Many interventions with ethical implications will never be studied in randomized controlled trials because it is difficult for a team of investigators to offer the intervention to one group of patients without influencing the care of the control group. If, for example, a diversity training study involves an educational program for clinicians at a primary care clinic, any clinicians who receive the training must have all their patients assigned to the intervention group, because it would be hard for clinicians to treat some of their patients according to the newly taught approach and other patients according to the older approach. If it is the clinicians who are assigned to intervention and control groups, it might also be difficult to teach a new approach to the clinicians in the intervention group without their influencing those colleagues in the control group in the course of their daily interactions. These difficulties may be avoided in multisite studies, but such studies are extraordinarily complex and expensive and present other problems due to differences among sites.

If investigators choose to design a study with intervention and control groups to which study subjects are not randomly assigned, several minimum criteria should be met (Weiss 1996): (a) control and intervention subjects must be clearly defined and enumerated; (b) eligibility criteria should be explicit and identical for intervention and control subjects; (c) in planning the study the two groups should be selected to be as similar as possible to minimize factors other than the intervention that would influence the outcome of interest; and (d) the tools for monitoring the outcome of interest should be identical for both study groups. In nonrandomized studies, intervention and control subjects might be matched on important variables, such as gender or educational attainment, or selected from similar geographic or service settings. The investigator must recognize that when historical controls are used in a study with prolonged follow-up, other secular trends or changes in health care delivery may affect the outcome. For example, the use of advance directives is steadily increasing over time in the United States. Therefore, a study comparing rates of advance directive use before and after an institutionwide educational program will be strengthened if the investigators include information on advance directive use in a larger geographic area that can show the impact of these secular trends over the time frame of their study.

DESIGNING THE INTERVENTION

Once a study design has been selected, the design of the intervention becomes the focus. In designing the intervention, the investigator should consider (a) existing evidence for the effect of the proposed intervention, (b) practical concerns about generalizability, (c) selection of control or comparison groups, and (d) whether to conduct an efficacy or effectiveness trial.

In designing an intervention, the investigator needs to decide how much to subsume under the label of one intervention. As an example, consider an educational intervention to teach medical students about informed consent. Review of the literature might suggest many possible educational methods: discussion groups, presentation of panels of patients or research subjects who discuss their perceptions of the value of informed consent, role plays in which students take on the roles of clinicians and patients, or modeling of informed consent by senior physicians working with the students. If the primary research question is whether one can improve medical students' knowledge of the principles and practice of informed consent, the investigators might wish to use several approaches in an effort to make the intervention as potent as possible. Their intervention might include as many of these strategies as possible as a combination of curricular materials presented in all four years of medical education. Alternatively, the investigators' review of the literature might suggest that two strategies—role playing and modeling by senior physicians—are the most effective educational methods. They might then combine these two techniques as the study intervention in the belief that a more defined intervention would be more practically incorporated into any medical school's curriculum. Alternatively, if prior successful trials had used varied methods to improve knowledge, the investigators might design a study to test one educational method against another or to test whether educational efforts could be concentrated in preclinical courses. For this study, investigators would use existing studies to select a single teaching method with the best evidence of success.

If an intervention is to benefit patients in general (i.e., outside of a research setting), it needs to be designed so that it can be feasibly reproduced in practice. Consider, for example, a randomized controlled trial of a multidisciplinary team to promote the autonomy of stroke patients with speech deficits. If the intervention requires intensive hours of speech and physical therapy but yields only modest benefit for patients, it is likely that the intervention will be considered too cumbersome and costly and not sufficiently portable or useful for other clinicians and patients. Thus, in designing an intervention that one hopes will be generally useful it ought to be as simple, inexpensive, and easy to export to other settings as possible.

The investigators must also design the control or comparison group's experience. For example, randomized controlled trials of decision aids to improve informed consent may allocate controls to usual clinical informed consent discussions or to one-on-one counseling without the decision aid (Green et al. 2004; Whelan et al. 2004). The choice should depend on the standard of care for the condition under study. The ethical acceptability of having a control group that receives no intervention or a placebo can be quite controversial. In clinical trials opponents of placebos consider their use unethical when a standard, proven treatment exists (Rothman and Michels 1994; Freedman, Glass, and Weijer 1996). Those who endorse placebos suggest that placebo-controlled trials may be ethical when deferral of therapy will not harm a patient (Temple and Ellenberg 2000). Safeguards that are recommended to make the use of placebos ethically acceptable involve the adherence to certain standards for their use, including minimization of risk, informed consent for study subjects, and optimization of treatment at the conclusion of a study (Miller 2000, 2008). The possibility of a control group that receives no intervention, or less than the standard of care, becomes even more complex when international research involves communities with differing standards of care. Which community standard to follow is a matter of intensive debate (Angell 1997; Varmus and Satcher 1998) that has been repeatedly addressed in revisions of the Declaration of Helsinki (Holm and Harris 2008).

In standard clinical trials two groups are being compared, but if the investigator chooses to study two interventions, then subjects may be randomized to one of two possible intervention groups with a third group serving as a control. One must consider the impact of this choice on the power of the study to detect differences between groups. Study power—the probability of detecting an intervention's effect in the study sample, if it exists in the population at large—is determined by the number of subjects in each group and the magnitude and variability of the difference in outcome between intervention and control groups. If a fixed number of potential subjects are divided into three groups, it will diminish the power of the study to detect differences between groups.

Intervention studies may be designed as either efficacy or effectiveness trials. In an efficacy trial, investigators wish to know whether an intervention has impact on the outcome of interest under optimal circumstances. Efficacy trials are generally used when an intervention is relatively unproven and are designed to maximize the impact of the intervention. They examine the outcome of an intervention under idealized circumstances. Efficacy trials may exclude patients who are less likely to benefit. The intervention is designed to be as powerful as possible.

Once efficacy has been demonstrated, investigators may then design an effectiveness trial in which they set out to examine whether the benefits endure under nonideal conditions. Thus, if one has completed an efficacy trial that demonstrates that an educational intervention to promote cultural sensitivity improves minority access to medical services, one might design an effectiveness trial to determine whether the intervention can work in a pressured work environment where clinic employees see patients in brief visits and where there is rapid staff turnover.

DEFINING OUTCOME MEASURES

Each intervention is designed with a goal in mind—a plan to influence some outcome of interest because it reflects an aspect of ethical reasoning or behavior. Thus, the outcome is as important as the intervention itself. Why else conduct the study? Defining the outcome of interest and deciding how to measure it is crucial. It may be difficult to find tangible measures of morally relevant outcomes because complex human beliefs and behaviors are not easily captured by quantitative measures. Investigators will begin with a broad concept of benefit, such as patient satisfaction with pain management. In the design of a study, they must consider whether, for example, family surrogates' satisfaction can substitute as an outcome measure for patients incapable of response (Sulmasy et al. 1998) and how to adjust for the strongly positive bias in most satisfaction scales (Hays and Ware 1986).

Clinical outcome measures may be usefully divided into process measures and patient-centered outcomes (Donaldson and Field 1998). Process measures are intermediate steps or easily identified components of care that may be used as proxies for the true outcomes of interest. Patient-centered outcomes are the best measures of successful clinical interventions, since the primary aim of most clinical research is to improve patient care. However, researchers may choose process measures when they lack the resources for extensive follow-up or interviews with patients. For example, in a study of medical student education on informed consent, the investigators might hope these students will do a better job with informed consent once they enter into practice. Since it would be impractical to conduct the study long enough to measure this endpoint, the investigator must measure other, more proximate endpoints. Any process measure should be selected based on some evidence that it is a good predictor of the ultimate outcome of interest. Thus, one might observe medical students obtaining informed consent during an Objective Structured Clinical Examination (OSCE), a standardized assessment tool used to evaluate examination skills (Roberts and Norman 1990). Other process measures, such as the students' knowledge and attitudes about informed consent and patient autonomy, might be measured to evaluate the short-term effects of the educational intervention.

Given the longitudinal nature of an intervention study, an investigator might give careful thought to the timing between the intervention and measurement of the outcome. For example, a study testing the merits of a weekend retreat to teach medical students about ethics, which measured the difference in the students' knowledge before and after the weekend, may show a substantial gain from Friday to Sunday, but one wouldn't want to rely on these results if one was hoping for retained knowledge in the long term. In all intervention studies it is important to measure and account for other factors that might influence the study outcome of interest. Thus, once the outcome measure is defined, data collection will need to include variables that could concurrently influence that outcome. In the example of the informed consent study, a survey might assess cultural background and demographic information of students that might influence their attitudes toward autonomy or communication with patients. If these other factors are equally distributed between treatment arms, as is usually the case in a randomized design, they should have negligible effect on the outcome.

Part of the definition of outcome measures entails the selection of study instruments. In conducting a trial related to an ethical issue, it is quite likely, for instance, that the attitudes of research participants will be an important outcome measure. Questionnaires therefore will be necessary to measure these attitudes. The selection of the instrument to use for this purpose raises issues that are addressed elsewhere in this volume (see chapter 14). When possible, investigators benefit from the use of survey instruments that have been previously developed and validated so that the investigator need not devote energies to instrument design, which entails a study in itself (Pequegnat and Stover 1995).

SELECTION OF STUDY PARTICIPANTS

To conclude that the results of an experiment are generalizable to other populations, the participants who form the study sample must be similar to a larger population, or target population, for whom the intervention might be useful. Although it is rarely possible to derive the study sample as an exact subset of the proposed clinical population, it is important to have the study sample be as similar to the population of interest as possible. If, for example, one wishes to learn about the effect of written advance directive materials on elderly individuals with low literacy, then studying the materials' impact on college students is not helpful. Even after selecting an appropriate study sample, it remains important to collect information from participants about sociodemographic characteristics such as their age, chronic disease experience, and education so that others then may compare their situation to the study sample when they are considering whether the study results might be applicable to them.

In selecting study participants, the investigator should define inclusion and exclusion criteria. It is important to appreciate that doing so can have opposing effects on the efficacy and generalizability of the study. If, for example, one is trying to teach cultural sensitivity to clinic staff to improve access to care for minority patients, one might specify in the inclusion criteria that study participants be able to read and write so that one can easily prepare written materials to offer them in clinic and survey them at the completion of the study by use of a written questionnaire. But patients who can read and write may be the easiest patients to help gain access, since health literacy has a substantial impact on health outcomes (Baker et al. 1998). By including only such patients, one has a higher likelihood of demonstrating that the intervention is effective. However, if the vast majority of clinics serving minority populations have patients who are not literate, then the exclusion of illiterate patients reduces the generalizability of the study results.

The selection of study participants also raises questions of fairness. Investigators should avoid underrepresentation of minority and elderly individuals who have often been left out of studies in the past while avoiding exploitation of economically disadvantaged populations, such as the uninsured, when they are enrolled (Pace, Miller, and Danis 2003; Meltzer and Childress 2008).

DETERMINATION OF THE SAMPLE SIZE

Aside from defining the characteristics of the study subjects, the number of study subjects must be determined. To set the sample size, the investigator must identify the hypothesis to be tested; select a statistical test that will be used to test whether the hypothesis has been proven; choose an effect size, indicating how much of a difference between the treatment and control group will be considered clinically important; and decide how much one is willing to tolerate making an error about the results (how acceptable it would be to have either a falsely positive study result, referred to as a type I error, or to have a falsely negative result, referred to as a type II error) (Cohen 1988; Hulley and Cummings 2006). The larger the sample size the greater the statistical power will be to detect a significant difference between the groups. One strategy for guaranteeing an adequate number of study subjects while minimizing the cost of conducting a study is to alter the sampling ratio so that the number of subjects in the control group exceeds the number of subjects in the intervention group (Morgenstern and Winn 1983).

SELECTION OF THE STUDY SITE

A variety of other decisions are involved in the design of an experimental trial. Should the trial be multicentered or located at one study site? If one is studying a fairly complex intervention, such as a whole course or various additions to the curriculum, it may be difficult to reproduce the intervention in more than one site. One advantage of a single site is that it can provide more reliably consistent data collection because the same staff collects all the data (Chow and Liu 1998). An advantage of a multisite study, when one is examining ethically charged issues, is that individual study sites can remain unidentified during reporting, leaving institutions less susceptible to being labeled "ethically deficient" as a result of their participation in a study. Use of multiple study sites permits the inclusion of geographically dispersed sites or sites that include ethnically and religiously diverse populations. Given the relationship of moral values to culture and religion, this can be an important consideration in a study of an intervention intended to have an ethically meaningful outcome. When using more than one site, ideally randomization should occur within each site. However, there are occasions when randomization needs to occur by site rather than by individual subject to avoid contamination of the intervention or ethical issues of withholding the intervention within a site as exemplified by a study of informed consent (Lavori, Wilt, and Sugarman 2007). Although this is a less desirable study design, to mitigate differences between sites, sites should be paired by comparable subject and site characteristics. Then each pair of sites is randomized to a treatment site and a control site (Yudkin and Moher 2001; Jordhøy et al. 2002).

Since research is commonly conducted across international boundaries, the possibility of conducting ethics research internationally arises. Here researchers are faced with a particularly complicated task of being attentive to the reality that ethical norms vary in different societies. One must be very cautious and wary about studying ethical interventions across cultures that have different ethical beliefs and practices.

SUBJECT RECRUITMENT

To facilitate maximal recruitment, investigators are advised to follow a number of rules, including identifying the actual and potential pool of subjects, developing a recruitment strategy, devising methods to optimize this strategy, developing alternative strategies, and writing the trial protocol with some sensitivity to its impact on recruitment (Spilker and Cramer 1992).

THE CONDUCT OF THE TRIAL

Given the complicated nature of many clinical trials, detailed procedures are required to ensure correct conduct of the trial. A thorough strategy for the conduct of a clinical trial has been well outlined by Good (2006).

ANALYSIS

A number of crucial steps are involved in understanding the significance of experimental results. Understanding the results of a trial includes three types of evaluation: data analysis, interpretation, and extrapolation (Spilker 1991). Data analysis involves a determination of the statistical significance of the study results and involves the use of statistical procedures and evaluations. Statistical significance does not automatically imply that the results are clinically important. Interpretation involves a determination of the clinical significance of the results based on clinical judgment. To determine that the results of a trial are clinically significant, it is best to establish criteria for significance before the trial begins. One must decide how large a response in the most important outcome measured in the study would be necessary to convince the relevant audience to use the intervention. One might decide beforehand that students should demonstrate a 25 percent difference in scores in order to consider the intervention to be an educational success. Extrapolation requires the use of judgment and logic to determine relevance of the study results for practice settings or circumstances beyond the precise circumstances created in the trial.

Data analysis

The ability to analyze study results is a crucial ingredient in conducting and understanding experimental research. For the interested reader, we venture here to explain the strategy for selecting a statistical approach to experimental research because it is difficult to locate a logical and concise strategy for statistical analysis in the literature.

The responses of research subjects to the intervention provide the clinical endpoints or data that will require analysis before the investigator can assess the effectiveness of the study intervention. The data may be either qualitative (nonnumeric data) or quantitative (numerical data). Qualitative data can be analyzed using standardized methods to discover, code, and categorize themes within text responses. Coded qualitative data may be reported descriptively or may be further classified and counted in categories and hence are labeled categorical data. For example, Roter and colleagues (1995) used qualitative analysis to code audiotaped clinical encounters to identify communication behaviors after a physician communication intervention. The frequency of codes during encounters was then used as a categorical measure of the impact of the training on behaviors. If the categories can be ordered then they may be called ranked or ordered categorical data. For example, in our hypothetical study of medical student education to obtain informed consent, we may use as our endpoint patients' satisfaction with the consent discussion as determined by interview following the consent process. These interviews may be analyzed with qualitative analytic techniques. Patients' responses may be placed in categories—such as unsatisfied, somewhat satisfied, and very satisfied—depending upon their comments about the student's ability to discuss the consent with them. Alternatively, we may ask patients to rank the interview on a numerical scale. The resulting data will be numerical data. If there are numbers with gaps between them, then the variables are discrete variables. If there are no such gaps, then the data are considered continuous.

To aid in our discussion of data analysis, we refer the reader to three diagrams, developed by Garrett, which provide a guide to the use of the most common statistical tests for data analysis. Figures 15.1, 15.2, and 15.3 provide decision strategies for selecting tests when performing an analysis with one (univariate), two (bivariate), or many variables (multivariable analysis), respectively. In general the strategy for selecting a statistical test is based on the characteristics of the variables, whether the variables are categorical or continuous, as defined above. In general the analytic approach one takes should be justified based on the character of the data and is best selected before the data are in hand to be certain that the analytic approach is not chosen to yield some desired result.

Before using statistical tests it is important to examine the values of each variable in order to assess for inaccurate, missing, or extreme data values and to determine the most appropriate form in which to use these variables in further analysis. Since one is dealing at this stage with one variable at a time, it is appropriate to use univariate methods (figure 15.1).

If the independent variable, X, is designated to represent whether or not the study subject received the intervention, then X is a categorical variable. If the dependent variable, Y, is the outcome of the study, it may be categorical or continuous. If it is continuous, it further may be classified as normally or not normally distributed. By normally distributed, we mean that the values are distributed in a fashion (called a probability distribution function) that looks like a bell-shaped curve. To analyze the effectiveness of the study intervention, one would use the test statistic that is appropriate for the particular type of variable with which one is dealing.

If the study is uncontrolled, the baseline and follow-up measurements of the outcome variable are considered repeated measures on the same sample of study subjects. Here the investigator would choose a paired t-test or McNemar's test to compare the baseline and follow-up measurements, depending upon whether the dependent variable is continuous and normally distributed, or categorical (figure 15.2).

If the study is a controlled trial, then it is appropriate to carry out a bivariate analysis, with X representing the independent variable (whether the subject was in the control or intervention group) and Y representing the outcome. Take, for example, a hypothetical study to determine whether a pain assessment as a "vital sign" (i.e., asking patients whether and how much pain they have every time their usual vital signs of blood pressure, pulse, respiratory rate, and temperature are checked) leads to improved pain management. The independent variable, X, represents whether or not the patient received the pain assessment. Thus, X is categorical with two categories. Our dependent variable, Y, is a pain score. If the patients' responses to the pain score divide cleanly into two groups—those patients whose pain is satisfactorily relieved and those whose pain is not satisfactorily relieved—then we can consider our outcome measure a categorical variable. Alternatively, we may choose to group the responses into several categories—very unsatisfactory, somewhat unsatisfactory, somewhat satisfactory, and very satisfactory. Yet another option, if the responses to the summary pain score seem to range along a continuum, would be to consider our outcome as a continuous variable. Ultimately, the selected analytic approach must be justified to the reader. If the interpretation of the results differs with use of different analytic approaches, the investigator can include these differing interpretations in publication of the results.

In this case a test statistic is appropriate when X is categorical. If we choose to handle the outcome data as categorical and the scores are divided into two categories, we use Pearson's Chi-square or alternatively Fisher's exact test if the sample is quite small (figure 15.2). If we choose to divide the pain scores into more than two categories, we use Pearson's chi-square or the Mantel-Haenzel test for trend. If the pain scores are continuous and have a normal distribution, we would select a two-sample t-test. If the pain scores are continuous but not normally distributed, we pick the Wilcoxon rank-sum test. Had we designed our study to have more than two treatment arms, it would be appropriate to use one-way analysis of variance (if Y is normally distributed) or the Kruskal-Wallis test (if Y is nonnormal).

If we wish to examine the joint contribution of sets of variables, to see the independent contribution of each variable or to control for bias when characteristics of

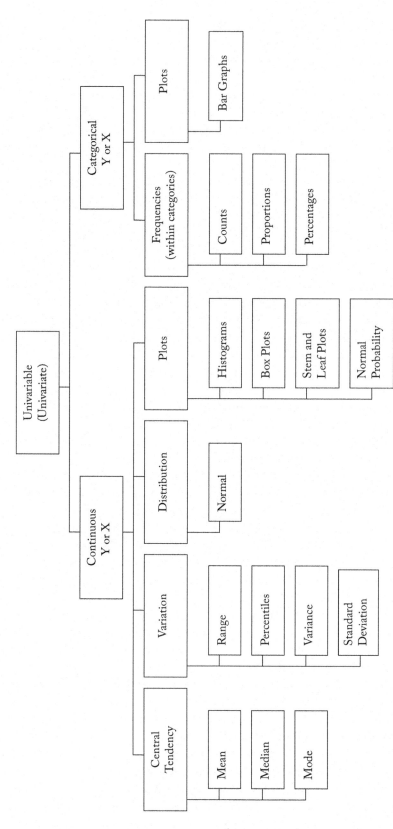

FIGURE 15.1 Analysis Plan for Univariate Data

Note: Y = outcome; X = independent variable

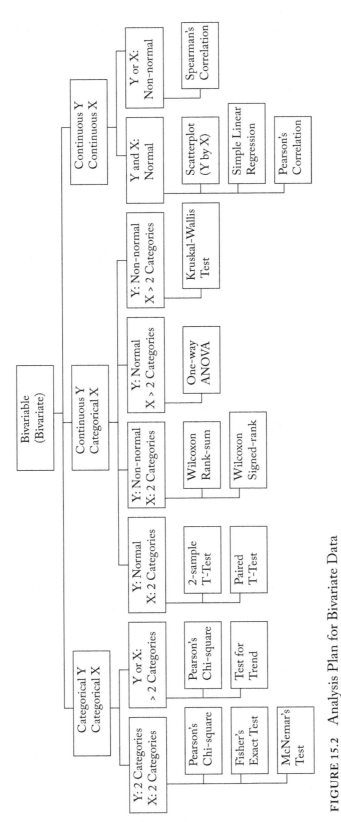

FIGURE 15.2 Analysis Plan for Bivariate Data

Note: Y = outcome; X = independent variable

subjects differ by intervention arm, then we would use multivariable analysis (figure 15.3). The X variable in any of the models depicted in figure 15.3 can be categorical or continuous. The analysis we choose is determined by the distribution of the outcome variable, Y.

Evaluating treatment efficacy in subgroups of the study. Study subjects are not all the same and may respond to a study intervention differently. We may wonder if their responses are a function of some particular characteristic. In our pain assessment study the overall results may be negative, but we may notice that children participating in the study tend to show different outcomes in the control and intervention groups. We may therefore choose to perform a subgroup analysis, separating out and analyzing results exclusively for children.

Alternatively, we may be disappointed with the overall negative results and wish to look for patient characteristics that would be associated with greater efficacy of the intervention but not have any one characteristic in mind. Thus, we may choose to perform a multivariable analysis. If the original study was not powered to find significance in a subgroup, an observed important effect, even if not statistically significant, could suggest hypotheses for future studies focusing on that subgroup.

Interpretation of clinical significance. One judges the clinical significance of the study results according to the expectations one sets out at the beginning of the trial. A statistically significant difference in outcomes between the intervention and control groups may not necessarily be clinically meaningful. Using the example of our hypothetical study of the use of a pain assessment item along with the usual vital signs, if the patients in the intervention group had statistically significantly more pain relief than the control group, as judged by responses to pain scores measured two hours after checking vital signs in the morning, but were no more comfortable by midday or evening and reported being no more satisfied with their care, one might judge that the intervention was not effective from the clinical standpoint, despite the statistical results.

Extrapolation

Another important outcome is the influence of the study results upon ethical theory. While SUPPORT failed to show an effect of the intervention, as mentioned above, it was an informative study that had a profound effect upon medical ethicists' thinking about life-sustaining treatment decision making. The study provided an impetus to find other approaches to improve care at the end of life. Thus, while the study intervention did not have its intended effect, the study certainly served to advance understanding of the ethical aspects of end-of-life care (Schroeder 1999).

Additional analytical issues

Whether in a randomized controlled trial or a nonrandomized trial, study subjects may fail to receive the intervention, and the investigator must decide, when analyzing the data, how to handle subjects who failed to receive the intervention. This may

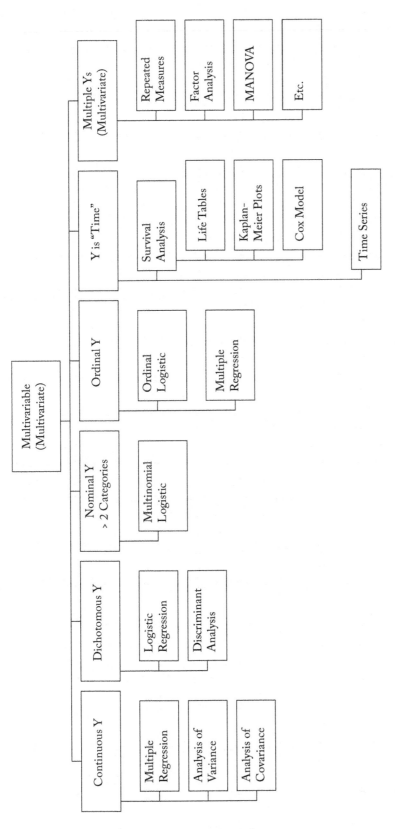

FIGURE 15.3 Analysis Plan for Multivariate Data

Note: Y = outcome; X = independent variable

happen because the execution of the intervention may not have occurred as intended during its design; the intervention may have been withheld or withdrawn because of some anticipated or actual adverse consequence of the intervention for a particular study subject; or the subject may have chosen not to undergo the intervention after agreeing to participate in the study. In analyzing a randomized control trial, the investigator chooses one of three options: to include the subject in the intervention arm, to include the subject in the control group, or to exclude the subject from the analysis altogether. It is generally preferable to take the first approach, called intention to treat analysis, since it avoids the possibility of bias or distortion of the results that may occur because of subjects with certain characteristics shifting from one group to another. One might imagine, for example, that medical students who are uncomfortable discussing difficult topics with patients might be less enthusiastic about learning the informed consent process and thus avoid the educational intervention. If they were analyzed with the control group, the participants in the intervention group would appear to demonstrate more capability in offering informed consent than they would have had these reluctant students been included among them. The intervention thus will look more effective than it would have had the data been analyzed by intention to treat. If the investigator chooses to include the subject in the control group, this undermines the randomized nature of the study design but reduces misclassification, which would underestimate the effect of the intervention (Fisher, Dixon, and Herson 1990). If the investigator removes a subject from analysis because the subject was placed in the intervention arm but did not receive the intervention, the benefit of randomization diminishes, since the subjects remaining in the two arms are no longer similar.

Finally, an experimental study is a longitudinal study in which the occurrence of outcome events may be studied over time. In our hypothetical study of the impact of teaching about cultural sensitivity on access to care among minority patients, these patients may be at risk for illness that requires care and be followed over a two-year time period. We might choose to follow patients with regular phone calls and chart reviews and compare the duration of time until the occurrence of some undesirable outcome, such as an illness during which some needed care was not provided. We could compare the length of time until the occurrence of such adverse events in the intervention and control groups using a technique called survival analysis (Peto et al. 1977).

REPORTING RESULTS

If the investigator conducts an excellent trial but does not report it well, the quality of the study will not be appreciated. Balas and colleagues have developed a tool for evaluating the quality of RCTs (Balas et al. 1995). It is worth utilizing their criteria as one prepares to report the study results.

❧ Critique of Experimental Methods

Experimental methods are appropriate for addressing only a select number of questions and have both advantages and limitations.

APPROPRIATE QUESTIONS

Experimental research methods can provide answers to empirical questions—questions that are amenable to measurable answers. Normative questions will never be answered by empirical examination. Thus, a philosopher who asks whether it is acceptable ethically to make health care decisions for comatose patients by relying on those patients' previously written instructions for care will answer this question by examining the theoretical arguments about whether or not the conscious individual who wrote the directive is still the same person when he is in a coma, whether it is best to have such a written advance directive speak for the comatose individual, or whether it is ethically preferable for someone else to make treatment decisions on that person's behalf. The philosopher establishes such an argument on theoretical grounds. However, having made that a philosophical claim, there are many questions about the impact of such an approach on patients and their significant others that can and ought to be examined.

Not all empirical questions that one might be interested in asking are amenable to investigation by an experimental trial. Given the enormous effort needed to conduct such a trial, the intervention that the investigator wishes to test ought to be at a certain stage in its evolution to warrant its examination in a clinical trial. The decision to test an intervention should be based not simply on sound theoretical arguments but also on some prior empirical evidence. Such an intervention would be one that is based on a matured idea for which some preliminary empirical evidence exists. At the same time, one ought to still have sufficient doubt about the efficacy of an intervention to warrant conducting the study. Thus, it might be an idea that ethicists have begun to debate and about which there are coherent opposing arguments. The scholarly community ought to be in a position of equipoise in which one is in genuine doubt about the likely outcome of the study in order to proceed with a randomized trial (Freedman 1987).

STRENGTHS AND WEAKNESSES

The experimental method has the potential to provide definitive evidence of the effectiveness of an intervention. While one may have anecdotal experiences, or a series of observations that influence one's belief in the efficacy of a particular practice, such unsystematic observations are notoriously susceptible to biases. Interventional studies, therefore, provide an invaluable check upon one's beliefs. While this is true for experimental studies in general, some research methodologists consider randomized controlled trials to provide a uniquely impeccable demonstration of effectiveness. Those who promote the use of evidence-based medical practice—recommending that practice be based on effectiveness that has been demonstrated in scientific studies—consider randomized controlled trials the sine qua non of definitive evidence (Guyatt et al. 2008). By controlling differences between the intervention and control groups, the likelihood of finding differences that are not truly due to the intervention can be eliminated.

The reader should be aware however of the critiques of the lofty place of randomized controlled trials in evidence-based practice (Borgerson 2009) and the acknowledgment by champions of evidence-based medicine of the need for flexibility in judging what evidence counts (Sackett et al. 1996). The reader should also recognize the significant drawbacks to conducting intervention trials. They are expensive. Aside from monetary expense, they require the expenditure of untold hours of personnel time. At the conclusion of a study, the results may be negative for a variety of reasons unrelated to the merit or the veracity of the hypothesis itself. The intervention as designed by the investigators may not have been as effective as it possibly could be; the design might have been excellent but the execution of the intervention during the conduct of the study might not have been successful; the sample size might not have been large enough to demonstrate a significant difference between the intervention and control group. These and other reasons may lead to the false conclusion that the tested intervention is not effective.

At the other extreme, study findings may be positive and yet the intervention may not have any practical value by the time the study is done (Dupont 1985; Fletcher 1989). This may be because the subjects selected for the trial may differ from typical persons seen in clinical practice; the end points measured in the trial may be of minimal clinical importance; or the intervention tested in the trial may be obsolete by the time the trial is over.

❧ Concluding Comments

An increasing number of experiments examining questions of ethical import demonstrate how valuable testing one's assumptions can be. While arguments about how we should conduct ourselves may not always be settled by demonstration of empirical evidence of consequences, for those who wish to make consequentialist arguments, it is important to demonstrate that the outcomes one expects to see from a recommended course of action really do occur. Beyond this, experiments at times provide new and surprising insights into human attitudes and behavior that are relevant to anyone with an interest in ethics. Ethicists do well to pay attention to such empirical findings as they conduct conceptual work.

❧ Notes on Resources and Training

The many skills that contribute to the conduct of a well-done clinical trial are not the domain of any single discipline. Rather, a multidisciplinary team with individuals trained in several fields is appropriate. An indispensable ingredient is an understanding of ethics with sufficient understanding of theory to generate a plausible hypothesis. Additional skills include: study design, grant writing, questionnaire design, project management, interviewing, chart review, data editing, data entry, computer programming, data analysis, and manuscript preparation. Principal investigators would do well to be familiar with the medical ethics research literature and will also have research training for a substantial duration of time, such as a two- or three-year fellowship. They may combine an interest in ethics with skills in health services research or epidemiology.

An excellent text for acquiring a general understanding of the design of experimental research is the textbook *Designing Clinical Research* (Hulley et al. 2006). Several textbooks provide valuable resources for the investigator engaged in the conduct of clinical trials (Spilker 1991; Spilker and Cramer 1992; Weiss 1996; Chow and Liu 2004; Good 2006), although several of these texts provide advice for clinical trials of pharmacologic agents. The investigator who wishes to test an intervention to alter an ethically important outcome is testing something far more complex than a medication or most other clinical interventions and should therefore be cautious in extrapolating from these texts to one's own work.

The conduct of a well-designed, well-conducted, and carefully analyzed experimental study is a costly endeavor that requires designated funds that are not usually available in an institution's usual operating budget. To seek funds from outside of their institution or to carefully justify the expenditure of their own organizational funds requires investigators to prepare a grant proposal. Several authors have written useful guides for doing so (Pequegnat and Stover 1995; Yang 2005). The U.S. Department of Health and Human Services provides on-line advice about grant preparation (www.hhs.gov/asrt/og/grantinformation/apptips.html). Originating from the Federal Financial Assistance Management Improvement Act of 1999, in 2002 the U.S. federal government created the site Grants.gov as a central storehouse for information on more than one thousand grant programs that provide access to approximately $500 billion in annual awards. A useful source of information about foundation grants is available at www.foundation-grants.com/.

☙ Note

This chapter is not subject to U.S. copyright.

☙ References

Angell, M. 1997. The ethics of clinical research in the third world. *New England Journal of Medicine* 342:967–69.

Baker, D. W., R. M. Parker, M. V. Williams, and W. S. Clark. 1998. Health literacy and the risk of hospital admission. *Journal of General Internal Medicine* 13:791–98.

Balas, E. A., S. M. Austin, B. G. Ewigman, G. D. Brown, and J. A. Mitchell. 1995. Methods of randomized controlled trials in human services research. *Medical Care* 33:687–99.

Borgerson K. 2009. Valuing evidence: Bias and the evidence hierarchy of evidence based medicine. *Perspectives in Biology and Medicine* 52:218–33.

Chow, S.-C., and J. Liu. 2004. *Design and analysis of clinical trials: Concept and methodologies.* Hoboken, NJ: Wiley-Interscience.

Cohen, J. 1988. *Statistical power analysis for the behavioral sciences.* 2nd ed. Hillsdale, NJ: Lawrence Erlbaum Associates.

Danis, M., L. I. Southerland, J. M. Garrett, J. L. Smith, F. Hielema, G. Pickard, D. M. Egner, and D. L. Patrick. 1991. A prospective study of advance directives for life-sustaining care. *New England Journal of Medicine* 324:882–88.

Donaldson, M. S., and M. J. Field. 1998. Measuring quality of care at the end of life. *Archives of Internal Medicine* 158:121–28.

Dupont, W. D. 1985. Randomized vs. historical clinical trials. *American Journal of Epidemiology* 122:940–46.

Fisher, L. D., D. O. Dixon, and J. Herson. 1990. Intention to treat in clinical trials. In *Statistical issues in drug research and development,* ed. K. E. Peace. New York: Marcel Dekker.

Fletcher, R. H. 1989. The cost of clinical trials. *Journal of the American Medical Association* 262:1842.

Freedman, B. 1987. Equipoise and the ethics of clinical research. *New England Journal of Medicine* 317:141–45.

———. 1990. Placebo-controlled trials and the logic of clinical purpose. *IRB* 12:1–6.

Freedman, B., K. C. Glass, and C. Weijer. 1996. Placebo orthodoxy in clinical research: II: Ethical, legal, and regulatory myths. *Journal of Law, Medicine, and Ethics* 24:252–59.

Good, P. I. 2006. *A manager's guide to the design and conduct of clinical trials.* 2nd ed. Hoboken, NJ: Wiley-Liss.

Green, M. J., S. K. Peterson, M. W. Baker, G. R. Harper, L. C. Friedman, W. S. Rubenstein, and D. T. Mauger. 2004. Effect of a computer-based decision aid on knowledge, perceptions, and intentions about genetic testing for breast cancer susceptibility: A randomized controlled trial. *JAMA* 292:442–52.

Guyatt, G., D. Rennie, M. Maureen Meade, and D. Cook. 2008. *Users' guides to the medical literature: A manual for evidence-based clinical practice.* 2nd ed. New York: McGraw-Hill.

Hays, R. D., and J. E. Ware Jr. 1986. My medical care is better than yours: Social desirability and patient satisfaction ratings. *Medical Care* 6:519–24.

Holm, S., and J. Harris. 2008. The standard of care in multinational research. In *The Oxford textbook of clinical research ethics,* eds. Emanuel et al. Oxford: Oxford University Press.

Hulley, S. B., S. R. Cummings, W. S. Browner, D. G. Grady, and T. B. Newman. 2006. *Designing clinical research.* 3rd ed. Philadelphia: Lippincott, Williams, and Wilkins.

Jordhøy, M. S., P. M. Fayers, M. Ahlner-Elmqvist, and S. Kaasa. 2002. Lack of concealment may lead to selection bias in cluster randomized trials of palliative care. *Palliative Medicine* 16:43–49.

Lavori, P., T. Wilt, and J. Sugarman. 2007. Quality assurance questionnaire for professionals fails to improve the quality of informed consent. *Clinical Trials* 4:638–49.

Meltzer, L. A., and J. F. Childress. 2008. What is fair participant selection? In *The Oxford textbook of clinical research ethics,* eds. Emanuel et al. Oxford: Oxford University Press.

Miller, F. G. 2000. Placebo-controlled trials in psychiatric research: An ethical perspective. *Biological Psychiatry* 47:707–16.

———. 2008. The ethics of placebo-controlled trials. In *The Oxford textbook of clinical research ethics,* eds. Emanuel et al. Oxford: Oxford University Press.

Morgenstern, H., and D. M. Winn. 1983. A method for determining the sampling ratio in epidemiologic studies. *Statistics in Medicine* 2:387–96.

Pace, C., F. Miller, and M. Danis. 2003. Enrolling the uninsured in clinical trials: An ethical perspective. *Critical Care Medicine* 3 (Supplement): S121–S125.

Pequegnat, W., and E. Stover. 1995. *How to write a successful research grant application: A guide for social and behavioral scientists.* New York: Plenum Press.

Peto, R., M. C. Pike, P. Armitage, N. E. Breslow, D. R. Cox, S. V. Howard, N. Mantel, K. McPherson, J. Peto, and P. G. Smith. 1977. Design and analysis of randomized clinical trials requiring prolonged observation of each patient II: Analysis and examples. *The British Journal of Cancer* 35:1–39.

Roberts, J., and G. Norman. 1990. Reliability and learning from the objective structured clinical examination. *Medical Education* 24:219–23.

Roter, D. L., J. A. Hall, D. E. Kern, L. R. Barker, K. A. Cole, and R. P. Roca. 1995. Improving physicians' interviewing skills and reducing patients' emotional distress: A randomized clinical trial. *Archives of Internal Medicine* 155:1877–84.

Rothman, K. J., and K. B. Michels. 1994. The continuing unethical use of placebo controls. *New England Journal of Medicine* 33 (1): 394–98.

Sackett, D. L., M. C. Rosenberg, J. A. Muir Gray, R. B. Haynes, and W. S. Richardson. 1996. Evidence-based medicine: What it is and what it isn't. *British Medical Journal* 312:71–72.

Schneiderman, L. J., R. A. Pearlman, R. M. Kaplan, J. P. Anderson, and E. M. Rosenberg. 1992. Relationship of general advance directive instructions to specific life-sustaining treatment preferences in patients with serious illness. *Archives of Internal Medicine* 152:2114–22.

Schroeder, S. A. 1999. The legacy of SUPPORT: Study to understand prognoses and preferences for outcomes and risks of treatment. *Annals of Internal Medicine* 131:780–82.

Spilker, B. 1991. *Guide to clinical trials.* New York: Raven Press.

Spilker, B., and J. A. Cramer. 1992. *Patient recruitment and clinical trials.* New York: Raven Press.

Sulmasy, D. P., P. B. Terry, C. S. Weisman, D. J. Miller, R. Y. Stallings, M. A. Vettese, and K. B. Haller. 1998. The accuracy of substituted judgments in patients with terminal diagnoses. *Annals of Internal Medicine* 128:621–29.

SUPPORT Principal Investigators. 1995. A controlled trial to improve care for seriously ill hospitalized patients: The study to understand prognoses and preferences for outcomes and risks of treatments (SUPPORT). *Journal of the American Medical Association* 274:1591–98.

Temple, R., and S. S. Ellenberg. 2000. Placebo-controlled trials and active-controlled trials in the evaluation of new treatments. *Annals of Internal Medicine* 133:455–63.

Varmus, H., and D. Satcher. 1998. Ethical complexities in conducting research in developing countries. *New England Journal of Medicine* 18:1331–32.

Weiss, N. S. 1996. *Clinical epidemiology: The study of the outcome of illness.* 2nd ed. Oxford: Oxford University Press.

Whelan, T., M. Levine, A. Willan, A. Gafni, K. Sanders, D. Mirsky, S. Chambers, M. A. O'Brien, S. Reid, and S. Dubois. 2004. Effects of a decision aid on knowledge and treatment decision making for breast cancer surgery: A randomized trial. *JAMA—Journal of the American Medical Association* 292:435–41.

Yang, O. O. 2005. *Guide to effective grant writing: How to write a successful NIH grant application.* New York: Kluwer Academic Press.

Yudkin, P. L., and M. Moher. 2001. Putting theory into practice: A cluster randomized trial with a small number of clusters. *Statistics in Medicine* 20:341–49.

CHAPTER 16

Economics and Decision Science

DAVID A. ASCH

I doubt that many health economists or medical decision scientists believe they are making contributions to the fields of medical ethics in the course of their work.

The methods used by scholars in these fields are attractive in part because they appear highly quantitative and value free. Those characteristics might make these approaches seem out of place within a list of tools to address problems in ethics, since ethical problems are so often seen as conflicts of value. Some economists and decision scientists probably take refuge in the view that their methods are ostensibly silent on the issue of values. But even if these fields really are value free at the level of their methodology, their contribution to the manipulation and analysis of values provided from other sources still offers much to empirical work in medical ethics. Moreover, at a very fundamental level, these fields take an implicit value-laden stance—one based largely on some form of utilitarianism. Sometimes that stance is obscured by the methodology that overlays it, but understanding what values may lurk underneath these seemingly sterile approaches will help scholars and policymakers understand both the applications and the limitations of these methods.

The applications are potentially profound. In this chapter I will focus on certain popular and normatively appealing techniques, such as decision analysis broadly, and cost-effectiveness analysis and related forms of clinical economics more specifically. However, there is much more to decision sciences than just decision analysis. For example, decision analysis is a technique for choosing among alternatives in the face of uncertainty. It is designed to produce an answer to the question, "what ought to be done?" and so it focuses on normative goals. But many who consider themselves decision scientists focus on descriptive observational or experimental studies of decision processes in an attempt to understand how clinicians and patients actually make medical decisions, to uncover biases in those processes (against some normative standard) and, more prescriptively, to de-bias or in other ways improve them.

Similarly, there is much more to health economics than cost-effectiveness analysis or cost-benefit analysis. Health economists also address the social and clinical implications of changes in health care financing, such as the introduction of new insurance products or modifications in the incentive structure for health systems or clinicians. Or they may study the implication of changes in clinician labor force (size, specialty, geographic distribution, for example) or related changes in projected patient demand, given changing demographics or the introduction of new medical technologies. These fields are broad, and much that health economists or medical decision scientists do is beyond the scope of this chapter.

☙ Description of Methods of Economics and Decision Science

This chapter focuses on those techniques of economics and decision science designed to evaluate alternative clinical approaches and in other ways determine best practices when the best choice is not already known.

AN ABBREVIATED PRIMER ON DECISION ANALYSIS

Imagine a physician who has just begun to set up her office but does not yet have the ability to perform diagnostic tests. With some frequency she sees patients who complain of urinary symptoms (burning on urination, a sense of urgency, and the like) that might signal a urinary tract infection (UTI) that could be treated with antibiotics. Since the physician does not yet have the ability to perform any diagnostic tests, such as an examination or culture of the urine that might help her make the diagnosis, she recognizes that she must decide on her own how likely it is that each patient with symptoms like this has a UTI. Although much judgment is involved, the task is not too difficult: Young women are much more likely to have urinary tract infections than young men; people who have had them before are more likely to get them again; some symptoms are particularly representative of urinary tract infections. Given her experience and judgment, she can assign a probability to each patient she sees that reflects her judgment that the patient has a urinary tract infection.

However, this physician now faces the question of deciding what probability of urinary tract infection is high enough to justify treatment with an antibiotic or, conversely, what probability is too low to justify such treatment. She reasons that this decision must reflect some combination of factors including the risks or costs of treating patients with antibiotics when they do not have an infection, the risk or costs of not treating patients when they do, and, if she had been able to use a test to help her with the diagnosis, the risks, costs, and accuracy of the test. Experienced clinicians do this intuitively, though they may never try to assign a numeric probability or develop explicit thresholds. They hear a set of symptoms and clinical circumstances that might be a UTI and use their judgment to decide if the diagnosis is plausible enough to justify treatment.

Decision analysis is a structured approach designed to help incorporate these different kinds of information more formally than using simple intuitions, and so identify the best choice when the best choice is otherwise uncertain. Figure 16.1 displays one way a decision analyst might represent the clinical problem of the UTI. As the tree is read left to right, the square node on the left indicates a choice the physician makes, between treating the symptoms with antibiotics or not. The circular nodes represent chance events, over which the physician has no control. In this case, the chance event is whether or not the patient indeed has a UTI, represented here with a probability, p, and this chance event and its associated probability are the

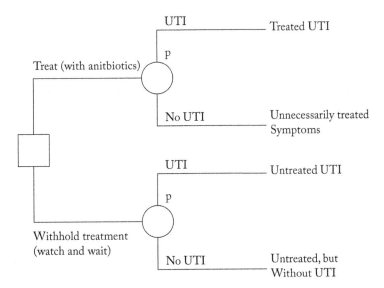

FIGURE 16.1 Sample Decision Tree for the Management of Suspected Urinary Tract Infection

Note: The square node represents a choice to be made. Circular nodes represent chance events, in this case at probability, *p*. UTI = urinary tract infection.

same regardless of the choice the physician makes. At the end of each branch is some reflection of the outcome, for example, a treated UTI.

More thorough descriptions of the techniques and methods of decision modeling are available elsewhere, including techniques based on trees, like the UTI example, or those based on Markov models or other simulations (Detsky, Naglie, Krahn, Naimark et al. 1997; Detsky, Naglie, Krahn, Redelmeier et al. 1997; Naglie et al. 1997; Krahn et al. 1997; Naimark et al. 1997; Weinstein and Fineberg 1980; Sox et al. 1988). Even so, the simple structure of the UTI example follows many of the steps and contains many of the elements essential to all of these models:

1. Imagine the model and draw the tree.
2. Identify the probabilities.
3. Identify the outcome variables.
4. Calculate the expected values.
5. Perform sensitivity analyses.

The first step is to structure the clinical problem and represent it in a tree format so that the consequences of alternative choice and chance events can be understood. Both science and art are necessary to structure trees well. Real clinical problems are complex, but useful clinical models simplify and constrain circumstances and choices. In the UTI example, only the choices to treat or withhold treatment were presented. However, real clinicians might see other options. For example, they might wait a day or two to see if the symptoms resolve on their own, and then treat only if they do not. Individual branches on a tree must be mutually exclusive, so that there is no overlap or confusion. Moreover, they must be exhaustive—meaning that together they encompass all of the important possibilities. However, how many "twigs" ought to be included on each branch, or how finely detailed the model ought to be is a matter of judgment, which is to say that the choices often reflect the values of the decision analyst. Skilled decision analysts find themselves pruning the trees of their students, who tend to include too much detail. Those who miss the big picture are often accused of missing the forest for the trees. In decision analysis the risk is missing the tree because of the branches.

The second step is to identify the probabilities that various chance events will occur. In figure 16.1, a circular chance node reflects the mutually exclusive and exhaustive possibilities that a UTI is present or not. In this example, the source of that probability could be the physician's judgment. For example, the physician might estimate that there is a 40 percent chance that a twenty-two-year-old woman has a UTI, given that she complains of new urinary frequency and burning on urination, but she is sexually inactive and has no prior history of UTI. Accurate or not, that estimate of probability, if it really is the physician's best estimate, ought to influence her management of the patient—whether it is incorporated into a formal decision analysis or not. In more legitimate analyses the best sources of this information are well-conducted studies published in the medical literature. Such studies are often unavailable for some or many parts of a model, and so investigators often rely on practical but less credible sources, such as expert opinions.

The third step is to identify the outcomes and assign values to them. The UTI example expressed in figure 16.1 includes only four outcomes reflecting that the patient either has a UTI or does not, and is treated with antibiotics or not. Many of the ethically relevant issues in a decision analysis are concentrated in choices about how these outcomes are valued. Because of their importance, these issues will be discussed more extensively in a later section. In the meantime, these outcomes might be ranked, from best to worst, in the following order:

1. The patient does not have a UTI and is not treated [0]
2. The patient does not have a UTI and is treated with antibiotics [−10]
3. The patient has a UTI and is treated with antibiotics [−20]
4. The patient has a UTI and is not treated [−50]

This order reflects that some outcomes are clearly better than others. For example, if we consider only the outcomes in which the patient does not have a UTI (1 and 2), it is better to be untreated than treated, so 1 > 2. Similarly, if we consider only the outcomes in which the patient has a UTI (3 and 4), it is better to be treated than untreated, and so 3 > 4. Finally, if we consider only the outcomes in which the patient receives antibiotics (2 and 3), it is better not to have a UTI than to have one, and so 2 > 3.

For a decision analysis, these outcomes must be given some relative values, not just a rank ordering, and some potential relative values are included in brackets in the list. These values might be considered as utilities, which are abstract representations of some amount of good. Or they could be expressed in dollars or some other value metric. In this example, the first outcome was given a value of 0, to reflect that the patient neither has the disease nor receives any treatment. The last was given a value of –50, reflecting that sometimes an untreated UTI can get worse and cause other problems, and that symptoms might persist longer than with treatment. These values, and the ones in between, were assigned somewhat arbitrarily. More formal, rigorous, and methodologically defensible techniques for assigning values to outcomes are described in a variety of sources but are conceptually and procedurally complex (Torrance 1986; Redelmeier and Detsky 1995; Froberg and Kane 1989). Some sources catalog utility measures for many different health states (Fryback et al. 1993).

The fourth step is to calculate the expected values. This step is a mathematical exercise in which the values of the outcomes (from step 3) are weighted by the probabilities that they will occur (from step 2). In the UTI example, given a 40 percent chance of a UTI (which means there is a 60 percent chance of no UTI), the expected value of following the upper branch of figure 16.1 and providing treatment is:

$$EV(\text{Treatment}) = 0.4 \times (-20) + 0.6 \times (-10) = -14.$$

The expected value of following the lower branch of figure 16.1 and withholding treatment is:

$$EV(\text{Withhold Treatment}) = 0.4 \times (-50) + 0.6 \times (0) = -20.$$

Because the expected value of treating this patient (–14) exceeds the expected value of withholding treatment (–20), this decision analysis suggests that treatment is the preferred option. The calculation of expected value is a mathematical approach with consequentialist goals, which are to achieve the highest expected value.

The final step is to perform a sensitivity analysis. In this example, the values assigned to the outcomes were not well justified and might plausibly be quite different. A decision analyst might ask whether the conclusion to prescribe antibiotics would be sustained under alternative plausible assumptions about these values. Similarly, in this example the probability of a UTI was estimated at 40 percent. However, this physician might want to know whether antibiotics are appropriate if the probability of a UTI falls to 10 percent or, more generally, what level of probability represents the threshold between prescribing antibiotics or not. A sensitivity analysis tests the stability of the conclusions across alternative assumptions about one or more variables in the model; it determines how sensitive the conclusions are to certain model assumptions, alone or in combination. For example, figure 16.2 reveals a sensitivity analysis for the UTI example and shows the expected value of the Treat and Withhold strategies over all probabilities of UTI, from 0 to 1. The two lines intersect at a probability of 0.25, meaning that given the structure of the tree and the assumptions about the value of the outcomes, patients whose likelihood of UTI is less than 25 percent should not be treated with antibiotics, and patients whose likelihood of UTI exceeds 25 percent should be treated.

The UTI example is simplistic in many ways, but it illustrates decision analysis' main purpose of structuring choices and analyzing them systematically. Indeed, a central advantage of decision analysis is that through its formal process, one can

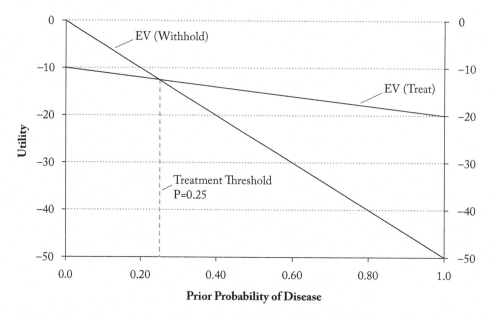

FIGURE 16.2   One-way Sensitivity Analysis for the UTI Example

Note: The expected value (EV) of the Treat and Withhold strategies is shown. For any probability of disease indicated on the horizontal axis, the best strategy can be found by identifying which strategy provides the highest expected utility. At probabilities less than .25, withholding treatment provides the greatest expected value. At probabilities exceeding .25, treating provides the greatest expected value.

avoid many of the emotional pitfalls that accompany conventional decision making. Nevertheless, decision analysis is not value free. Not only are the choices one makes in creating a decision analysis often questions of value, but decision analysis can also be used to structure ethical questions. The next section discusses the question of valuing outcomes. The section after that provides an example of using decision analysis to explore an ethically charged area.

A CLOSER LOOK AT THE ISSUE OF VALUING OUTCOMES

In the previous section, the valuations of the outcomes in the UTI example were presented without much explanation, merely to move the example forward. However, the choices made in valuing these outcomes reflect underlying beliefs about what issues are important. To the extent that decision analyses are sensitive to these valuations—as they often are—these beliefs determine the results of the analysis and, in turn, what advice is given to patients or policy makers. For this reason, the methods used in valuing outcomes need some special attention.

For example, decision analysts are nearly always interested in clinical outcomes, like serious illness or death. However some clinical outcomes do not reflect serious illness or death but nevertheless are associated with pain or anxiety. Although these symptoms are often very important to patients, they are included only in some decision analyses—largely because they are so difficult to measure. In deciding what aspects of each outcome to account for—for example, that effects on mortality will be included but effects on anxiety or patient worry will not—decision analysts in effect determine what considerations are seen as important. One potential advantage of chorionic villus sampling over amniocentesis for prenatal diagnosis is that the former can be performed earlier during a pregnancy and so the results can be available sooner. A decision analysis comparing amniocentesis with chorionic villus sampling that looks only at how accurately the test performs, or how well it identifies abnormalities in the fetus, may fail to reflect the concerns of women and couples if diagnostic delay is something to be avoided.

Decision analysts also must decide whether to include economic costs in addition clinical outcomes when they evaluate alternatives. Cost-effectiveness analyses and cost-benefit analyses, for example, are decision analyses that include as measured outcomes not just the clinical outcomes but also the economic outcomes of alternative clinical strategies. Incorporating costs into a decision analysis is as ethically value laden as incorporating considerations of costs into real time clinical decisions. First, some people are uncomfortable incorporating costs into a clinical decision because they believe, rightly, that this approach implicitly puts a monetary value on human life.

The only reason to compare the cost-effectiveness of two clinical approaches, for example, is to help one later decide whether the increased costs of the more expensive approach are justified by any increased health benefits. However, they might not be—either because the more expensive approach does not convey any additional benefits (which makes decision making easy: use the cheaper approach because it is at least no worse) or because the additional benefits provided by the more expensive approach just aren't worth the additional cost. Those who feel that no price can be put on life are implicitly supporting an impossible position. If one fails to put a finite price on the value of saving a life, then one effectively commits unlimited resources to saving lives, and becomes bankrupt. If, instead, one puts a finite price on saving a life then there will be some costs that will exceed that limit (Asch 1995).

A second fundamental ethical challenge to clinical economics is that the answer to the question, "How much does it cost?" depends critically on who is asked. A patient with full insurance coverage bears no additional charge when a more expensive option is chosen over a cheaper one. The insurance company may see greater charges or may not if it has previously negotiated an arrangement with the physician or health system to provide either one at the same rate. But in the latter case, the health system might face greater costs if indeed the more expensive option consumed more resources (staff time, equipment) that could have been put to other use. Costs and charges are different (Finkler 1982). Charges measure the cost only to those who pay those charges.

Most economists argue that costs should be viewed from the societal perspective when performing economic assessments, where the societal perspective reflects the consumption of resources regardless of who pays the bill (Gold et al. 1996). There are advantages to this approach, in that it is less susceptible to manipulation and because most of these analyses are designed to take societal perspectives into consideration in the first place. Nevertheless, the results of a cost-effectiveness analysis that measures costs from the societal perspective will misrepresent the interests of individual patients who may see costs very different from those seen by society as a whole.

Clinicians who choose a less costly, less effective alternative because the additional benefit of the more expensive alternative is not worth it, need to recognize that they may not be saving their patient's money, but someone else's (Asch et al. 2003). How comfortable we feel about those decisions is inherently a question of values.

Several resources provide more thorough descriptions of the techniques of clinical economics (Drummond, Stoddard, and Torrance 1987; Eisenberg 1989; Gold et al. 1996; Sox et al. 1988). The next section provides an illustration of how these techniques can be used in an ethically charged clinical area.

CARRIER SCREENING FOR CYSTIC FIBROSIS

Asch and colleagues used cost-effectiveness analysis to evaluate several alternative strategies for screening couples for the genetic mutations responsible for cystic fibrosis (CF).[1] Approximately one in twenty-five Caucasians in the United States carries the genetic mutation for CF, and approximately one in twenty-five hundred babies born is affected. Cystic fibrosis is an autosomal recessive disease that means that if both reproductive partners are carriers, one in four of their children will have CF. Most children with CF are born to couples without a family history who learn they are carriers only through the birth of an affected child. Although the CF gene has been identified, the hundreds of distinct mutations of this gene make it impractical to screen for all of them. For this reason most DNA-based screening tests for only five or ten of the most common mutations representing in aggregate about 85 percent of carriers (U.S. Congress 1992).

Population-based CF carrier screening is controversial, in part because genetic screening in the setting of reproductive planning raises important ethical issues and also because even very good tests perform poorly when applied to low prevalence conditions.

The application of CF carrier screening is further complicated because many different screening strategies may be constructed that use different decision rules for proceeding to further testing or deciding whether to continue a pregnancy (Asch et al. 1996). For example, one screening strategy might screen both partners in a couple for the presence of the gene. Those couples for whom both partners are found to carry the gene (which causes no problems in those who merely carry one copy) might then proceed to prenatal diagnosis using amniocentesis or chorionic villus sampling to determine if the fetus has inherited both mutations and therefore might be affected. Alternatively, partners within a couple might be screened in sequence: the second partner is screened only if the first partner is found to carry the mutation, and the fetus is tested only if both partners in the couple are carriers. Many other permutations of tests are possible, varying the breadth of the screen used, or combinations with other tests. Altogether, Asch and colleagues examined sixteen different strategies, each likely to lead to different clinical and economic outcomes. Thus, the clinical and economic questions are not only whether widespread CF carrier screening should be done but how it should be done.

Several representative branches of the overall decision tree are shown in figures 16.3 and 16.4. All branches end with a clinical outcome reflecting a pregnancy that is delivered, miscarried, or terminated. In addition, each pregnancy represents a fetus that is affected with CF or not. These outcomes under consideration distinguish this kind of cost-effectiveness analysis from many others. Most analyses target few and relatively uncontroversial goals. For example, policies toward childhood immunization, prostate cancer screening, or dietary fat reduction have as explicit goals the reduction of disease and disability, the promotion of health, or related goals easy to share. Typically, these policies become controversial only when these clinical goals conflict with other goals to reduce costs.

In contrast, genetic carrier screening for the purposes of reproductive planning leads to clinical outcomes that are more controversial. These strategies often raise issues concerning abortion, eugenics, contraception, and reproductive choice—issues that can incite or challenge strong feelings (Wilfond and Fost 1992). More important, the kinds of economic evaluations these analyses address can seem unusual.

Table 16.1 displays the distribution of a hypothetical cohort of 500,000 pregnancies over these six clinical outcomes (delivery, miscarriage, or termination × CF or not CF) for selected strategies from the original analysis. Strategy A reflects the no screening option and is used for comparison. A description of the other strategies is not essential for this illustration but can be found elsewhere (Asch et al. 1998).

These results reveal much about the consequences and trade-offs of different policies. Fewer children are born with CF with Strategy C than Strategy A (no screening), but one of the nonfinancial costs of achieving this goal is that more total abortions are performed, and these tend to be terminations of pregnancies that would have resulted in the delivery of unaffected children had the pregnancies been continued. The reason for the large number of abortions in Strategy C is that the identification of each additional affected pregnancy requires tests of lower and lower specificity used on pregnancies of only intermediate risk. The result is an increasing rate of false positive tests. The rate of miscarriages increases in this strategy as well because more couples undergo prenatal diagnosis, and this procedure induces a small but tangible risk of miscarriage. Costs also differ considerably among the strategies—whether these costs are considered as a whole or as a ratio of the cost per CF birth avoided.

If one were interested only in avoiding as many CF births as possible, one would choose Strategy E. However, this strategy comes with many abortions of pregnancies that would not result in the delivery of a child affected with CF, a higher rate of miscarriages attributable to the risks of prenatal diagnoses, the highest total costs, and second highest cost per CF birth avoided. If, in addition, one wanted to avoid abortions of unaffected pregnancies, Strategy F might seem attractive, but it is much more costly than Strategy N. More generally, even if the goal of CF carrier screening is to reduce the number of children born with this condition, many would want to balance that goal with the outcomes reflected in other cells of the table.

Table 16.1 illustrates the genuine trade-offs that exist in this clinical situation. The economic and decision analytic approach that produces this table helps make these trade-offs explicit, but it does not clearly point to a best strategy or, in general, a way to resolve these trade-offs. Moreover, the reporting of the results in table 16.1 itself reflects a series of value-laden choices about what outcomes are useful to measure and track. Some might believe that costs or abortions ought not to matter.

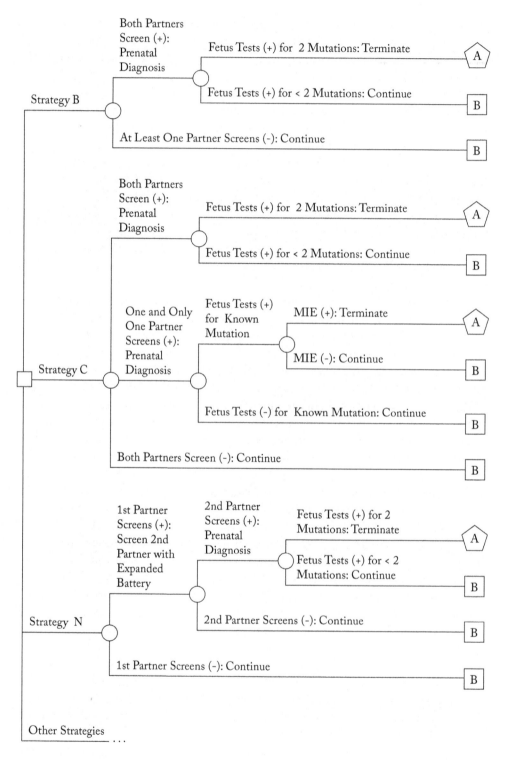

FIGURE 16.3

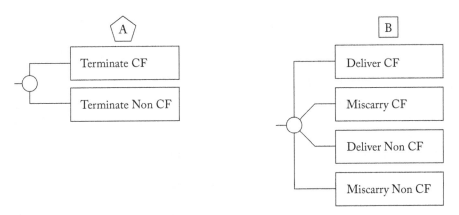

FIGURE 16.4

FIGURES 16.3 and 16.4   Selected Branches of the Tree and Subtree for the CF Carrier Screening Problem

Note: Each pregnancy can either be terminated (subtree A) or continued (subtree B). If it is terminated, it might have led to the birth of a child with CF or without CF. If it is continued, it might lead to a miscarriage or to delivery and, in either case, might be affected with CF or not. MIE = microvillar intestinal enzyme analysis, a biochemical test that could be used to improve diagnosis of CF but is now no longer used. (Adapted from D. A. Asch, J. C. Hershey, M, L. DeKay, M. V. Pauly, J. P. Patton, M. K. Jedrziewski, F. X. Frei, R. Giardine, J. A. Kant, and M. T. Mennuti. Carrier screening for cystic fibrosis: Costs and clinical outcomes. *Medical Decision Making* 18 [1998]: 202–12.)

Others might believe that certain outcomes currently not reflected in this table (such as the amount of anxiety couples face while they are awaiting the news of prenatal diagnosis) ought to be included or featured prominently.

PROBLEMS WITH VALUES

Table 16.1 also introduces a different set of concerns related to the economic evaluation of these clinical strategies (Asch et al. 1996). In a cost-benefit analysis, all outcomes are evaluated in monetary terms and compared to the additional costs incurred. Strategies producing an excess of benefits over costs are desirable. In a cost-effectiveness analysis, clinical outcomes are measured and related to a measure of costs. Often the analysis is expressed as a ratio of the cost incurred while achieving these clinical goals—for example, dollars per year of life saved. Even in a cost-effectiveness analysis, however, one must eventually have some sense of how many dollars saving a year of life is worth, or strategies in the end are unevaluable.

Nevertheless, many clinicians are uncomfortable with economic analyses because they do not believe the measures of value are valid, because they find difficult or offensive the requirement that clinical outcomes be evaluable in monetary terms, or because they think costs ought not to matter. Even those comfortable with economic analysis in the main may have special problems evaluating outcomes in the case of genetic screening. In a conventional screening strategy for breast cancer, for example, one evaluates strategies that help individuals present at earlier and more easily treated stages. With genetic carrier screening, one evaluates strategies that prevent the births of individuals with the disease, rather than the disease in people already born. From

TABLE 16.1 Base-Case Analysis for Selected Alternative CF Carrier Screening Strategies

Strategy	CF			Non-CF			CF Births Avoided (rel. to A)	Total Cost	Cost per CF Birth Avoided (rel. to A)
	Births	Abortions	Miscarriages	Births	Abortions	Miscarriages			
A	195	0	5	487,305	0	12,495	0	$1,530,313,000	—
B	57	142	1	487,302	0	12,498	138	$1,623,710,000	$676,000
C	8	191	0	486,787	340	12,673	187	$1,641,185,000	$594,000
E	6	194	0	486,737	358	12,705	189	$1,694,522,000	$867,000
F	39	160	1	487,300	0	12,499	156	$1,627,544,000	$625,000
N	49	150	1	487,301	0	12,499	146	$1,583,972,000	$367,000
O	49	150	1	487,301	0	12,499	146	$1,607,352,000	$527,000
P	32	167	1	487,045	169	12,586	163	$1,593,807,000	$391,000

Note: Selected from: D. A. Asch, J. C. Hershey, M. L. DeKay, M. V. Pauly, J. P. Patton, M. K. Jedrziewski, F. X. Frei, R. Giardine, J. A. Kant, and M. T. Mennuti. 1998. Carrier screening for cystic fibrosis: Costs and clinical outcomes. *Medical Decision Making* 18:202–12. The figures represent the results of a strategy applied to a cohort of 500,000 pregnancies that have survived through 16-weeks' gestation. Birth outcomes are rounded to the nearest 1, and costs to the nearest $1,000, in 1995 dollars.

a population perspective, the two approaches can yield identical results but from an individual perspective conventional screening strategies work by preventing or treating disease, and reproductive genetic screening strategies work by preventing the births of persons who might develop the disease. Absent specific therapy, genetic screening in the reproductive setting at best replaces individuals with genetic conditions with those without them. It does nothing positive for the individuals who are affected or those who would be.

How does one measure the value of avoiding a delivery that would have resulted in the birth of a child with CF? Presumably, if the parents attach a positive value to the birth they would not terminate a pregnancy even at high risk. Conversely, a couple that chooses to terminate such a pregnancy reveals a set of values for which the birth of an affected child would be worse than an abortion. Such a decision would not imply, however, that should a child with CF be born to these parents, having that child survive is worse than having that child die. Most children with CF are deeply loved by their families. More likely the decision to terminate a pregnancy is based on an expectation that the abortion will be followed by a new pregnancy and a second chance at delivering an unaffected child.

In theory, for a specific couple or a specific individual one could engage in an exercise to assess the value, in monetary or nonmonetary terms, of each of the six clinical outcomes represented in table 16.1 in the context of an overall reproductive plan spanning several pregnancies. Such an exercise might help individuals make choices, which is the purpose of policy analysis applied to the individual case. But in this case, great individual variation in values is likely, so it is virtually certain that no general policy could be ideal for everyone. In the case of conventional screening for breast cancer, all are likely to agree that more years of health are better than fewer, though they probably do not agree on how much better they are, and at how much cost in money, pain, or disfigurement. But as hard as it is to set a national policy for breast cancer screening, it is probably impossible and not very useful to set a uniform policy for genetic screening where values are likely to be even more varied.

∾ Critique

This chapter began with the assumption that most health economists or medical decision scientists probably do not believe they are making contributions to the fields of medical ethics in the course of their everyday work. For what questions in medical ethics, then, might these approaches be useful?

These techniques have their greatest application in domains of medical ethics when understanding the *consequences* of alternative choices is likely to define the most appropriate path. Many ethical questions surround the use of CF carrier screening in the reproductive setting. Some of these center on ethical principles of reproductive choice or concerns about eugenics or the social construction of disease. Others are based on a legitimate desire to understand the likely clinical and economic consequences of screening, to help understand what trade-offs are involved, and whether those trade-offs are worth it.

More generally, questions amenable to clinical economic analysis are also inherently rife with political conflict. That is so in part because considerations of the appropriateness of cost in clinical decisions are deeply divisive. Those divisions occur at two levels. The first is ideological: Many believe that cost should not matter when human life is at stake, and they hold to that belief even in the face of arguments that such approaches are economically unsustainable. Such individuals might be content with a cost-effectiveness analysis revealing that one clinical strategy is cheaper than another and achieves the same or better outcomes—that just saves money—but they would never be comfortable with results suggesting that a more effective approach ought to be abandoned because it is too costly. Cost-effectiveness has little persuasive power for these individuals. To those who are ideologically against putting a price on human life, cost-effectiveness analysis is a method that is appropriate only when it provides certain kinds of answers.

The second political divide is not ideological but appears to be self-interested. At this writing, in the milieu of the 2009–10 U.S. health reform activities, considerable attention has focused on the promise of comparative effectiveness research. Similarly, in the economic stimulus package of the American Recover and Reinvestment Act, considerable financial resources were targeted to advance this research. Many see threat, not promise, from this approach. They see comparative effectiveness research as code for cost-effectiveness research, with the word "cost" euphemistically and disingenuously omitted. Some of those seeing threat may be ideological opponents—worried that comparative effectiveness research will lead to the identification and elimination of beneficial health strategies because they are costly. Others perhaps drape their concerns in those words, but in fact their concerns are more self-centered, such as some of those who are in the business of selling pharmaceuticals, devices, or procedures that might be determined to be too costly. Their practices might fail tests of comparative effectiveness and might be at particular risk of failing tests of cost-effectiveness. For these individuals the use of cost-effectiveness analysis raises narrow concerns that reflect self-interest rather than ideology.

But in either case, the approach can be divisive because issues of cost are divisive. Certainly many issues in medical ethics are politically divisive without any clear connection to cost. For example, discussions about abortion and reproductive freedom were once—in the 1960s and 1970s—considered part of the substance of medical ethics but have since largely been considered issues of politics. Approaches that blend economic considerations with moral considerations are almost always judged in part by political motivations because money is at stake.

For those reasons efforts like the National Institute for Health and Clinical Excellence (NICE, www.nice.org.uk/) in the United Kingdom, which has its charge to assess the value of medical processes and technologies and approaches to public health, has been simultaneously praised for its efforts to rationalize care and criticized for its efforts to ration care. Contemporary debates in the United States seem to follow the same pattern, with critics concerned either about the idea of using cost or the personal consequences of those analyses. As a result, some of the important conflicts in the use of these approaches to address ethical concerns reflect their acceptability against ideology and personal interest.

The next two sections outline the strengths and weaknesses of these approaches in more detail, but the basic focus of these approaches is on understanding the consequences of choices, when the best choice is not otherwise clear.

STRENGTHS

The fundamental power of decision analytic and economic approaches to clinical problems or issues in medical ethics is that these approaches are explicit, formal, and systematic. The tradition in these fields, and the nature of the work, demands that individual assumptions are specified and, in the best case, open to view. Similarly, the results can be presented following the same explicit rules. For example, the CF analysis, reported in table 16.1, provides an organized view of the consequences of several alternative ethically charged choices. Sometimes these consequences are unanticipated or make sense only in retrospect.

The second strength of these approaches is that the process used to construct a model may be a useful end in itself. Scholars willing to go through the exercise of structuring a decision tree may find that the process helps clarify their own thinking because of the regimented steps required. Formalizing a problem in this way enforces discipline and helps to distance scholars from their visceral reactions to a problem in medical ethics. That distance can be useful if those visceral reactions are not defensible by clearer heads.

A third strength of these approaches is that the need to assign values to the outcomes encourages careful attention to these critical items. People generally want to avoid a miscarriage but making good decisions often requires a more detailed sense of exactly how that outcome is valued. As with other elements, the process of decision analysis enforces disciplined thinking in essential areas.

Finally, modeling provides tremendous power in its opportunity to support sensitivity analyses. Sensitivity analyses allow scholars to test the impact of alternative plausible assumptions about all aspects of the problem. What if the risk of miscarriage following amniocentesis were higher? What if the test has a higher rate of false positives? What if we decided that we need to understand the impact of couples' anxiety? These analyses are useful in two ways. First, they can indicate what assumptions, when changed, critically alter the results, so that one would choose a different approach after viewing those results. When a sensitivity analysis shows this, and the alternative assumptions are plausible, then it is time to return to the literature, the laboratory, the clinic, or wherever necessary to get more precise information about those particular assumptions.

Or, as in the CF case, perhaps it means that if different values would lead to vastly different management strategies, then developing an appealing uniform policy across individuals would be impossible. Second, sensitivity analyses can indicate what assumptions, even when changed substantially, leave the overall conclusions unaffected. Such a finding indicates that those assumptions are simply not important to the situation, and certainly that no more work should go into increasing the precision of their estimates.

WEAKNESSES

There is a vast and growing literature on the weaknesses of economic approaches to evaluating health care programs. The aim of much of this literature is to refine methods to address problems and thereby move the field forward. Much of the literature also addresses ways to standardize approaches across investigators, to make studies comparable, and to increase the confidence that results are not subject to manipulation by idiosyncratic accounting procedures. For example, critical issues in the use of these methods include ways to incorporate life expectancy and quality of life into economic models, whether public or patient values are most appropriate in evaluating health states, distinguishing between fixed and variable costs and allocating the costs of infrastructure, appropriate techniques in the temporal discounting of costs or health benefits, clear ways to reflect uncertainty in model results, and so on.

These specific challenges to the field reflect technical advances or choices and are summarized well elsewhere (Gold et al. 1996). However, there are weaknesses in these methods that are more specific to bioethical applications. Underlying these weaknesses is the fundamental issue that decision analytic reasoning is inherently utilitarian. Although one can think of modifications to decision analyses that might incorporate notions of individual rights (for example, one might simply not structure decision trees with branches that violate important individual rights), decision analyses evaluate strategies only by the outcomes they produce and not how they get there. This consequentialist approach may conflict with the approach of many theoretical medical ethicists.

Asch and Hershey have examined one particular tension that can arise in the conduct of these analyses (1995, 1998). Most decision analyses, when they take a population perspective, inherently aggregate the outcomes of individuals across the population. In this way, although some individuals may realize bad outcomes, these may appear to be offset by the good outcomes realized by other individuals. More generally, these analyses often present the central tendency of the analysis, or the average result, without giving much attention to the distribution of outcomes across individuals in the population. If programs are evaluated only on the basis of the average outcome, they may be misevaluated—because most individuals will not bear the average outcome, but some other outcome that will be like the average only when viewed in combination with what happens to everyone else.

Tsevat and colleagues calculated the gains in life expectancy attributable to reducing various coronary heart disease risk factors. They found that reducing serum cholesterol to 200 mg/dl for thirty-five-year-old men would result in a population-wide increase in individual life expectancy of 0.7 years. The authors were careful and correct to note that individual gains could be much more substantial (Tsevat et al. 1991). If everyone bore the average burden of a health intervention and received the average benefit, many might jump at the chance to give up 0.7 years of life in exchange for the comfort of eating high fat foods with abandon. Of course many of these patients would give up nothing, and some would suffer very early mortality. The population-based perspectives of the boardroom often miss the point that clinicians and patients care about the distribution of outcomes, as well as the central tendency (Asch 1999).

Some forms of utilitarianism shy away from interpersonal comparisons, but other forms are premised on the idea that the good outcomes achieved by some individuals offset the bad outcomes achieved by others. In contrast, rights-based or deontological theories of justice get their support in part from the view that by averaging outcomes across individuals, utilitarian perspectives elide important distinctions between persons (Rawls 1971). Those who want to use the techniques of clinical economics or decision analysis to help them address bioethical problems need to be keenly aware of the implicit philosophical assumptions that underlie these methods.

❧ Concluding Comments

Ethical values are inherent to cost-effectiveness analyses and other forms of quantitative decision analysis, despite the seeming objectivity and value-neutrality of these techniques. These techniques embody a form of utilitarianism that can contrast with other systems of justice based on rights, for example. For these reasons, the decision to adopt the results of a decision analysis in addressing a question of health policy is in part the adoption of that moral framework.

Indeed, the utilitarian framework is one of the virtues of decision analysis in that the utiles or other units of these analyses can be summed and compared—at least mathematically. Arguments based on rights, for example, often lose their heuristic appeal when different rights compete—or at least the solution to such conflicts is often not clear. When two rights compete, which one trumps? Decision analyses provide a structured approach to examining such conflicts, and the insistence on common metrics of value makes it easier to resolve what otherwise might become shouting matches.

❧ Notes on Training and Resources

Because of the breadth of these methods, training is available from many different sources and comes in many forms. At one extreme, those aiming to pursue original scholarship in these fields can enter doctoral programs in economics, public policy, operations research, epidemiology, and the like. Some specialized programs focus on health economics.

Master's level training in these areas is often available in schools of public health and related programs. Some universities offer joint degrees, pairing clinical training with methodologic training in medical decision making or clinical economics. Popular combinations are MD or RN programs paired with a PhD in economics, MPH, or MBA programs. Many universities offer master's training specific to epidemiology, health policy, or health services research.

Many scholars who are interested in these areas, but not sufficiently interested to justify long, degree-granting programs, might do well to investigate the short courses offered by the Society for Medical Decision Making (www.smdm.org/) during its annual national meeting. Half-day and full-day courses are typically offered in basic and advanced decision analysis, Markov modeling, clinical economics, decision psychology, and the like. Attending the remainder of the scientific meeting and reading through the journal, *Medical Decision Making* (http://mdm.sagepub.com/), can provide additional insights.

RESOURCES

Many of the papers and books cited in the bibliography were chosen because they represent useful tutorials or guides for those interested in these methods. As mentioned in the previous section, the journal *Medical Decision Making* often contains technical notes and other review articles that can help scholars use these methods. Because these fields are so quantitative, a variety of software programs exist to perform decision analyses. One of the most popular and easy to use programs is available for Windows or Macintosh platforms (TreeAge Software, Inc.; Williamstown, MA; www.treeage.com/).

⚘ Notes

This chapter is not subject to U.S. copyright, excluding the following material for which the publisher attained permission to reprint:

D. A. Asch, J. C. Hershey, M. L. DeKay, M. V. Pauly, J. P. Patton, M. K. Jedrziewski, F. X. Frei, R. Giardine, J. A. Kant, and M. T. Mennuti, "Carrier Screening for Cystic Fibrosis: Costs and Clinical Outcomes," *Medical Decision Making* 18 (1998): 202–12.

D. A. Asch, J. C. Hershey, M. V. Pauly, J. P. Patton, M. K. Jedrziewski, and M. T. Mennuti, "Genetic Screening for Reproductive Planning: Methodologic and Conceptual Issues in Policy Analysis," *American Journal of Public Health* 86 (1996): 684–90. © 1996 by the American Public Health Association.

1. Much of the material in this section has been taken from two sources: D. A. Asch, J. C. Hershey, M. V. Pauly, J. P. Patton, M. K. Jedrziewski, and M. T. Mennuti, "Genetic Screening for Reproductive Planning: Methodologic and Conceptual Issues in Policy Analysis," *American Journal of Public Health* 86 (1996): 684–90; and D. A. Asch, J. C. Hershey, M. L. DeKay, M. V. Pauly, J. P. Patton, M. K. Jedrziewski, F. X. Frei, R. Giardine, J. A. Kant, and M. T. Mennuti, "Carrier Screening for Cystic Fibrosis: Costs and Clinical Outcomes," *Medical Decision Making* 18 (1998): 202–12.

⚘ References

Asch, D. A. 1995. Basic lessons in resource allocation: Sharing, setting limits, and being fair. *Pharos* 58 (2): 33–34.

———. 1999. From boardroom to bedside: Bioethical implications of policy research for clinical practice. *Journal of Investigative Medicine* 47:273–77.

Asch, D. A., and J. C. Hershey. 1995. Why some health policies don't make sense at the bedside. *Annals of Internal Medicine* 122:846–50.

———. 1998. Avoidable errors in health policy analysis. *Journal of General Internal Medicine* 13:762–67.

Asch, D. A., J. C. Hershey, M. L. DeKay, M. V. Pauly, J. P. Patton, M. K. Jedrziewski, F. X. Frei, R. Giardine, J. A. Kant, and M. T. Mennuti. 1998. Carrier screening for cystic fibrosis: Costs and clinical outcomes. *Medical Decision Making* 18:202–12.

Asch, D. A., J. C. Hershey, M. V. Pauly, J. P. Patton, M. K. Jedrziewski, and M. T. Mennuti. 1996. Genetic screening for reproductive planning: Methodologic and conceptual issues in policy analysis. *American Journal of Public Health* 86:684–90.

Asch, D. A., C. Jepson, J. C. Hershey, J. Baron, and P. A. Ubel. 2003. When money is saved by reducing health care costs, where do us primary care physicians think the money goes? *American Journal of Managed Care* 9:438–42.

Detsky, A. S., G. Naglie, M. D. Krahn, D. Naimark, and D. A. Redelmeier. 1997. Primer on medical decision analysis: Part 1—Getting started. *Medical Decision Making* 17:12325.

Detsky, A. S., G. Naglie, M. D. Krahn, D. A. Redelmeier, and D. Naimark. 1997. Primer on medical decision analysis: Part 2—Building a tree. *Medical Decision Making* 17:12635.

Drummond, M. F., G. L. Stoddard, and G. W. Torrance. 1987. *Methods for the economic evaluation of health care programmes*. New York: Oxford.

Eisenberg, J. M. 1989. Clinical economics. A guide to the economic analysis of clinical practices. *JAMA* 262:2879–86.

Finkler, S. A. 1982. The distinction between costs and charges. *Annals of Internal Medicine* 96:306–10.

Froberg, D. G., and R. L. Kane. 1989. Methodology for measuring health-state preferences—I. Measurement strategies. *Journal of Clinical Epidemiology* 42:345–54.

Fryback, D. G., E. J. Dasbach, R. Klein et al. 1993. The beaver dam health outcomes study: Initial catalog of health-state quality factors. *Medical Decision Making* 13:89–102.

Gold, M. R., J. E. Siegel, L. B. Russel, and M. C. Weinstein. 1996. *Cost-effectiveness in health and medicine*. New York: Oxford.

Krahn, M. D., G. Naglie, D. Naimark, D. A. Redelmeier, and A. S. Detsky. 1997. Primer on medical decision analysis: Part 4—Analyzing the model and interpreting the results. *Medical Decision Making* 17:142–51.

Naglie, G., M. D. Krahn, D. Naimark, D. A. Redelmeier, and A. S. Detsky. 1997. Primer on medical decision analysis: Part 3—Estimating probabilities and utilities. *Medical Decision Making* 17:136–41.

Naimark, D., M. D. Krahn, G. Naglie, D. A. Redelmeier, and A. S. Detsky. 1997. Primer on medical decision analysis: Part 5—Working with Markov processes. *Medical Decision Making* 17:152–59.

Rawls, J. 1971. *A theory of justice*. Cambridge, MA: Harvard University Press.

Redelmeier, D. A., and A. S. Detsky. 1995. A clinician's guide to utility measurement. *Primary Care* 22:271–78.

Sox, H., M. A. Blatt, M. C. Higgins, and K. I. Marton. 1988. *Medical decision making*. London: Butterworth.

Torrance, G. W. 1986. Measurement of health state utilities for economic appraisal: A review. *Journal of Health Economics* 5:1–30.

Tsevat, J., M. C. Weinstein, L. W. Williams, A. N. Tosteson, and L. Goldman. 1991. Expected gains in life-expectancy from various coronary heart disease risk factor modifications. *Circulation* 83:1194–201.

U.S. Congress, Office of Technology Assessment. 1992. *Cystic fibrosis and DNA tests: Implications of carrier screening*, OTA-BA-532. Washington, DC: U.S. Government Printing Office, August, ch. 2.

Weinstein, M. C., and H. V. Fineberg. 1980. *Clinical decision analysis*. Philadelphia: Saunders.

Wilfond, B. S., and N. Fost. 1992. The introduction of cystic fibrosis carrier screening into clinical practice: Policy considerations. *Milbank Quarterly* 70:629–59.

PART III

Applications

Appendix

CHAPTER 17

Research in Medical Ethics

Scholarship in "Substituted Judgment"

DANIEL P. SULMASY

The purpose of this chapter is to explore a single topic that has been investigated by a number of scholars who use many of the methods presented in this book. While this exploration necessarily entails a review of the literature, the aim of this review is not so much to be exhaustive as illustrative. In contrast to the kind of review article one finds in the medical literature, the main focus of the chapter will be on the methods, not the results, of research. That is, this chapter will show what methods have been used, how various disciplines have interacted with each other, and what general lessons can be learned about methodology and medical ethics by exploring the scholarly work that has revolved around a single, important question in the field of medical ethics.

The topic of advance directives, and in particular the concept of substituted judgment, provides an excellent paradigm for the purposes of this chapter.[1] This topic has been of sustained interest to medical ethicists over several decades of research. The concept arose out of legal scholarship, was amplified and supported by normative philosophical theory, and has been subjected to intense study from a variety of empirical disciplines. It is one of the few topics in medical ethics that has engendered enough empirical investigation to warrant the publication of what is called a meta-analysis—a quantitative review that sums up all of the quantitative studies that have investigated a single question using a single empirical method.

The theory of substituted judgment arose out of legal theory and moral philosophy's stress on the importance of respect for the autonomy of individuals regarding medical decision making. According to this approach, when patients lose their decision-making capacity, they do not thereby forfeit all of their autonomy. What the patient thinks and feels might not be directly known, but one might still express respect for the patient's autonomy if one were to make the decision that one thought the patient would have made were he or she fully capable of making a decision. Thus, in the clinical setting, one is instructed to ask not, "What would you like us to do for your mother?" but rather, "What do you think your mother would have wanted if she had been able to tell us herself?" Decisions made in the spirit of the latter question are made according to the theory of substituted judgment (Buchanan and Brock 1986).

This chapter will explore how scholarship in medical ethics has shaped, refined, and reflected upon this theory and practices related to it.

❧ Origins

As late as the 1970s, thorny ethical questions arose about the best way to treat patients who were unable to speak for themselves. Patients with decision-making capacity had only recently acquired a strong say in treatment decisions, especially establishing their right to refuse unwanted medical interventions. New advances such as improved respirator care, cardiopulmonary resuscitation, and the introduction of the intensive care unit had burst upon the scene. Contemporaneously, the legal doctrine of informed consent had become enshrined as clinical, ethical, and legal dogma. Accordingly, clinicians faced a burgeoning number of vexing cases in which powerful technologies provided the possibility of prolonging the lives of patients who could not, because of their medical conditions, give informed consent or refusal for themselves. These cases provoked great consternation for all parties concerned. In some cases families requested the forgoing of these interventions, but physicians were uncertain that either traditional medical ethics or the law would permit the withholding or withdrawing of life-sustaining treatments for patients without decision-making capacity.

Many of these cases went to court. Thus it was legal scholars who first struggled to find ways to address these ethical quandaries. The now very famous cases included, among others, *In re Quinlan* (1976), *Superintendent of Belchertown State School v. Saikewicz* (1977), *In re Dinnerstein* (1978), *In re Spring* (1980), *In re Eichner* (1981), and *In re Storar* (1981).

Prior to these cases concerning care at the end of life, the doctrine of substituted judgment had been invoked in a pair of cases regarding organ donation for relatives by individuals lacking decision-making capacity. These cases appear to have been the points of entry by which the notion of substituted judgment gained a place in legal decision-making regarding ethical quandaries in contemporary medical care. In the case of *Strunk v. Strunk* (1969), the doctrine was invoked by a court in justifying its decision to authorize a kidney donation by a mentally retarded man to his brother. By contrast, in the case of *Lausier v. Pescinski* (1975), a Wisconsin appellate court denied that a chronic schizophrenic with a mental age of twelve years could act as a kidney donor for his sister on the basis of the substituted judgment argument proposed by his guardian. Although the court did not permit the transplant on the basis of substituted judgment in the case of Mr. Pescinski, the standard was defended vigorously by Robertson (1976).

As a legal matter, substituted judgment is a relatively recent development in the common law of the United States and the UK (Robertson 1976; Weber 1985–86; Harmon 1990). It can be traced to the cases of *Ex parte Whitbred* (1816) in England and *In re Willoughby* (1844) in the United States. These cases concerned whether persons who lacked capacity but had inherited estates could be construed as authorizing that some of their inheritance go to other members of the family to whom they owed no duty of support. According to this doctrine, the court was to substitute itself for the incompetent person, donning the "mental mantle" of the person who could not speak for himself or herself, deciding according to the motives and considerations that the person would have had were he or she able to make the decision. Courts were subsequently permitted to construe on the part of incompetent persons motives such as charity, altruism, self-interest, and even an interest in minimizing taxes in making decisions regarding the disposition of their estates (Robertson 1976; Weber 1985; Harmon 1990).

Robertson (1976) argued forcefully that the same doctrine should be applied in the case of medical decisions by persons lacking decision-making capacity, such as the decision about whether a retarded man should be allowed to donate an organ. For centuries before the era of contemporary medical ethics, legal scholars have looked to philosophy for theoretical support for their jurisprudential claims. Robertson sought support for the legal theory of substituted judgment by appeal to the liberal philosophical ethics of Mill, Rawls, and Dworkin. Robertson argued that while it might be difficult to "choose as the incompetent would, if competent," nonetheless, "the determinative factor appears to be consent or choice. Respect for persons requires that incompetents be similarly treated. We should treat incompetents as they would choose to be treated in a given situation." Substituted judgment, he argued, was the best means by which to do that, rather than following a "paternalistic" legal alternative of "best interests."

Courts soon began to invoke the doctrine of substituted judgment in decisions regarding care at the end of life. In some cases, such as *Superintendent of Belchertown State School v. Saikewicz* (1977), this doctrine was invoked even on behalf of persons who had never had capacity. While it might seem peculiar that substituted judgments would be invoked on behalf of persons who were without decision-making capacity from birth, one must recognize that this legal doctrine had effectively been called upon to do just that in settling estate cases for over a century (Harmon 1990).

Nonetheless, substituted judgment was not uniformly embraced by all scholars in the field of medical ethics. As the courts began to apply the doctrine, not even all legal scholars agreed that it was the best way to settle the ethical problem of deciding for those unable to speak for themselves. Annas (1980) called it "an invention from fantasyland." Gutheil and Appelbaum (1983) called it "best interests in disguise." Weber (1985) warned that the rights of the vulnerable were at risk once society condoned the invocation of altruistic motives on behalf of persons lacking in capacity in order to justify the withdrawal of treatment. Most legal scholars, however, quickly embraced the notion (Davis 1978; Dunphy and Cross 1987). Others simply accepted it as the new legal norm (Suber and Tabor 1982a, 1982b).

Some philosophers also began to comment on how to decide for those who could not decide for themselves, but in the 1970s and early 1980s, the only options they seem to have considered were the preexisting legal options that judges were attempting to fit to this novel circumstance. The menu was limited to a choice between the "reasonable person," "best interests," or "substituted judgment" standards.

Freedman (1978) was an early philosophical critic. He not only argued that providing an actual substituted judgment might well be empirically impossible, he also argued that what matters most about human freedom is not so much the achievement of the results of free choice as the exercise of free choice. Since, by definition, the decisionally incapable person cannot exercise free choice, it is nonsensical to try to construct a legal apparatus by which they might do so.

Some philosophers supported the notion of substituted judgment in only a quali-fied way. O'Neil (1983), for instance, suggested that asking "what the patient would have chosen" would be a reasonable approach only insofar as one were to understand that it is really the most expedient way of determining the patient's best interests.

By contrast, most philosophers working in the field of medical ethics embraced the concept of substituted judgment full-throttle. Buchanan (1979) first proposed what would later become the familiar three-tiered system of decision making. Prior-ity should go to "a clear and reliable prior expression of the patient's preferences when he or she was competent (for example, a bona fide 'living will')." Barring such evi-dence, decision making should rest with the family who should "do what the patient would choose, if he or she were competent, or, where this cannot be ascertained, what is, in their opinion, in the patient's best interests."

Most other philosophers concurred. Dworkin (1993) developed a sophisticated theory of autonomy to support the making of substituted judgments, based on three distinctions. First, he argued that the real meaning of respect for autonomy is respect for autonomy as integrity, rather than as welfare—that is—respect for our capacity to express ourselves and create our character through our choices rather than respect for the making of the choices that are best for us. Second, he argued that critical interests (based on deeply held and persistent values) are more important than experiential interests (e.g., the pleasure or pain we might experience at a given moment). Third, he argued that we can exercise this "integrity" type of autonomy with respect to our critical interests through "precedent" autonomy, either by making clear expressions about how we ought to be treated in the future, or by having others choose for us in a way that fully respects our autonomy, not by considering past choices as evidence of present choices, but by making present choices on our behalf that are consistent with our character and values.

Reading through the various editions of Beauchamp and Childress's famous textbook, *Principles of Biomedical Ethics*, one is provided a view of how the concept of substituted judgment rapidly evolved. These authors shifted from not mentioning substituted judgment in the first edition (1979), to criticizing its use by the courts and prioritizing best interests over substituted judgment in the second edition (1983), to a qualified endorsement of the concept as "an appropriate guideline for previously competent patients whose relevant prior preferences can be discerned" in the third edition (1989), to considering substituted judgment so obviously correct in cases in which a relevant prior autonomous judgment can be known that it collapses into a mere corollary of the fundamental principle of respect for autonomy in the fourth, fifth and sixth editions (Beauchamp and Childress 1994, 2001; 2009, 135–40).

In the early years of scholarly discussion about substituted judgment, physicians, for the most part, merely awaited the outcomes of judicial decisions and either hailed them or complained about them in occasional editorials (see, e.g., Relman 1978). Few scholars from other disciplines had much to say about substituted judgment early on, especially in the 1970s and early 1980s as the concept was being introduced into medical decision making.

The President's Commission (1983, 136) explicitly prioritized the substituted judgment standard over the best interests standard for surrogate decision making but offered only a brief theoretical justification based on the need to promote self-determination. The theoretical case for substituted judgment was soon thereafter made quite vigorously by two of the commission's staff members, Allen Buchanan and Dan Brock, first in an influential article (Buchanan and Brock 1986), and subsequently in book form (Buchanan and Brock 1990). Following Robertson (1976), they argued that the moral duty to respect the fundamental value of the right of self-determination of persons requires that when a patient cannot exercise self-determination, if that patient's preferences can reasonably be inferred, then substituted judgment is the appropriate technique for respecting the patient's self-determination. They criticized courts that had used the substituted judgment standard to decide cases in which the patient had never been competent or in which there was almost no contact between the family and the patient during a previous period of competency. In such cases, they argued, there is no reasonable basis for knowing the patient's preferences, and a best-interests standard should be applied. In these two works they formalized the now-familiar tripartite hierarchy of decision making on behalf of those incapable of speaking for themselves: treatment directives if the patient expressed explicit treatment preferences, whether verbal or written; substituted judgments if there are no explicit preferences but the preferences of the patient who once had capacity can reasonably be inferred; and best-interests decisions for those who have no explicit directives and there is no basis for inferring preferences due to long-standing mental incapacity or social isolation. This hierarchy has become canonical in bioethics textbooks (Ahronheim, Moreno, and Zuckerman 2000; Jonsen, Siegler, and Winslade 2006) and in professional codes (American College of Physicians 2005; American Medical Association 2009).

Also in the early 1980s, more likely in response to the recommendations of judges in court cases than to theoretical ethical arguments, state legislatures began to enact laws codifying durable powers of attorney for health care and health care proxies (Martyn and Jacobs 1984). Legal scholars took up the task of surveying what was happening in various jurisdictions across the United States. In 1983 the President's Commission made a recommendation promoting the Durable Power of Attorney for Health Care (DPAHC) as an alternative to the living will, and specified substituted judgment as the preferred standard by which such proxies should make decisions (President's Commission 1983, 151). The commission even proposed a model statute. Although the term "living will" appears to date to the late 1960s, only twenty-two states had enacted living will legislation by 1984, and only Delaware (1982) and California (in 1983) had passed DPAHC laws. The Patient Self-Determination Act (1990) gave further emphasis to advance directives and indirectly to the notion of substituted judgment embedded in concept of a durable power of attorney for health care. Research, education, and policy efforts were directed not towards questioning how advance directives ought to be used but to improving the implementation of respect for precedent autonomy through such legal instruments, expanding the use of advance directives, and assuring that patients' preferences were being honored (see, for example, Hammes and Rooney 1998; Tolle et al. 1998). Eventually, every state (and the District of Columbia) had enacted DPAHC legislation, and almost all of these statutes instruct proxies to make substituted judgments rather than basing decisions upon best-interests judgments (Sabatino 1999).

❧ Empirical Studies

Keenly aware of the ways that descriptive techniques could contribute to debates about theory and policy, empirical research on the subject of substituted judgment began in the late 1980s (Sugarman 1994). Investigators began to note that the theory of substituted judgment yielded an empirically testable hypothesis: could surrogates accurately predict the wishes of their loved ones? A sustained program of investigation over twenty years has answered that question (Uhlmann, Pearlman, and Cain 1988; Ouslander et al. 1989; Zweibel and Cassel 1989; Tomlinson et al., 1990; Seckler et al. 1991; Hare, Pratt, and Nelson 1992; Pearlman, Uhlmann, and Jecker 1992; Gerety et al. 1993; Suhl et al. 1994; Sulmasy, Haller, and Terry 1994; Layde et al. 1995; Libbus and Russell 1995; Matheis-Kraft and Roberto 1997; Marbella et al. 1998; Sulmasy, Terry et al. 1998; Principe-Rodriguez et al. 1999; Smucker et al. 2000; Coppolino and Ackerson 2001; Ditto et al. 2001; Fagerlin et al. 2001; Houts et al. 2002). In fact, a sufficient number of empirical studies accumulated regarding this topic that a meta-analysis (a statistical technique for pooling all of the results of various studies of a single research question) has been performed (Shalowitz Garrett-Mayer, and Wendler 2006). The answer to the question is that surrogates' substituted judgments are about 68 percent accurate—that is—surrogates correctly predict the patient's wishes about two-thirds of the time. Fifty percent accuracy would be expected by chance alone. This degree of accuracy is statistically better than chance, but far less than perfect. Surrogates are more accurate than the patients' physicians, whose accuracy statistics approximate chance alone (Uhlmann, Pearlman, and Cain 1988; Tomlinson et al. 1990). More recent studies have shown that this degree of surrogate inaccuracy also obtains for treatment decisions in clinical situations other than at the end of life, such as those regarding cataract surgery (Mantravadi et al. 2007) and dialysis (Pruchno et al. 2005), and that surrogates in a culture with more closely knit families (i.e., Japan) are no more accurate than surrogates in the United States (Miura et al. 2006). Further, attempts to improve the accuracy of surrogates' substituted judgments have proven unsuccessful (Ditto et al. 2001).

Qualitative empirical techniques (see chapters 12 and 13) have been used in concert with quantitative techniques (see chapter 14) to address questions about substituted judgment. For instance, the stress that decision making places on loved ones who are asked about whether to limit life-sustaining treatments for patients lacking in decision-making capacity had not widely been appreciated. Qualitative interviews with surrogate decision makers reveal very high levels of stress (Vig et al. 2007; Braun et al. 2008; Handy et al. 2008). Psychometric instruments used to predict post-traumatic stress disorder have shown that the stress levels among surrogates who have been asked about limiting treatment for a loved one are equivalent to those seen in persons who have just survived house fires or similar catastrophes (Sulmasy, Sood et al. 2006). Similarly high stress levels persist for months after the patient has died (Tilden et al. 2001). It is not known whether being directed to perform a substituted judgment ameliorates or worsens this stress, although prior communication with the patient about end-of-life decisions appears to diminish surrogates' stress (Tilden et al. 2001; Vig et al. 2007; Handy et al. 2008).

Despite legislative and ethical directives that have instructed surrogates, where possible, to practice substituted judgment when deciding on behalf of patients, several qualitative studies have demonstrated that surrogates often rely exclusively on their own judgments about the patient's best interests when making decisions and that most surrogates use complex mixtures of their own judgments about what would be best for the patient, what they think the patient would have wanted, and the advice of health care professionals and loved ones in arriving at a decision (Hirschman, Kapo, and Karlawish 2006; Vig et al. 2006). It is especially important to note that substituted judgments are frequently overridden even when the surrogates have good evidence of the patient's prior wishes.

Ethical theory, as outlined above, has justified the standard decision-making hierarchy (i.e., treatment directives first, substituted judgments second, and best interests third), by appeal to the foundational importance of respect for individual autonomy. On the strength of this foundational premise, one might expect results such as those described above to be deeply troubling to patients, who might fear that their most fundamental value of self-determination would be in danger of being overturned in the event that they lost decision-making capacity. Empirical studies, however, have shown that while this is true for some patients, it appears to be true only for a minority. For instance, when asked whether, in cases of conflict, physicians should follow a theoretically perfect living will or the directions of loved ones in making treatment choices should they lose decisional capacity, a majority of patients prefer that the physicians follow the directions of loved ones (Terry et al. 1999). When asked how much flexibility loved ones should be given in interpreting their treatment directives, only 39 percent of a group of dialysis patients wanted their directives followed strictly, and 31 percent endorsed giving their loved ones complete "freedom to do what they think is best for you" (Sehgal et al. 1992). Hawkins et al. (2005) found only 9 percent of patients wanted their treatment directives followed strictly. Similarly, Puchalski et al. (2000) found that only 29 percent of hospitalized patients would want their directives against cardiopulmonary resuscitation (CPR) strictly interpreted. In this same report, among patients in intensive care, only 12 percent would want their directives followed strictly if they had a spouse to whom to defer. In a series of studies asking terminally ill patients more explicitly just how they would want treatment decisions to be made in the event of decisional incapacity, only a minority would prefer a strict substituted judgment, while the majority of patients appear to want decisions to be based on complex admixtures of varying degrees of their own preferences and the best-interests judgments of their loved ones and their health care professionals, with a minority deferring completely to the judgments of others (Nolan et al. 2005; Sulmasy et al. 2007). Similar findings have been found among ambulatory geriatric patients and the recently bereaved (Fins et al. 2005). These preferences for *how* decisions are to be made are generally stable over time, even in persons very close to death (Sulmasy et al. 2007).

❧ Further Theoretical Scholarship

Several philosophers have taken note of these empirical findings and have incorporated these data into their analyses of the ethics of deciding for those who have lost decisional capacity. High, for instance, began as a proponent of substituted judgment (High 1989) but soon thereafter changed his mind (High 1994). While a philosopher he had become engaged in several interdisciplinary empirical studies and found that elderly patients were much more interested in *who* was making the decision than in *what* the decision would be. This led him to question not only the importance of substituted judgment, but also the "atomistic" notion of autonomy which formed its philosophical foundation.

Brock, by contrast, remains a proponent of substituted judgment. Holding to the premise that self-determination is the preeminent foundational value, he notes that the data show that family proxies do better at predicting the patients' preferences than other parties, such as physicians. In an imperfect world in which respect for self-determination is the ideal ethical norm, he argues that substituted judgments by family members are still the best approximation we have of that ethical ideal (Brock 1996).

Nelson and Nelson (1994) built upon High's critiques and the empirical data cited above to take issue with Brock's persistent defense of substituted judgment, accusing him of a Hobbesian approach to the authority of the family, according to which familial authority is justified to the extent that patients have ceded to the family, as part of a micro-social contract, some of the autonomous decision-making authority that is rightfully theirs. They argue for a richer account of persons by which individuals come to see themselves "and their fulfillment in terms of constitutive social relationships." By such an understanding, the role of a surrogate would be much more than a channel for patient preferences, and the moral basis for the primacy of substituted judgment would be undermined.

PERSONHOOD AND SUBSTITUTED JUDGMENT

A second line of philosophical critique of substituted judgment does not question the importance of self-determination, but instead criticizes advance directives as not being able to ensure self-determination. The argument is that when the patient lacks capacity, the self to be determined in that situation is not the same self as the (formerly) competent self whose values and preferences constitute the basis upon which substituted judgment is being made. Rebecca Dresser, drawing upon Parfit's neo-Lockean, psychological continuity conception of a person (a being capable of thinking itself to be the same thing at two points in time), argued that the demented person was not the same person as the formerly competent person, and therefore only a best-interests judgment, not a substituted judgment, would be reasonable (Dresser 1986). She observed that the demented person has radically different interests and, depending upon the extent of the dementia, different preferences (Dresser 1995). Robertson soon joined her in that view, despite his early defense of substituted judgment (Dresser and Robertson 1989; Robertson 1991).

This view has drawn rebuttals. Rich (1997) supports Dworkin's notion of prioritizing critical interests over experiential interests and has suggested that the best policy solution would be to set a very low threshold for psychological continuity, so that all but the permanently vegetative would qualify as the same person. Blustein

(1999) proposed two possible solutions: similarly to Rich, a policy of setting a low threshold for the psychological continuity of persons; or revising the theory of personal identity to a theory of narrative continuity in which a person's interest in his or her whole life story could be carried out by other persons that he dubbed the "continuers" of the person now lacking in capacity. These arguments have not reached a definitive conclusion (Dresser 2003).

THE ROLE OF FAMILY

Substituted judgment has also been criticized because it fails to pay sufficient attention to the role and needs of the family. Hardwig (1990) has argued that family decisions should include the interests of the family and not just the values and preferences of the patient, as substituted judgment implies. Further, he argued, one should consider the counterintuitive implication that if the patient were a generous and self-sacrificing person, substituted judgment would lead the family to discontinue beneficial life-sustaining treatments when they might otherwise think it their duty to continue (Hardwig 1993). Kuczewski (1996) has asserted that bioethics, influenced by American individualism, has fallen into the trap of falsely conceiving of decision making as a disjunction—the competent patient is the sole proper decision maker; if capacity is lost, then the family decides as the patient would have decided. In clinical reality, he suggests, the decision-making roles are never so clearly compartmentalized. Levine and Zuckerman (1999) accuse health care institutions of sometimes using the substituted judgment standard to simplify the decision-making process and avoid the complexity of real family decision making. While all these arguments tend to undermine the basis for substituted judgment, these latter critiques are more in keeping with the philosophical anthropology of Nelson and Nelson (1994)—that human beings are essentially formed in relationship and characterized by relationships. Hardwig's arguments, by contrast, are driven by claims of distributive justice with respect to the family.

SUBSTITUTED JUDGMENT AND THE LOGIC OF COUNTERFACTUALS

One interesting line of philosophical investigation has been an exploration of the logic of the contrary-to-fact conditional statement upon which substituted judgment is based. Wierenga (1983) first noted that the form of the substituted judgment is: "If X had decision-making capacity, X would not want Y. X does not have decision-making capacity, therefore we should stop treatment Y." The problem Wierenga saw was that if X *did* have decision-making capacity, then X would not have the disease or condition that was making X both terminally ill and lacking in decisional capacity and therefore presumably would want treatment Y. Nagasawa (2008) agrees with this counterfactual analysis and argues further that the alternative philosophical approach of using possible world semantics instead of counterfactuals will not salvage the logic of substituted judgment because we have no way of locating a possible world in which an incompetent patient with a terminal illness has capacity.[2] Even if we did, we could not know with certitude what treatment preference the patient would have in that world.

RECENT PHILOSOPHICAL DEFENSES

Davis (2002, 2007) has offered a series of philosophical defenses of at least one aspect of substituted judgment—what he has called, after Dworkin, "precedent autonomy." He rejects the personal identity problem as a figure of speech rather than a genuine metaphysical claim. While he grants that those who offer the personal identity objection to advance directives are correct in their intuition that circumstances often change dramatically in morally relevant ways when a person loses decision-making capacity, he argues that we still think it is Grandma in the bed, not some other person, even if Grandma is demented. Yet, he finds the autonomy defenses mounted by Dworkin, Brock, and Buchanan inadequate, and the narrative defense offered by Kuczewski too vague. Despite his protestations that he is offering something new, his arguments rely on distinctions that are not unlike Dworkin's distinctions between critical interests and experiential interests and between welfare and integrity. Nonetheless, he does offer many fresh and interesting insights and develops the ideas much further than any previous defender of the autonomy-based defense of substituted judgment. He assumes that respect for autonomy is the value of paramount importance. He then argues that preferences are not only characterized by their content, but also by the reasons a person offers for them. These reasons, even the ability to offer reasons, commonly change for individuals who have lost capacity. Even if they have the same preference, it matters morally that they might not have that preference for the same reasons they previously did. Nonetheless, he argues that we are all aware of higher order resolution preferences, by which a person settles on a preferred hierarchy of preferences for making decisions when preferences clash. He notes that a person might seem to have a conflict between a previous preference (say, against life-sustaining treatment in the event of advanced dementia because of a loss of dignity) and a present preference (say, to continue treatment because simple things are now pleasurable). If that person has a resolution preference to prioritize the preservation of dignity over the enjoyment of simple pleasures, then the case can be made for respecting the precedent autonomy expressed in the advance directive to forgo life-sustaining treatments in that situation. Further, he argues that in addition to welfare interests such as air, food, water, and shelter, persons have investment interests in how they are seen, treated, and function in the world and that these interests can survive even as a person loses decision-making capacity. Thus we would not be acting against their interests to respect their precedent autonomy. This series of arguments does not address the epistemological objections to substituted judgment (i.e., how do we know the patient would have that interest if able to speak to us) nor the logical problems with counterfactuals nor the deeper metaethical arguments against the priority of autonomy. Nonetheless, there has not yet been a vigorous reply from those who object to the concept of precedent autonomy.

SOME RECENT CORRECTIVE PROPOSALS

Given all these problems and objections, both empirical and theoretical, several proposals have been made to salvage the substituted judgment approach to making decisions for those who lack decisional capacity by adjusting its theory and application. For instance, Tonelli (1997) proposed a sliding-scale approach. Holding firmly to the primacy of respect for autonomy, Tonelli called for a blending of best interests and substituted judgment—the more the substituted judgment corresponds to the clinicians' objective judgment of the patient's best interests, the less the evidence there must be that the substituted judgment is accurate; the more the decision seems to diverge from the patient's best interests, the higher the required standard of evidence should be set that the substituted judgment truly represents the patient's values and preferences. Braun, Naik, and McCoullough (2009) suggest an algorithm by which only surrogates who are highly certain about their loved ones' preferences should use substituted judgment, while all others pursue a best-interests model. Sabatino (1999) acknowledges many of the defects in substituted judgment and suggests various small changes that might help somewhat, but without abandoning the concept. He simply asks, in effect, is there any better alternative?

Brudney has argued that the mistake in theorizing about deciding for those who cannot decide has been to think that we are trying to respect patients' autonomy when we make substituted judgments (2009). Rather, he suggests, what we are looking for is not a simulacrum of the autonomous choice they are incapable of making, but an authentic choice that is consistent with, and expressive of, the distinctiveness and individuality of the person. While that authentic self results from the accumulation of multiple particular autonomous choices, what we are after is really not the answer to some particular question, such as, "Would Joe have chosen another attempt at weaning from the ventilator before consenting to an order not to be resuscitated?" Rather, we are after the choice that is most reflective of who Joe authentically is. The substituted judgment exercise is, at best, a heuristic device for getting at this deeper and more morally salient issue. Brudney's view is more nuanced, but similar to that of Kuczewski, who proposed a duty to respect the narrative self as a way to maintain a version of substituted judgment, overcome the personal identity critique, and leave some clinical flexibility in interpreting advance directives and prior patient statements (1999).

CALLS FOR ABANDONING SUBSTITUTED JUDGMENT ALTOGETHER

Fagerlin and Schneider (2004) have called for abandoning the use of the living will in favor of using health care proxies. In so doing, however, they made indirect reference to some of the problems associated with substituted judgment and did not endorse it as the favored decision-making model for proxies. This has left the door open for raising the question of whether, in the light of all the critiques raised above, substituted judgment in decision making at the end of life, as we have known it for the last forty years, should finally be put to rest. Several scholars have now explicitly called for a new approach to health care decision making at the end of life. Overall, they propose that (a) living wills should be used by a few people (such as those with no one who could speak for them); (b) health care proxies should be promoted as the preferable form of advance directive; (c) other surrogates, such as family members, should be empowered to make decisions in the absence of treatment directives or formally designated proxies; (d) the practice of asking these surrogates to provide substituted judgments should be abandoned and they instead should be invited to participate in health care decision making on behalf of the patient in a more complex but clinically, morally, and socially reasonable way.

The reasons given by these authors, which can almost serve as a summary of the critiques mentioned in this chapter, include the following:

(a) Data show that actual decision making is an admixture of models (Welie 2001; Berger, DeRenzo, and Schwartz 2008).

(b) Data show that surrogates often make best-interests judgments even when there is contrary evidence about the patient's wishes (Welie 2001; Berger, DeRenzo, and Schwartz 2008).

(c) Courts have been so confused that they even have applied the substituted judgment standard to patients who have never had decision-making capacity (Welie 2001).

(d) The autonomy/best interests dichotomy is false because one cannot know patients' best interests apart from their autonomy (Welie 2001).

(e) While the substituted judgment/best interests dichotomy is sometimes called the subjective/objective distinction, this confuses ontology with epistemology: the patient is always subjectively a person and the objective best interests of the patient are, in reality, intersubjectively knowable (Welie 2001).

(f) The judgment of the patient is perhaps the most critical function of the exercise of autonomy, and that is precisely what the patient without capacity cannot exercise and cannot be substituted (Drane and Coulehan 1995).

(g) That substituted judgment is a fiction because the patients' actual preferences cannot be known (Welie 2001).

(h) In support of this epistemological claim, data show that surrogates are often inaccurate in predictions of patientsí preferences (Torke, Alexander, and Lantos 2008; Berger 2009).

(i) Data show that patients' preferences change over time (Berger, DeRenzo, and Schwartz 2008; Torke, Alexander, and Lantos 2008).

(j) Data show that most patients don't want decisions to be made on their behalf by substituted judgment (Berger, DeRenzo, and Schwartz 2008; Torke, Alexander, and Lantos 2008).

(k) In an environment of increasing cultural diversity, the notion of autonomy as the fundamental moral norm and the use of substituted judgment as the mechanism for achieving this norm are foreign ideas to many people and it may be insensitive to impose this structure upon them (Berger, DeRenzo, and Schwartz 2008).

These critics offer a variety of suggestions for how to replace substituted judgment. Drane and Coulehan (1995) suggest a model based on a complex philosophical anthropology of the patient to support a revised version of best interests. Welie (2001) also suggests a best-interests model but explains that this notion incorporates the notion of the patient as a subject with attendant individuality and individual preferences, a model he calls intersubjective sympathy. Torke, Alexander, and Lantos (2008) suggest a model they argue is not a form of substituted judgment but is not unlike the modified substituted judgment models proposed by Kuczewski and Brudney, based on a narrative conception of the patient. Berger, DeRenzo, and Schwartz (2008) recommend prioritizing proxies over living wills, asking patients to indicate whether they want their specific care directives followed strictly or used as a general guide, all in the service of a "more robust, multi-dimensional notion of autonomy."

ॐ What Does This Body of Work Indicate about the State of Scholarship in Medical Ethics?

These forty years of scholarship on the topic of substituted judgment demonstrate a rich, complex, multidisciplinary commitment to research in medical ethics. The clinical situation at the heart of the matter—the need to decide for those who cannot decide for themselves—remains extremely common, yet extremely vexing both for clinicians and for patients' loved ones. The topic is perennially relevant and well deserving of the extensive attention it has received.

Substituted judgment has been examined through the disciplinary lenses of law, philosophy, medicine, nursing, social psychology, sociology, anthropology, and health services research. The normative perspectives have included, among others, philosophical liberalism, analytic philosophy, communitarianism, and narrative theory. The empirical techniques employed have included an array of quantitative methods, including surveys, experimental designs, and a number of qualitative techniques such as focus groups and qualitative interviews.

The empirical studies have been notable for their emphasis on moral psychology and their engagement with ethical theory. All too often, empirical work in medical ethics consists of opinion surveys, viz., "How many physicians think substituted judgment is a good idea?" By contrast, multiple descriptive ethics studies regarding substituted judgment have been characterized by research that touches upon fundamental values, cultural diversity, and the psychology of medical decision making on behalf of other persons. Empirical researchers, for instance, noted that the theory of substituted judgment depended, to some degree, on empirically testable premises, and these premises were subjected to scrutiny. This is the best that descriptive ethics can offer, and the sophistication of the empirical work about this topic has been exemplary, even if it is often atypical for much empirical research in medical ethics. Perhaps it is a sign that the field is coming of age.

Many of these studies have been conducted by interdisciplinary teams—combinations of clinicians, psychologists, anthropologists, sociologists, philosophers, and lawyers. Philosophers and law professors have found themselves coauthoring empirical papers. Empirical investigators have found themselves coauthoring theoretical papers with philosophers and law professors. Many philosophers and legal scholars have incorporated the empirical findings into their theoretical reflections even if they themselves were not part of any empirical study, showing that they are aware of and are reading the descriptive literature in medical ethics. Even those theorists who continue to defend the substituted judgment standard have grappled with the empirical data and have reacted to these data in their theoretical defenses. Notably, there has been little evidence that either descriptive or normative scholars have overstepped the limits of these data and violated the fact-value distinction. They all seem to be aware that even if the syllogism that "ought implies can" holds true, and it has been shown that surrogates do a poor job at what they are told that they "ought to do" (i.e., provide a substituted judgment), the norm has not thereby been refuted. Neither does the fact that most patients oppose pure substituted judgment refute the norm. These findings may provide serious reasons for questioning the norm, but they do not refute it. One can argue, for example, that the norm is still true and that patients who do not adhere to it are mistaken in their moral views and should be persuaded to want substituted judgment. One also can argue that the norm is true and so important that even if family members are often incorrect in their substituted judgments, they are the best approximation of the moral ideal. Further, one can argue that the norm is true and so important that there is a moral imperative to train potential surrogates so that they can do a better job of providing accurate substituted judgments. Still, the data are compelling, and many will see these counterarguments as either stubborn or unrealistic in light of the fact that ethics must always be the most practical branch of philosophy. Such dialogue between the empirical and the theoretical would be evidence of a mature interdisciplinarity.

Notably, some disciplines have not contributed very extensively to research on this topic. Somewhat surprisingly, for instance, substituted judgment has not seemed to have been a major topic of interest for theologians, at least not since a very early contribution by McCormick (1978). The textbook of theological bioethics by Ashley, deBlois, and O'Rouke (2006) simply endorses the notion in a single paragraph. Cahill (2005) takes a social justice approach to all of bioethics in her recent text, and even though she has two chapters on care at the end of life, she does not address this question. Lammers and Verhey assembled 128 theological essays on bioethics into a single edited volume (1998), but only a few of these essays even mention the issue of substituted judgment, and then, largely in passing, as a narrow idea that is inadequate to the theological dimensions of death and dying. While they often criticize the hegemony of the American conception of autonomy upon which the notion of substituted judgment is founded, theologians have seemed more interested in issues of substance than of process, concentrating on topics such as distinguishing euthanasia from withholding and withdrawing life-sustaining treatments, and the concept of death with dignity.

It may be too recent a development to have been a topic of great interest to historians of ethics, but it is still surprising that substituted judgment has not received more attention in the various histories of bioethics (Rothman 1991; Walter and Klein 2003; Baker and McCullough 2009). When these scholars discuss cases such as *Quinlan* and *Saikewicz*, they emphasize how novel the notion of allowing patients to die was in the 1960s and '70s and describe disputes about who should decide (physicians vs. courts vs. committees), not the standard by which decisions should be made. Jonsen mentions the influence of Robertson and explicitly uses the phrase "substituted judgment" but treats the matter in a somewhat cursory fashion over four pages (1998). One legal scholar, however, while not a professional historian, has provided a comprehensive history of the common law of England and the United States regarding substituted judgment and how this legal fiction came to prominence in thinking about care at the end of life (Harmon 1990).

The most surprising finding, however, is that all this rich discussion and research has not had a great deal of impact on public policy. After the idea was endorsed by the President's Commission (1983), no other U.S. federal commission addressed this issue until the President's Council (2005). The President's Council endorsed proxies over living wills and was mildly critical of the substituted judgment standard, but it made no firm policy recommendations about how proxies ought to decide. There has also been minimal activity on the state level. One notable exception is that the state of Maryland has introduced into its standard living will form a section to allow patients to designate whether they wish the document to be followed strictly or used as a general guide by decision makers (Md. Health-Gen. Code 2009).

Perhaps the lack of attention to this issue as a policy matter is due to the fact that the center of attention in public policy debates regarding bioethics has shifted to concerns about research ethics, such as embryonic stem cells, conflicts of interest for investigators, and the conduct of clinical trials in developing nations. Perhaps since the passage of the Patient Self Determination Act in 1990, policymakers and legislators have simply considered the matter settled. Perhaps it is because the politics of medical ethics in the United States has become so divisive and rancorous that no one wants to open the question for fear that matters might become worse. The fact that the enterprise of bioethics itself has become, in the view of certain lobbying groups, suspect as a movement to promote euthanasia may be deterring politicians from addressing any and all issues regarding care at the end of life. Nonetheless, the numerous questions raised about substituted judgment by both normative and empirical investigators suggest the need to reexplore its wisdom as a matter of public policy.

❧ Concluding Comments

This chapter demonstrates the methodological diversity, sophistication, and serious interdisciplinarity of the body of work on substituted judgment. Multiple disciplines, using an array of methods, have made substantial contributions. Medical ethics research regarding other important normative questions could benefit from the example of the kind of work that has transpired regarding substituted judgment, for the research regarding that topic has demonstrated the vast potential of the many methods of medical ethics.

❧ Notes

1. The first edition of this book explored two examples of scholarship in the field of bioethics: assisted suicide and genetic diagnosis. In this second edition we opted for a new example for several reasons. Assisted suicide and genetic diagnosis were much more topical a decade ago than they are now. This is not to say that no one is writing about these issues anymore or that there is not continued political and policy activity regarding them. Rather, it appears that the intensity of debate and volume of publications regarding these topics is less prevalent now than it was in 2001 (see Shalowitz and Emanuel 2004; also, chapter 2). In addition, as this chapter will show, substituted judgment gives a more robust sense of the potential depth and breadth of multidisciplinary work in medical ethics.

2. Possible world semantics refers to a concept introduced by Leibnitz in his *Theodicy* (and famously satirized by Voltaire), that has proven immensely useful in modal logic since the latter half of the twentieth century, especially in the work of Saul Kripke. One can investigate the meaning of a linguistic expression or the validity of an argument by conceiving of the expression or logical formula in possible worlds that differ from the actual world (see Adams 1995).

❧ References

Adams, R. M. 1995. Possible worlds. In *The Cambridge Dictionary of Philosophy*, ed. R. Audi, 633–34. New York: Cambridge University Press.

Ahronheim, J. C., J. D. Moreno, and C. Zuckerman. 2000. *Ethics in clinical practice*. 2nd ed. Gaithersburg, MD: Aspen, 23–28, 39.

American College of Physicians. 2005. *Ethics manual*. 5th ed. www.acponline.org/running_practice/ethics/manual/ethicman5th.htm#making. Last accessed September 21, 2009.

American Medical Association. 2009. *Code of medical ethics*, Opinion 8.081—Surrogate Decision Making. www.ama-assn.org/ama/pub/physician-resources/medical-ethics/code-medical-ethics/opinion 8081.shtml. Last accessed September 21, 2009.

Annas, G. J. 1980. Quality of life in the courts: Earle Spring in fantasyland. *Hastings Center Report* 10 (4): 9–10.

Ashley, B. M., J. deBlois, and K. D. O'Rourke. 2006. *Health care ethics: A theological analysis*. 5th ed. Washington, DC; Georgetown University Press, 192.

Baker, R. B., and L. B. McCullough, eds. 2009. *The Cambridge world history of medical ethics*. New York: Cambridge University Press.

Beauchamp, T. L., and J. F. Childress. 1979. *Principles of biomedical ethics*. 1st ed. New York: Oxford University Press.

———. 1983. *Principles of biomedical ethics*. 2nd ed. New York: Oxford University Press, 137–41.

———. 1989. *Principles of biomedical ethics*. 3rd ed. New York: Oxford University Press, 173.

———. 1994. *Principles of biomedical ethics*. 4th ed. New York: Oxford University Press, 170–78.

———. 2001. *Principles of biomedical ethics*. 5th ed. New York: Oxford University Press, 103.

———. 2009. *Principles of biomedical ethics*. 6th ed. New York: Oxford University Press.

Berger, J. T. 2009. Patients' concerns for family burden: A nonconforming preference in standards for surrogate decision making. *Journal of Clinical Ethics* 20 (2): 158–61.

Berger, J. T., E. G. DeRenzo, and J. Schwartz. 2008. Surrogate decision making: Reconciling ethical theory and clinical practice. *Annals of Internal Medicine* 149:48–53.

Blustein, J. 1999. Choosing for others as continuing a life story: The problem of personal identity revisited. *Journal of Law Medicine and Ethics* 27:20–31.

Braun, U. K., R. J. Beyth, M. E. Ford, and L. B. McCullough. 2008. Voices of African American, Caucasian, and Hispanic surrogates on the burdens of end-of-life decision making. *Journal of General Internal Medicine* 23:267–74.

Braun, U. K., A. D. Naik, and L. B. McCullough. 2009. Reconceptualizing the experience of surrogate decision making: Reports vs. genuine decisions. *Annals of Family Medicine* 7:249–53.

Brock, D. W. 1996. What is the moral authority of family members to act as surrogates for incompetent patients? *Milbank Quarterly* 74:599–618.

Brudney, D. 2009. Choosing for another: Beyond autonomy and best interests. *Hastings Center Report* 39 (2): 31–37.

Buchanan, A. 1979. Medical paternalism or legal imperialism: Not the only alternatives for handling Saikewicz-type cases. *American Journal of Law and Medicine* 5 (2): 97–117.

Buchanan, A., and D. W. Brock. 1986. Deciding for others. *Milbank Quarterly* 64 (Suppl 2): 17–94.

———. 1990. *Deciding for others: The ethics of surrogate decision making*. New York: Cambridge, 87–126.

Cahill L. 2005. *Theological bioethics: Participation, justice, change*. Washington, DC: Georgetown University Press.

Coppolino M., and L. Ackerson. 2001. Do surrogate decision makers provide accurate consent for intensive care research? *Chest* 119:603–12.

Davis, J. K. 2002. The concept of precedent autonomy. *Bioethics* 16:114–33.

———. 2007. Precedent autonomy, advance directives, and end-of-life care. In *Oxford handbook of bioethics*, ed. B. Steinbock, 349–74. New York: Oxford University Press.

Davis, K. 1978. Constitutional law—right of privacy—qualified right to refuse medical treatment may be asserted for incompetent under doctrine of substituted judgment. *Emory Law Journal* 27 (2): 425–60.

Ditto, P. H., J. H. Danks, W. D. Smucker, J. Bookwalla, K. M. Coppola, R. Dresser, A. Fagerlin, R. M. Gready, R. M. Houts, L. K. Lockhart, and S. Zynanski. 2001. Advance directives as acts of communication: a randomized controlled trial. *Archives of Internal Medicine* 161:421–30.

Drane, J. F., and J. L. Coulehan. 1995. The best-interest standard: Surrogate decision making and quality of life. *Journal of Clinical Ethics* 6 (1): 20–29.

Dresser, R. 1986. Life, death, and incompetent patients: Conceptual infirmities and hidden values in the law. *Arizona Law Review* 28 (3): 373–405.

———. 1995. Dworkin on dementia: Elegant theory, questionable policy. *Hastings Center Report* 25 (6): 32–38.

———. 2003. Precommitment: A misguided strategy for securing death with dignity. *Texas Law Review* 81:1823–47.

Dresser, R. S., and J. A. Robertson. 1989. Quality of life and non-treatment decisions for incompetent patients: A critique of the orthodox approach. *Law Medicine and Health Care* 17 (3): 234–44.

Dunphy, S. M., and J. H. Cross. 1987. Medical decisionmaking for incompetent persons: The Massachusetts substituted judgment model. *Western New England Law Review* 9 (1): 153–67.

Dworkin, R. 1993. *Life's dominion: An argument about abortion, euthanasia, and individual freedom.* New York: Alfred A. Knopf, 222–33.

Ex parte Whitbred, a lunatic, 2 Mer. Rep. 99 (1816).

Fagerlin A., P. H. Ditto, J. H. Danks, R. M. Houts, and W. D. Smucker. 2001. Projection in surrogate decisions about life-sustaining medical treatments. *Health Psychology* 20:166–75.

Fagerlin, A., and C. E. Schneider. 2004. Enough: The failure of the living will. *Hastings Center Report* 34 (2): 30–42.

Fins, J. J., B. S. Maltby, E. Friedmann, M. G. Greene, K. Norris, R. Adelman, and I. Byock. 2005. Contracts, covenants and advance care planning: An empirical study of the moral obligations of patient and proxy. *Journal of Pain and Symptom Management* 29:55–68.

Freedman, B. 1978. On the rights of the voiceless. *Journal of Medicine and Philosophy* 3:196–210.

Gerety, M. B., L. K. Chiodo, D. N. Kanten, M. R. Tuley, J. E. Cornell. 1993. Medical treatment preferences of nursing home residents: Relationship to function and concordance with surrogate decision-makers. *Journal of the American Geriatrics Society* 41:953–60.

Gutheil, T. G., and P. S. Appelbaum. 1983. Substituted judgment: Best interests in disguise. *Hastings Center Report* 13 (3): 8–11.

Hammes, B. J., and B. L. Rooney. 1998. Death and end-of-life planning in one Midwestern community. *Archives of Internal Medicine* 158:383–90.

Handy, C. M., D. P. Sulmasy, C. K. Merkel, and W. A. Ury. 2008. The surrogate's experience in authorizing a do not resuscitate order. *Palliative and Supportive Care* 6 (1): 13–19.

Hardwig, J. 1990. What about the family? *Hastings Center Report* 20 (2): 5–10.

———. 1993. The problem of proxies with interests of their own: Toward a better theory of proxy decisions. *Journal of Clinical Ethics* 4 (1): 20–27.

Hare, J., C. Pratt, and C. Nelson. 1992. Agreement between patients and their self-selected surrogates on difficult medical decisions. *Archives of Internal Medicine* 152:1049–54.

Harmon, L. 1990. Falling off the vine: Legal fictions and the doctrine of substituted judgment. *Yale Law Journal* 100 (1): 1–71.

Hawkins, N. A., P. H. Ditto, J. H. Danks, and W. D. Smucker. 2005. Micromanaging death: Process preferences, values, and goals in end-of-life medical decision making. *Gerontologist* 45 (1): 107–17.

High, D. M. 1989. Caring for decisionally incapacitated elderly. *Theoretical Medicine* 10:83–96.

———. 1994. Families' roles in advance directives. *Hastings Center Report* 24 (6): S16–S18.

Hirschman, K. B., J. M. Kapo, and J. H. Karlawish. 2006. Why doesn't a family member of a person with advanced dementia use a substituted judgment when making a decision for that person? *American Journal of Geriatrics Psychiatry* 14:659–67.

Houts, R. M., W. D. Smucker, J. A. Jacobson, P. H. Ditto, and J. H. Danks. 2002. Predicting elderly outpatients' life-sustaining treatment preferences over time: The majority rules. *Medical Decision Making* 22:39–52.

In re Dinnerstein, 6 Mass. App. Ct. 466, 380 N.E.2d 134 (1978).

In re Eichner, 52 N.Y.2d 363, 420 N.E.2d 64, 438 N YS.2d 266 (1981).

In re Quinlan, 70 N.J. 10, 355 A.2d 647, *cert. denied*, 429 U.S. 922 (1976).

In re Spring, 380 Mass. 629, 405 N.E.2d 115 (1980).

In re Storar, 52 N.Y.2d 363, 438 N YS.2d at 266, 420 N.E.2d 64 *cert. denied*, 454 U.S. 858 (1981).

In re Willoughby, a Lunatic, 11 Paige 257 (N.Y. 1844).

Jonsen, A. R. 1998. *The birth of bioethics*. New York: Oxford University Press, 266–69.

Jonsen, A. R., M. Siegler, and W. J. Winslade. 2006. *Clinical ethics: A practical approach to ethical decisions in clinical medicine*. 6th ed. New York: McGraw-Hill, 89–91.

Kuczewski, M. G. 1996. Reconceiving the family. The process of consent in medical decisionmaking. *Hastings Center Report* 26 (2): 30–37.

———. 1999. Commentary: Narrative views of personal identity and substituted judgment in surrogate decision making. *Journal of Law Medicine and Ethics* 27 (1): 32–36.

Lammers, S. E., and A. Verhey, eds. 1998. *On moral medicine: Theological perspectives in medical ethics*. 2nd ed. Grand Rapids, MI: Wm. B. Eerdmans.

Lausier V. Pescinski 67 Wisc. 2d 4, 226, N.W.2d. 180 (1975).

Layde, P. M., C. A. Beam, S. K. Broste et al. 1995. Surrogates' predictions of seriously ill patients' resuscitation preferences. *Archives of Family Medicine* 4:518–23.

Levine, C., and C. Zuckerman. 1999. The trouble with families: Toward an ethic of accommodation. *Annals of Internal Medicine* 130:148–52.

Libbus, M. K., and C. Russell. 1995. Congruence of decisions between patients and their potential surrogates about life-sustaining therapies. *Image: The Journal of Nursing Scholarship* 27:135–40.

Mantravadi, A. V., B. P. Sheth, R. S. Gonnering, and D. G. Covert. 2007. Accuracy of surrogate decision making in elective surgery. *Journal of Cataract and Refractive Surgery* 33:2091–97.

Marbella, A. M., N. A. Desbiens, N. Mueller-Rizner, and P. M. Layde. 1998. Surrogates' agreement with patients' resuscitation preferences: effect of age, relationship, and support intervention: Study to understand prognoses and preferences for outcomes and risks of treatment. *Journal of Critical Care* 13:140–45.

Martyn, S. R., and L. B. Jacobs. 1984. Legislating advance directives for the terminally ill: The living will and durable power of attorney. *Nebraska Law Review* 63:779–809.

Md. Health-Gen. Code Ann. § 5-603 (2009).

Matheis-Kraft, C., and K. A. Roberto. 1997. Influence of a values discussion on congruence between elderly women and their families on critical health care decisions. *Journal of Women and Aging* 9:5–22.

McCormick, R. A. 1978. Freedman on the rights of the voiceless. *Journal of Medicine and Philosophy* 3:211–21.

Miura, Y., A. Asai, M. Matsushima, S. Nagata, M. Onishi, T. Shimbo, T. Hosoya, and S. Fukuhara. 2006. Families' and physicians' predictions of dialysis patients' preferences regarding life-sustaining treatments in Japan. *American Journal of Kidney Disease* 47 (1): 122–30.

Nagasawa, Y. 2008. Proxy consent and counterfactuals. *Bioethics* 22 (1): 16–24.

Nelson, H. L., and J. L. Nelson. 1994. Preferences and other moral sources. *Hastings Center Report* 24 (6): S19–S21.

Nolan, M. T., M. T. Hughes, D. P. Narenda, J. R. Sood, P. B. Terry, J. Kub, R. Thompson, and D. P. Sulmasy. 2005. When patients lack capacity: The roles that patients with terminal diagnoses would choose for their physicians and loved ones in making medical decisions. *Journal of Pain and Symptom Management* 30:342–53.

O'Neil, R. 1983. Determining proxy consent. *Journal of Medicine and Philosophy* 8:389–403.

Ouslander, J. G., A. J. Tymchuk, and B. Rahbar. 1989. Health care decisions among elderly long-term care residents and their potential proxies. *Archives of Internal Medicine* 149:1367–72.

Patient Self-Determination Act. Omnibus Budget Reconciliation Act of 1990, Pub. L. No. 101–508 §§ 4206, 4751.

Pearlman, R. A., R. F. Uhlmann, and N. S. Jecker. 1992. Spousal understanding of patient quality of life: Implications for surrogate decisions. *Journal of Clinical Ethics* 3:114–23.

President's Commission for the Study of Ethical Problems in Medicine and Biomedical and Behavioral Research. 1983. *Deciding to forgo life-sustaining treatment: Ethical, medical, and legal issues in treatment decisions.* Washington, DC: U.S. Government Printing Office.

President's Council on Bioethics. 2005. *Taking care: Ethical caregiving in our aging society.* Washington, DC: Government Printing Office, 63–65, 215–16.

Principe-Rodriguez K., W. Rodriguez-Cintron, A. Torres-Palacios, and J. Casal-Hidalgo. 1999. Substituted judgement: Should life-support decisions be made by a surrogate? *Puerto Rico Health Sciences Journal* 18:405–9.

Pruchno, R. A., E. P. Lemay Jr., L. Feild, and N. G. Levinsky. 2005. Spouse as health care proxy for dialysis patients: Whose preferences matter? *Gerontologist* 45:812–19.

Puchalski, C. M., Z. Zhong, M. M. Jacobs, E. Fox, J. Lynn, J. Harrold, A. Galanos, R. S. Phillips, R. Califf, and J. M. Teno. 2000. Patients who want their family and physician to make resuscitation decisions for them: Observations from SUPPORT and HELP. Study to understand prognoses and preferences for outcomes and risks of treatment. Hospitalized elderly longitudinal project. *Journal of the American Geriatrics Society* 48 (5 Suppl): S84–S90.

Relman, A. S. 1978. The Saikewicz decision: Judges as physicians. *New England Journal of Medicine* 298:508–9.

Rich B. A. 1997. Prospective autonomy and critical interests: A narrative defense of the moral authority of advance directives. *Cambridge Quarterly of Healthcare Ethics* 6 (2): 138–47.

Robertson, J. A. 1976. Organ donations by incompetents and the substituted judgment doctrine. *Columbia Law Review* 76 (1): 48–78.

———. 1991. Second thoughts on living wills. *Hastings Center Report* 21 (6): 6–9.

Rothman, D. J. 1991. *Strangers at the bedside: A history of how law and bioethics transformed medical decision making.* New York: Basic Books.

Sabatino, C. P. 1999. The legal and functional status of the medical proxy: Suggestions for statutory reform. *Journal of Law Medicine and Ethics* 27 (1): 52–68.

Seckler, A. B., D. E. Meier, M. Mulvihill, and B. E. Cammer-Paris. 1991. Substituted judgment: How accurate are proxy decisions? *Annals of Internal Medicine* 115:92–98.

Sehgal, A., A. Galbraith, M. Chesney, P. Schoenfeld, G. Charles, and B. Lo. 1992. How strictly do dialysis patients want their advance directives followed? *Journal of the American Medical Association* 267:59–63.

Shalowitz, D., and E. Emanuel. 2004. Euthanasia and physician-assisted suicide: Implications for physicians. *Journal of Clinical Ethics* 15:232–36.

Shalowitz, D. I., E. Garrett-Mayer, and D. Wendler. 2006. The accuracy of surrogate decision makers: A systematic review. *Archives of Internal Medicine* 166:493–97.

Smucker, W. D., R. M. Houts, J. H. Danks, P. H. Ditto, A. Fagerlin, and K. M. Coppola. 2000. Modal preferences predict elderly patients' life-sustaining treatment choices as well as patients' chosen surrogates do. *Medical Decision Making* 20:271–80.

Strunk v. Strunk, 445 S.W. 2d 145 (1969).

Suber, D. G., and W. J. Tabor. 1982a. Withholding of life-sustaining treatment from the terminally ill, incompetent patient: Who decides? Part I. *Journal of the American Medical Association* 248:2250–51.

———. 1982b. Withholding of life-sustaining treatment from the terminally ill, incompetent patient: Who decides? Part II. *Journal of the American Medical Association* 248:2431–32.

Sugarman, J. 1994. Recognizing good decisionmaking for incapacitated patients. *Hastings Center Report* 24 (6): S11–S13.

Suhl, J., P. Simons, T. Reedy, and T. Garrick. 1994. Myth of substituted judgment: Surrogate decision making regarding life support is unreliable. *Archives of Internal Medicine* 154:90–96.

Sulmasy, D. P., K. Haller, and P. B. Terry. 1994. More talk, less paper: Predicting the accuracy of substituted judgments. *American Journal of Medicine* 96:432–38.

Sulmasy, D. P., M. T. Hughes, R. E. Thompson, A. B. Astrow, P. B. Terry, J. Kub, and M. T. Nolan. 2007. How would terminally ill patients have others make decisions for them in the event of decisional incapacity? A longitudinal study. *Journal of the American Geriatrics Society* 55:1981–88.

Sulmasy, D. P., J. R. Sood, K. Texeira, R. McAuley, J. McGugins, and W. A. Ury. 2006. Prospective trial of a new policy eliminating signed consent for do not resuscitate orders. *Journal of General Internal Medicine* 21:1261–68.

Sulmasy, D. P., P. B. Terry, C. S. Weisman, D. J. Miller, R. Y. Stallings, M. A. Vettese, and K. B. Haller. 1998. The accuracy of substituted judgments in patients with terminal diagnoses. *Annals of Internal Medicine* 128:621–29.

Superintendent of Belchertown State School v. Saikewicz, 373 Mass. 728, 370 N.E.2d 417 (1977).

Terry, P. B., M. Vettese, J. Song, J. Forman, K. B. Haller, D. J. Miller, R. Stallings, and D. P. Sulmasy. 1999. End-of-life decision making: When patients and surrogates disagree. *Journal of Clinical Ethics* 10: 286–93.

Tilden, V. P., S. W. Tolle, C. A. Nelson, and J. Fields. 2001. Family decision-making to withdraw life-sustaining treatments from hospitalized patients. *Nursing Research* 50 (2): 105–15.

Tolle, S. W., V. P. Tilden, C. A. Nelson, and P. M. Dunn. 1998. A prospective study of the efficacy of the physician order form for life-sustaining treatment." *Journal of the American Geriatrics Society* 46: 1097–1102.

Tomlinson, T., K. Howe, M. Notman, and D. Rossmiller. 1990. An empirical study of proxy consent for elderly persons. *The Gerontologist* 30: 54–64.

Tonelli, M. R. 1997. Substituted judgment in medical practice: evidentiary standards on a sliding scale. *Journal of Law Medicine and Ethics* 25 (1): 22–29, 2.

Torke, A. M., C. G. Alexander, and J. Lantos. 2008. Substituted judgment: The limitations of autonomy in surrogate decision making. *Journal of General Internal Medicine* 23 (9): 1514–17.

Uhlmann, R. F., R. A. Pearlman, and K. C. Cain. 1988. Physicians' and spouses' predictions of elderly patients' resuscitation preferences. *Journal of Gerontology* 43: M 115–21.

Vig, E. K., H. Starks, J. S. Taylor, E. K. Hopley, and K. Fryer-Edwards. 2007. Surviving surrogate decision-making: What helps and hampers the experience of making medical decisions for others. *Journal of General Internal Medicine* 22:1274–79.

Vig, E. K., J. S. Taylor, H. Starks, E. K. Hopley, and K. Fryer-Edwards. 2006. Beyond substituted judgment: How surrogates navigate end-of-life decision-making. *Journal of the American Geriatrics Society* 54:1688–93.

Walter, J. K., and E. P. Klein, eds. 2003. *The story of bioethics: From seminal works to contemporary explorations.* Washington, DC: Georgetown University Press.

Weber, W. M. 1985–86. Substituted judgment doctrine: A critical analysis. *Issues in Law & Medicine* 1:131–59.

Welie, J. V. 2001. Living wills and substituted judgments: A critical analysis. *Medicine Health Care and Philosophy* 4 (2): 169–83.

Wierenga, E. 1983. Proxy consent and counterfactual wishes. *Journal of Medicine and Philosophy* 8 (4): 405–16.

Zweibel, N. R., and C. K. Cassel. 1989. Treatment choices at the end of life: A comparison of decisions by older patients and their physician-selected proxies. *Gerontologist* 29:615–21.

CHAPTER 18

Reading the Medical Ethics Literature

A Discourse on Method

DANIEL P. SULMASY

W hat constitutes a good paper or book in medical ethics? This important question cannot be decided merely by whether or not one agrees with the conclusion of a paper or a book! As the previous chapters should make clear, there are many fine works in medical ethics written by talented authors who employ a wide variety of methods. The best of these works genuinely expand knowledge, expose hidden assumptions, challenge prevailing convictions, make rigorous arguments, enrich understanding, or illuminate contentious issues in fresh ways. However, frankly speaking, the medical ethics literature is also filled with chaff—often sincere chaff—but chaff nonetheless. The aim of this chapter is to provide an overview on how to read the medical ethics literature critically, separating the golden grains of wheat from the inconsequential chaff.

The many methods of medical ethics make this a very challenging task. Many readers of the literature of medical ethics are not trained in the particular research disciplines of the authors. Clinicians, for example, are often keenly interested in medical ethics, yet their training rarely equips them to read studies about ethics sensibly and critically. Many scholars in the field of medical ethics read research studies conducted by scholars in other disciplines, often examining the same questions they themselves are examining. However, they may be unfamiliar with the methods and disciplinary assumptions of their colleagues across the campus and unsure how to apply this work to their own inquiry. In addition, many people who are neither clinicians nor scholars are interested in the writings of medical ethicists. Since the issues of medical ethics affect the lives of almost everyone, all readers of the medical ethics literature have an interest in distinguishing sound bites from sound scholarship.

Editors and peer reviewers for journals in medicine and medical ethics have a special need to understand how to judge the quality of scholarship in medical ethics.

The editors of medical journals are often scientists for whom any paper that does not present empirical data in numerical form is considered opinion. They might have little experiential basis for distinguishing an editorial from a philosophical essay or a qualitative empirical study, let alone judging whether these are good or bad pieces of scholarship. In such cases editors generally rely upon the judgments of peer reviewers. However, without sufficient background, they might even have difficulty determining who should play the role of peer. For instance, many editors of medical journals seem not to value advanced training in medical ethics as an important qualification for reviewers of submissions in medical ethics (Schulman, Sulmasy, and Roney 1994; Landy et al. 2009).

This chapter provides suggestions about aspects of medical ethics research that readers, editors, and reviewers might want to look for in assessing the quality of scholarship in the field. If there is to be a genuinely interdisciplinary exchange in medical ethics research, readers must know at least the rudiments of how to critically read the work of colleagues in other disciplines. Otherwise, discourse about medical ethics will remain fragmented and much less helpful than it might be otherwise. At the risk of creating a false dichotomy, the discussion is divided into two categories: humanities research and descriptive research.[1] Each category is discussed in turn.

∿ Judging Good Humanities Research in Medical Ethics

The authors of chapters 3 though 10 all have offered some insights into what counts as good quality scholarship in their respective disciplines. Nonetheless, it is helpful to collate these rules, customs, suggestions, and fallacies and expand upon them. Some of these are widely applicable to all scholars working in the humanities, not just medical ethicists. For example, DeGrazia and Beauchamp (2001) have outlined some of the features they believe are evidence of excellent work in philosophical medical ethics, such as the importance of the topic, the clarity of the writing, the strength of the arguments, and the novelty of the ideas presented. McCullough, Coverdale, and Chervenak (2004) suggest several important questions to ask in assessing a normative ethical argument: Is the ethical question clear, focused, and important? Are the arguments valid? Is the literature reviewed comprehensively, used appropriately in the argument, and cited accurately? Will the conclusions be useful in policy or practice? In addition, in chapter 1, Jeremy Sugarman and I describe in detail a set of logical fallacies to be avoided, such as arguments based on brute biological facts, appeals to authority, majority opinion, historical precedent, and the fact that a practice is legal. These criteria can be useful to assess the quality of scholarship in medical ethics that employs many of the methods of the humanities.

Other features of good scholarship will be particular to a specific humanistic discipline or areas of research. Pellegrino (chapter 6), for instance, explains how codes of ethics can figure in moral arguments legitimately without falling into the logical fallacy of the argument from authority. Lederer (chapter 9) criticizes the use of historical relativism in works of medical ethics and history. Chambers (chapter 10) warns against excessive reliance on the literary scholar's technique of interpreting the world as a text, which can degenerate into an all-consuming fetish.

Nonetheless, it would seem that there are some rules, customs, suggestions, and fallacies that are common to excellent humanities research in medical ethics that have not been addressed elsewhere in the medical ethics literature or in this book. Some of these may seem obvious, but precisely because they are so obvious they may be overlooked. Others concern the ways in which scholarship in medical ethics crosses disciplinary boundaries and must therefore be addressed not in individual chapters about particular methods, but only in a chapter that surveys work in medical ethics as a whole. This first section of this chapter proposes standards by which one can be a critical reader of the humanities literature in medical ethics. This section draws upon well-established standards for essay composition (e.g., Strunk and White 1959; Crews 1974), as well as works on philosophical writing (Watson 1992; Martinich 1996). Even if everything proposed in this chapter is not endorsed wholeheartedly by all scholars, this chapter will provide at least a point of departure for future discussion and refinement of these standards.

STRUCTURE

The contribution of the humanities to medical ethics is frequently to make normative arguments, and normative arguments have a customary structure. Good normative writing usually requires a beginning, a middle, and an end; that is, an introduction stating the thesis, an argument to prove it, and a conclusion. This more or less has been the structure of a good argument since the time of Aristotle (1941). Of course, the very best writers manage to do this in such an effortless way that the underlying structure is not so apparent. But this structure will be expected by most serious readers of a normative argument, just as a clinician expects a chief complaint at the beginning of a case presentation, or a scientist expects that a description of the methods will follow the introduction to a scientific paper. Readers who fail to find such a structure will be either confused or forced to conclude that the author is trying to hide something or is confused.

ASSUMPTIONS

Second, since scholarship in medical ethics is generally concerned with arguments, good humanities writing in this field will move from premises to conclusions. Yet it is important to recognize that all of these arguments are based upon assumptions. Arguments cannot start from scratch. Therefore, a well-written paper in medical ethics using the methods of the humanities will include an explicit discussion of the underlying assumptions. If the assumptions are not given directly, the critical reader will need to arrive at them inferentially after having read the whole paper. For example, philosophers often have particular theoretical orientations. They therefore should acknowledge explicitly that their analysis is utilitarian or Rawlsian or libertarian or based upon some other theoretical orientation. It is difficult to evaluate a non-empirical paper critically without knowledge of the underlying assumptions and the author's theoretical orientation.

Further, as Brody (1990) has pointed out, the work is better if it also acknowledges that the assumptions of the author may not be shared by all readers, and attempts to show how other theoretical orientations might lead to similar conclusions. Quality scholarship in medical ethics is aware of and in dialogue with moral traditions other than those of the author.

DEFINITIONS

Third, medical ethics research by scholars in the humanities often makes use of technical terms or employs ordinary words in technical ways. Good research in the humanities defines the terms used in the book or article. This may be done up front, early in the work. Alternatively, terms may be defined as they are introduced. Critical readers will look for such definitions.

Sometimes entire arguments turn upon how the terms are defined. The informal logical fallacy of *petitio principi* ("begging the question") means that the conclusion of the argument is already contained in the premises (Copi 1982). For example, if one defines killing as morally unjustified, then defines euthanasia as killing, and then concludes that euthanasia is morally unjustified, one has begged the question. This fallacy is very common in published arguments about medical ethics. It often goes unnoticed because the terms have not been clearly defined. The definitions are simply assumed, are obliquely acknowledged, or are separated by long strings of additional but unnecessary premises. When the terms are defined clearly, however, the logical error becomes obvious.

Of note, the term "begging the question" is itself often misconstrued and misused. It does not mean "this question cries out for an answer" but refers to an argument that has assumed its conclusion at the outset. Definitions clearly count, even for words or phrases like "begging the question" that proscribe the improper use of definitions.

INTERNAL CONSISTENCY

Fourth, arguments must be internally consistent. One can disagree with an author's premises, but this does not mean that the argument is wrong, unless one can prove that the premises are wrong. Regardless of whether one agrees with the premises or the conclusion, to show that one part of an argument contradicts another is to show that the argument is invalid. Good arguments (sound arguments) are at least internally consistent.

FACTUAL CORRECTNESS

Fifth, work in the humanities in medical ethics must not employ any factual misconceptions. It is sometimes the case that a philosophical or theological or legal argument in medical ethics is based upon misconceptions about the medical facts. This provides an easy way to refute the argument. Such a refutation can be a genuine embarrassment to the author.

In pointing to the importance of correct medical facts, however, it must be acknowledged that some medical "facts" are in dispute and open to interpretation. When this is the case, authors should be careful to consider alternative interpretations of the scientific or medical data and the ways in which this might affect the arguments, even in a work employing methods from the humanities to address issues in medical ethics.

FIRM GRASP OF THE LITERATURE

Sixth, the author should demonstrate a firm grasp of the relevant literature. This often is demonstrated by citation of these other works, but citation alone does not suffice to establish either that the author has truly grasped this literature, or that the author has been able to situate his or her work within this wider discourse. Sometimes, particularly in medical journals, authors seem to feel that since they have no "data," they must prove that they have been rigorous by citing dozens, even hundreds of books and papers in preparing their own essays. One should be cautious about such essays. Citing 150 books and papers can be a poor substitute for demonstrating the type of genuine grasp of the relevant literature that is necessary to make a good nonempirical argument. Sometimes, for example, whole books are cited in support of very specific points, yet the relevant page number may not be included in the citation. Quite often, authors engage in what has been dubbed "proof-texting," plucking isolated quotes out of the context of the larger body of work of a classical or renowned scholar in order to claim an authority in support of the author's own thesis. Sometimes, it seems as if the author has only read the online abstract of a work yet has cited the entire paper or book. The arguments made in the humanities are usually complex and subtle; they need to be read carefully and understood fully before they can be cited properly. The point is that a good essay in casuistry or history or theology or law, for example, must demonstrate either a grasp of the subtleties of the extant literature or a profound, sweeping, "forest-for-the-trees" interpretation of this literature as an integrated body of work. Otherwise, it is not very good scholarship.

COUNTERARGUMENTS

Seventh, it is important to be sure that the authors of a humanities work in medical ethics have considered counterarguments. Good scholars know that others may disagree with them or have differing arguments. These arguments must be weighed carefully, and major objections to the author's own position ought to be considered and addressed in a nonempirical paper. Works that do this well are stronger works. One should be wary, however, of counterarguments that unfairly represent the position of those who hold the opposite view or present only the weakest sort of counterarguments that no serious opponent would endorse. These weak counterarguments are called "straw man" arguments. Critical readers of humanities studies in medical ethics should be alert to the use of such arguments.

∾ Judging Good Descriptive Research in Medical Ethics

Chapters 12 through 16 describe many of the empirical methods used in descriptive medical ethics. Obviously, some studies in descriptive medical ethics are better than others. The authors of these chapters on empirical methods have described in detail how to conduct excellent studies in descriptive ethics. But what should a reader of the medical ethics literature look for in attempting to separate the wheat from the chaff in these disciplines?

As the chapters in this volume make clear, descriptive medical ethics is remarkably multidisciplinary. Each of a multitude of disciplines contributes a set of methods and criteria for scholarly excellence. These methods are applied to the investigation of moral questions and are to be judged according to the criteria for scholarly excellence proper to the discipline. The methods may be quantitative or qualitative. They may be unique to a particular discipline or shared by several. But the work that results is to be judged according to how well it meets the criteria for scholarly excellence established for studies in its discipline. Thus, one judges an anthropological study in medical ethics according to the standards of the discipline of anthropology and an economic study according to the standards of the discipline of economics.

One factor complicates this situation tremendously. What draws all these scholars together is a common interest in the study of moral questions in medical practice. Medical ethics is a single field of inquiry, studied by many empirical disciplines, using a variety of methods. Yet no single scholar is capable of mastering all these various disciplines, each with its own proper methods, technical vocabulary, and standards. Thus, it is critical that these scholars be able to communicate their research in a way that emphasizes the rigors that are proper to their own disciplines but in a manner that is accessible to a very diverse audience. Since such communication skills are difficult to cultivate, this can be extremely challenging. Scholars in medical ethics should make an effort to understand the rudiments of the methods of the numerous other disciplines that contribute to this field. But no one can be the master of all these various trades. The onus really falls upon each scholar to communicate research results in jargon-free language without sacrificing the scholarly rigors of the field. This makes the multidisciplinary character of descriptive medical ethics research very challenging.

QUALITATIVE RESEARCH

Many topics in medical ethics are not readily amenable to quantitative research using surveys that consist of closed-ended questions with multiple-choice answers. Such a survey is appropriate when the researchers have a sufficient level of understanding of the research population that they can create a range of responses that will capture the opinions of the respondents. However, making such an assumption in the case of medical ethics could be presumptuous. This is one of the main reasons that researchers in descriptive ethics have begun increasingly to turn to qualitative methods.

Qualitative research does not simply consist of a group of well-intentioned researchers devising a few open-ended questions and then presenting their interpretation of the responses. Careful readers will want to be sure that the research has been conducted according to the standards of excellence delineated by Taylor, Hull, and Kass in chapter 12, and Marshall and Koenig in chapter 13. Such readers will look for evidence that the authors have used appropriate methods, such as observational studies, ethnographic interviews, focus groups, and Delphi panels.

Observational studies

The authors of qualitative studies in medical ethics that are based on observation should clarify whether they have used direct observation, or participant-observer techniques, as distinguished by Taylor, Hull, and Kass (chapter 12) and Marshall and Koenig (chapter 13). They should specify their methods of data collection (e.g., whether they have used field notes, tape recordings, or both). They should comment on the degree of engagement by participant–observer, as described by Marshall and Koenig (chapter 13). The length of time devoted to this type of study should typically be specified in the report. In good studies this time period is rather extended. For example, a report based on a weekend spent interviewing refugees in a border camp should be viewed with skepticism. Participant observation is very labor intensive. Studies that report having utilized this technique are preferred to studies that simply report anecdotal experiences or episodic observations.

Ethnographic interviews

Ethnographic interviews are another important type of qualitative research method used in medical ethics (Ventres and Frankel 1996). A research report of a study that used this technique and was well conducted will report whether interviews were structured or semistructured, and whether the subjects were chosen randomly, by convenience-sampling, or by key-informant methods, as Marshall and Koenig point out (chapter 13).

Good ethnographic interviews will clearly define the research question. The report of a well-conducted study will describe how the data were analyzed, using specific techniques such as saturation, triangulation, and "thick description" (chapters 12 and 13). Reports of these studies will also include frank acknowledgment of sources of bias in interpretation of the observations. Studies that include such methodological rigor can give excellent information about actual behavior, for example, how health care professionals act in settings of interest to medical ethics, or about medical ethics decision making in particular familial or cultural contexts.

Focus groups

Focus groups are a systematic method for gathering qualitative information in a setting in which individuals are able to generate ideas by discussing a defined topic in a group setting and to respond to the remarks of others in the group (Morgan 1997). There are many opportunities to make use of such techniques in descriptive medical ethics. However, critical readers will be wary of whether such studies have conformed to the methodologic rigor described by Taylor, Hull, and Kass (chapter 12) and by Marshall and Koenig (chapter 13). Good reports should describe the focus group technique employed, and this method should be appropriate to the goals of the study. For example, the Nominal Group Technique is designed to avoid dominance by any particular member and to generate a wide variety of ideas arranged in a hierarchy of importance (Delbecq, Van de Ven, and Gustafson 1975). Other kinds of focus groups can be run using techniques to achieve consensus. Like reports of good ethnographic analyses, reports of focus group research should describe the composition of the groups, who ran them, how the data were collected, and what method was used to generate themes from the data, and frankly acknowledge potential sources of bias in interpretation and steps taken to minimize this bias. Without such information, the reader should be skeptical of whether the research was well conducted.

Delphi panels

An important semiquantitative technique not discussed in either chapter 12 or 13 is the use of Delphi panels. A Delphi panel is a formal method for achieving a consensus opinion among a group of experts regarding a particular topic (Delbecq, Van de Ven, and Gustafson 1975). This technique is particularly useful when it is not feasible to bring the members of the group together in a single, face-to-face session. Experts are asked to respond to a question, rank their answers, and explain their answers in a written fashion. The responses are collated, kept anonymous, and circulated among the group through a series of iterations until consensus is reached. Sometimes this technique is used to provide information that is fed into formal decision analyses (see chapter 16).

QUANTITATIVE METHODS

Quantitative research can also play an important role in medical ethics scholarship. Two such approaches are survey research and experimental methods. When one uses quantitative methods, it is critical that the data are appropriately analyzed.

Survey research

In chapter 14 Pearlman and Starks describe how excellent survey research should be conducted in medical ethics. Since survey research is probably the most common type of research technique in descriptive medical ethics (see chapter 2), anyone interested in medical ethics should know the rudiments of how to read a report of a medical ethics survey in a careful, critical fashion. Surveys serve good purposes, pointing out both areas of disagreement and interesting associations between particular opinions and certain characteristics of the population under study. More sophisticated survey instruments try to elicit more basic underlying attitudes, psychological tendencies, cultural norms, or stages of moral development.

Careful readers ought to remember that while simple opinion surveys can be very important in identifying ethical controversies, the best studies do more than simply ask a few questions and count up the answers. In assessing the quality of descriptive ethics research using surveys, critical readers should expect that the authors will state clearly that they have designed the study according to the sorts of standards outlined by Pearlman and Starks (chapter 14). The authors of a research study should indicate the hypotheses that led them to design the survey. Questions should avoid framing bias (i.e., phrasing a question in such a way as to influence the response). Ideally, the exact wording of the most important question in the study should be reported in the paper, so that readers can judge for themselves whether the question was properly constructed. There should be some evidence that the questions validly reflect the information being sought. Better studies will report having done this by actual testing for face validity, criterion validity, and/or construct validity, as described in chapter 14. There should also be some mention that the questions were pilot tested before the actual survey was fielded.

The main outcome variable in a survey tends to be more valid if it is a scale based on several questions than if it is a single item on a survey (Neuman 1994). This is especially important if the researchers are trying to examine deep underlying attitudes, cultural norms, psychological tendencies, or stages of moral reasoning. As Pearlman and Starks discuss, these scales need to be checked for internal consistency. Research reports should indicate this using appropriate statistical tests such as Cronbach's α.

Certain factors that are often of interest in descriptive ethics research have been studied extensively by multiple other investigators who have developed valid and reliable instruments. Thus, there is generally no need for researchers to create new instruments to measure anxiety, depression, dementia, confusion, functional status, severity of illness, or quality of life. There are plenty of scales available to measure such factors. One should be wary of studies that include idiosyncratic measures of well-studied factors such as dementia and even more wary of studies that report on such complex phenomena on the basis of single questions rather than scales.

Of course, there may be valid reasons for descriptive ethics researchers to develop their own scales for such factors in particular circumstances, but the justification for doing so should be stated clearly. For example, there could be a priori reasons to suspect that severity-of-illness scales developed for unselected patients might differ from severity-of-illness scales for patients suffering from chronic, terminal conditions, leading researchers to develop and validate their own instruments particular to a group of patients who generate considerable ethical interest (Knaus et al. 1995).

Basic demographic characteristics of the respondents also should be presented in a good survey report. Response rates should be adequate (generally about 70 percent or more for patients, nurses, house officers, or students, and about 50 percent or more for practicing physicians). Some reporting on the characteristics of nonrespondents should be given to help to support the contention that there has been little response bias.

Survey research in descriptive ethics can be very helpful and very interesting, but there must be clear evidence in the research reports that the survey has been carefully constructed, administered, analyzed, and interpreted.

Experimental methods

The ability to introduce the experimental method into medical ethics could, as Thomasma (1985) noted, only enhance the field. Critical readers will want to be sure they know when experimental methods are appropriate in medical ethics. As described in detail by Danis, Hanson, and Garrett (chapter 15), experimental methods are best employed when ethical or legal theory has proposed a normative standard and one wishes to test whether or not that standard can be met in actual clinical practice. A program designed to promote a particular clinical behavior deemed morally praiseworthy (e.g., better informed consent practices) or designed to educate clinicians about a new law or about ethics in general can be tested by a controlled trial. As pointed out in chapter 15, all of the rigorous standards appropriate to the conduct of excellent randomized clinical trials in any field of medicine should be applied to the assessment of the quality of randomized clinical trials in medical ethics (see, for example, Meinert [1986]).

The analysis of quantitative data

Analysis of data in reports of research in descriptive ethics should follow standard procedures for statistical testing, as detailed in chapter 15. Readers who are unfamiliar with statistics but who are skeptical about a finding can ask colleagues who are skilled in this area to review the research report.

Readers should be particularly careful in evaluating studies that present correlations. Correlations between outcome variables and sociodemographic, clinical, or other respondent characteristics should be reported in a manner that takes into account multiple associations, using, for example, multivariable regression models (Concato, Feinstein, and Holford 1993). There should be adequate numbers of events so that any regression model reported is neither underfitted (too few events to detect important associations) nor overfitted (too many subjects with too few events). Correlations are not sufficient to infer causation, and authors should be very careful not to imply that this is so.

Systematic reviews and meta-analyses are becoming quite prevalent in the medical literature. When a sufficient number of studies has been conducted regarding a single question using equivalent methods, one can review all these studies in a rigorous and systematic way to assess the methodological quality of the studies and one may pool all of the results into a single overall analysis. These techniques are being used increasingly in bioethics, studying questions as diverse as the frequency with which biomedical researchers fabricate their data (Fanelli 2009), the prevalence of moral distress among nurses (Dierckx de Casterlé et al. 2008), and the accuracy of surrogates' substituted judgments (Shalowitz, Garrett-Mayer, and Wendler 2006). Very strict methodological criteria for conducting and reporting such studies have been promulgated (Liberati et al. 2009).

An additional issue is the difference between statistical significance and clinical or moral importance. For example, if one has ten thousand study subjects and wants to investigate factors associated with responses to a single question (e.g., Do you want to be resuscitated?), even the patient's shoe size might randomly show a statistically significant association. In these cases researchers bear important responsibility for justifying the sample size and for sorting out the important variables.

Subgroup analyses should reflect genuine preconceived hypotheses or be acknowledged explicitly as an exercise in hypothesis generation. "Data dredging" for statistically significant results is all too common and should be avoided. If the study was not designed to compare subgroups, such analysis may be misleading.

Interpretation of the data should scrupulously avoid normative conclusions. It may be interesting, for example, if one were to discover that 75 percent of physicians do not believe they are bound by the precepts of the Hippocratic Oath. It would be inappropriate, however, to suggest that this means that the Hippocratic Oath should no longer be considered normative for medical practice. That may or may not be the case, depending upon the strength of various normative arguments.

THEORETICAL FRAMEWORK

Empirical research in sociology, anthropology, and psychology is often judged on the basis of whether or not it specifies a particular theoretical framework. This will be true as well of empirical research in medical ethics that is approached from any of these disciplines. But while this is a necessary ingredient for the highest-quality research in descriptive ethics, it is not sufficient. Excellent descriptive research in medical ethics will not only specify the theoretical framework particular to the empirical discipline, it will also explicitly designate the ethical theory that undergirds the research. So, for example, a study on end-of-life decision making that employs a willingness-to-pay utility analysis and also acknowledges specifically that the moral theory undergirding the study is preference-based utilitarianism is superior to a study in which the authors do not appear to understand whether or not they are operating within the framework of any particular theory of ethics (see chapter 16).

As Brody (1993) has pointed out, even in the absence of a specifically acknowledged theoretical orientation, the investigators must be able to conceptualize the question from an ethical perspective in order to conduct solid projects in descriptive ethics. Failure to conceptualize the research adequately from an ethical point of view will make the study less ethically illuminating.

DETACHED DISINTEREST

These concerns about the quality of descriptive studies in medical ethics are important for all readers of the medical ethics literature, not just ethicists. Some studies will be published because they appear to support a particular point of view, regardless of their quality. Especially in ethics, a more detached and disinterested spirit would ideally be expected, but this does not always obtain in reality. Whether reviewers, editors, or readers agree with the position that appears to be supported by the study should not influence the decision to publish. If an editor or reviewer has a particular viewpoint regarding an issue, it should not be necessary that a paper persuade the editor or reviewer to change his or her mind on the issue in order for the paper to be deemed publishable. It pays to recall that no descriptive study ever answers a normative question. One should be more concerned about whether the results are of intrinsic interest, whether the study answers an empirical question relevant to a normative argument, or whether the study adequately tests the implementation of a normative standard. These studies should make no claims to answer any normative questions. Regardless of one's normative position on the issue under study, one should support quality in descriptive research.

CONFLICTS OF INTEREST

Conflicts of interest may distort the interpretation of empirical data (Sharpe 2002). Readers of reports of empirical research have no ready access to the primary data and must be able to trust in the integrity and objectivity of the investigators who have collected an analyzed these data. Even if the judgment of the investigators has not, in fact, been altered by the conflict, empirical investigators must realize that the mere appearance of a potential bias due to an apparent conflict of interest undermines trust in the integrity of their work and that of the entire scientific enterprise. For example, if an investigator owns stock in a biotech company conducting research with human embryonic stem cells and then conducts a survey about public attitudes regarding the ethics of such research, the investigator has a conflict of interest. Such conflicts should be subject to clear and effective policies. Most policies require disclosure of such conflicts to the editors and the publication of a notice of such competing interests with the publication of the article. With the advent of the "empirical turn" in medical ethics, this is now also required of empirical studies published in bioethics journals (International Working Group 2007). However, doubts remain about the effectiveness of a policy requiring mere disclosure rather than an outright ban on financial conflicts of interest (Elliott 2008). It has also been argued that such regulation of conflicts of interest ought not be applied to normative scholarship, since the "data" of a normative article are the arguments and the citations presented in the article itself, which are readily accessible to readers (Jansen and Sulmasy 2003).

❧ Conclusion

In this chapter I have tried to outline some of the indicators of quality scholarship in medical ethics, emphasizing that these quality indicators are largely the quality indicators of the methods and the disciplines that are being employed. Nonetheless, there are also some indicators of quality that are common to many methods and disciplines within the broad category of the "humanities" and within the broad category of "descriptive research." These factors have been delineated with the hope that this chapter will help ethicists, clinicians, journal editors, students, and lay readers to become more careful, critical readers of the vast literature of medical ethics.

❧ Note

1. I have used the word "humanities" despite its awkwardness. The methods employed by the disciplines represented in chapters 3 through 7 and chapter 10 all seem to fit together under this label, and to be distinguishable from the empirical methods and disciplines of chapters 12 though 16. However, labeling some of these fields is not easy. On the one hand, as the authors of chapters 8 and 9 point out, it is not quite proper to call either law or history nonempirical or nondescriptive. On the other hand, it would not be proper to call such studies theoretical, either. Casuistry (chapter 7) is descriptive in the sense that it starts from real cases and in this regard is like the law. Historical studies should not be labeled "normative," but in their interpretive aspect can be quite theoretical. Law and casuistry, like philosophy and theology, might make normative arguments. Overall, despite these caveats, it seems that "humanities" best covers the methods and disciplines of chapters 3 through 10, and distinguishes them from those in chapters 11 though 16. Admittedly, "humanities" may be too inclusive—implying the inclusion even of the arts—fields that might enhance discussions of medical ethics but might not properly be said to constitute research in medical ethics. But the word at least roughly divides the kind of writing that is generally done in medical ethics into two broad camps. In a field as diverse as medical ethics, achieving even this much clarity seems sufficient.

∾ References

Aristotle. 1941. Rhetoric. In *The Basic Works of Aristotle*, ed. R. McKeon, 1325–1454. New York: Random House.

Brody, B. A. 1990. The quality of scholarship in bioethics. *The Journal of Medicine and Philosophy* 15:161–78.

———. 1993. Assessing Empirical Research in Bioethics. *Theoretical Medicine* 14:211–19.

Concato, J., A. R. Feinstein, and T. R. Holford. 1993. The risk of determining risk with multivariable models. *Annals of Internal Medicine* 118:201–10.

Copi, I. M. 1982. *Introduction to logic.* 6th ed. New York: Macmillan, 107–8.

Crews, F. 1974. *The Random House handbook.* New York: Random House.

DeGrazia, D., and T. L. Beauchamp. 2001. Philosophy. In *Methods in medical ethics*, eds. J. Sugarman and D. P. Sulmasy, 31–46. Washington, DC: Georgetown University Press.

Delbecq, A. L., A. H. Van de Ven, and D. H. Gustafson. 1975. *Group techniques for program planning: A guide to nominal group and delphi processes.* Middleton, WI: Green Briar Press.

Dierckx de Casterlé, B., S. Izumi, N. S. Godfrey, and K. Denhaerynck. 2008. Nurses' responses to ethical dilemmas in nursing practice: Meta-analysis. *Journal of Advanced Nursing* 63:540–9.

Elliott, K. C. 2008. Scientific judgment and the limits of conflict-of-interest policies. *Accountability in Research* 15 (1): 1–29.

Fanelli, D. 2009. How many scientists fabricate and falsify research? A systematic review and meta-analysis of survey data. *PLoS One* 4 (5): e5738.

International Working Group on Ethical Standards in Bioethics Publication (The San Francisco Group). 2007. Ethical guidelines. http://www.springer.com/philosophy/philosophy+of+sciences/journal/11017. Last accessed September 24, 2009.

Jansen, L. A., and D. P. Sulmasy. 2003. Bioethics, conflicts of interest, and the limits of transparency. *Hastings Center Report* 33 (4): 40–43.

Knaus, W. A., F. E. Harrell, J. Lynn, et al. 1995. The SUPPORT prognostic model: objective estimates of survival for seriously ill hospitalized adults. *Annals of Internal Medicine* 122:191–203.

Landy, D. C., J. H. Coverdale, L. B. McCullough, and R. R. Sharp. 2009. Prepublication review of medical ethics research: Cause for concern. *Academic Medicine* 84:495–97.

Liberati, A., D. G. Altman, J. Tetzlaff, C. Mulrow, P. C. Gøtzsche, J. P. Ioannidis, M. Clarke, P. J. Devereaux, J. Kleijnen, and D. Moher. 2009. The PRISMA statement for reporting systematic reviews and meta-analyses of studies that evaluate health care interventions: Explanation and elaboration. *Journal of Clinical Epidemiology* 62 (10): e1–34.

Martinich, A. P. 1996. *Philosophical writing: An introduction.* 2nd ed. Oxford: Blackwell Publishing.

McCullough, L. B., J. H. Coverdale, and F. A. Chervenak. 2004. Argument-based medical ethics: A formal tool for critically appraising the normative medical ethics literature. *American Journal of Obstetrics and Gynecology* 191:1097–102.

Meinert, C. L. 1986. *Clinical trials.* New York: Oxford University Press.

Morgan, D. L. 1997. *Focus groups as qualitative research.* 2nd ed. Thousand Oaks, CA: Sage Publications.

Neuman, W. L. 1994. *Social science research methods: Qualitative and quantitative methods.* 2nd ed. Boston: Allyn and Bacon, 227–69.

Schulman, K., D. P. Sulmasy, and D. Roney. 1994. Ethics, economics, and the publication policies of major medical journals. *Journal of the American Medical Association* 272:154–56.

Shalowitz, D. I., E. Garrett-Mayer, and D. Wendler. 2006. The accuracy of surrogate decision makers: A systematic review. *Archives of Internal Medicine* 166:493–97.

Sharpe, V. A. 2002. Science, bioethics, and the public interest: On the need for transparency. *Hastings Center Report* 32 (3): 23–26.

Strunk, W., and E. B. White. 1959. *The Elements of Style.* New York: Macmillan.

Thomasma, D. C. 1985. Empirical methodology in medical ethics. *Journal of the American Geriatric Society* 33:313–14.

Ventres, W. B., and R. M. Frankel. 1996. Ethnography: A stepwise approach for primary care research-ers. *Family Medicine* 28:52–56.

Watson, R. A. 1992. *Writing philosophy: A guide to professional writing and publishing.* Carbondale: University of Illinois Press.

Contributors

David A. Asch, MD, MBA, Health Services Research, Philadelphia Veterans Affairs Medical Center and Leonard Davis Institute of Health Economics, University of Pennsylvania

Tom L. Beauchamp, PhD, Kennedy Institute of Ethics and Department of Philosophy, Georgetown University

Alison Boyce, MA, Berman Institute of Bioethics, Johns Hopkins University

Lisa Sowle Cahill, PhD, Theology Department, Boston College

Tod Chambers, PhD, Medical Humanities & Bioethics Program, Northwestern University, Feinberg School of Medicine

Marion Danis, MD, Section on Ethics and Health Policy, Department of Bioethics, National Institutes of Health

David DeGrazia, PhD, Department of Philosophy, George Washington University

Raymond De Vries, PhD, Bioethics Program, University of Michigan Medical School

Ruth Faden, PhD, MPH, Berman Institute of Bioethics, Johns Hopkins University

Joanne M. Garrett, PhD, Center for Women's Health Research, University of North Carolina, Chapel Hill

Diego Gracia, MD, PhD, School of Medicine, Complutense University of Madrid

Mark A. Hall, JD, Center for Bioethics, Health and Society, Wake Forest University

Laura Hanson, MD, MPH, University of North Carolina Palliative Care Program, Division of Geriatric Medicine, Center for Aging and Health, University of North Carolina, Chapel Hill

Sara Chandros Hull, PhD, Office of the Clinical Director, National Human Genome Research Institute; and Department of Bioethics, Clinical Center National Institutes of Health

Albert R. Jonsen, PhD, Medical History and Ethics, University of Washington

Nancy E. Kass, ScD, Department of Health Policy and Management, Johns Hopkins Bloomberg School of Public Health; and Berman Institute of Bioethics, Johns Hopkins University

Nancy M. P. King, JD, Department of Social Sciences and Health Policy, Wake Forest University School of Medicine, and Center for Bioethics, Health, and Society, Wake Forest University

Barbara A. Koenig, PhD, Department of Health Sciences Research, Mayo College

Susan E. Lederer, PhD, Medical History and Bioethics, University of Wisconsin School of Medicine and Public Health

Patricia A. Marshall, PhD, Department of Bioethics, Case Western Reserve University

Robert A. Pearlman, MD, MPH, VA Puget Sound Health Care System and National Center for Ethics in Health Care; and Department of Medicine, University of Washington

Edmund D. Pellegrino, MD, Center for Clinical Bioethics, Georgetown University

Helene E. Starks, PhD, MPH, Department of Bioethics and Humanities, University of Washington

Jeremy Sugarman, MD, MPH, MA, Berman Institute of Bioethics and Department of Medicine, Johns Hopkins University

Daniel P. Sulmasy, OFM, MD, PhD, Department of Medicine, Divinity School, and The MacLean Center for Clinical Medical Ethics, The University of Chicago

Holly A. Taylor, PhD, MPH, Department of Health Policy and Management, Johns Hopkins Bloomberg School of Public Health; and Berman Institute of Bioethics, Johns Hopkins University

Index

Page numbers followed by f indicate figures, those followed by t indicate tables.

CPSIA information can be obtained
at www.ICGtesting.com
Printed in the USA
BVOW09s1039080617
486345BV00010B/63/P

9 781589 017016